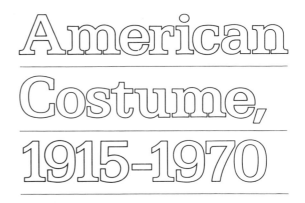

American Costume, 1915-1970

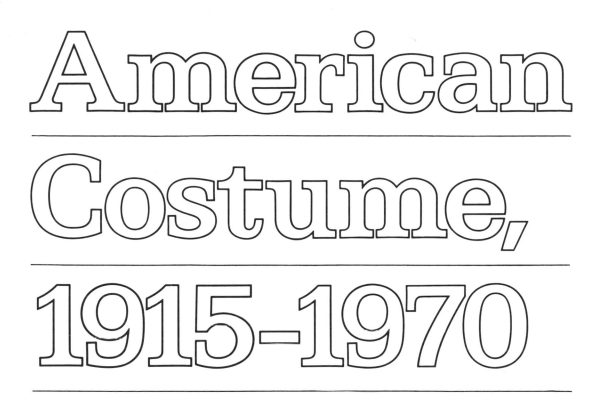

American Costume, 1915-1970

A Source Book for the Stage Costumer

SHIRLEY MILES O'DONNOL

 Indiana University Press / *Bloomington*

Manufactured in the United States of America

Library of Congress Cataloging in Publication Data

O'Donnol, Shirley Miles, 1915-
    American costume, 1915-1970.

    Bibliography: p.
    1. Costume — United States — History — 20th century.
I. Title.
PN2067.03   792'.026   81-48390
ISBN 0-253-30589-6   AACR2
    3 4 5 86 85 84

*To Paul Kozelka, who inspired
and guided so many theatre students*

CONTENTS

FOREWORD

DURING THE TWENTIETH century fashion in dress has become increasingly international. By "fashion" is meant not only the *haute couture* aspired to by some few in every country but the accepted appearance of both men and women in those countries we call "Western" — that is, Europe and the Americas. In the Slavic countries also urbanized people follow the Western trend, and many in Asia and Africa add "Western" clothes to their native wardrobes.

Even with all the sameness resulting from easy intercommunication, there are now and probably always will be national and even regional differences that lend variety to the overall uniformity. One can still tell, by their dress, English from French and Americans from either. Each country has preferences in fabrics, in tailoring, in colors, and particularly in accessories. Yet wherever there is home dressmaking, as, say, in Kansas City, Manchester, Lyon, or Hamburg, the same pattern book or some counterpart serves the woman who constructs her own wardrobe.

Therefore this book, which records, decade by decade, the preferred appearance of men and women in the United States, may be confidently used as a source book by the stage costumer who is dressing plays set in many countries. Here, in faithful detail, both pictorial and written, is recorded what is needed to recreate changes during those crowded years.

This book provides factual information needed by the costume designer that heretofore could be acquired only by time-consuming search among the files of old periodicals. More than that, for every decade the author has furnished a brief background, so necessary to a designer's understanding of his task. In addition, chapter-by-chapter suggestions have been given for productions pertinent to each decade.

Here is indeed a source book for that part of costume history so recent that it is hardly recognized as history, its characteristic ways of dressing not yet acknowledged as "costume." Plays written in or about those fateful six decades are indeed "costume plays." They will lose some of their significance if they are dressed in the fashions of "now." Many recent successes in reviving the classics may be proving that to present a timeless *Hamlet* in clothes like those the audience is wearing is more valid than to put our fashionable garb on characters in the Mayfair or Long Island society plays of the nineteen twenties and thirties — a vanished world whose interpretation calls for its own dress and decor as well as speech and deportment.

Here in this book the costumer will find well-documented material with which to put in visible form that world of the days just before yesterday.

LUCY BARTON

SANDWICH, MASSACHUSETTS

PREFACE

SINCE THE BEGINNING of the twentieth century, the mode of dress in the United States has undergone considerable change. The first decade of this era was characterized by a carry-over of Victorian modes and manners from the late nineteenth century. The ideal female was "a fine figger of a woman" — mature, voluptuous, and very feminine. During two world wars, women's fashions took on a tailored, mannish look and a free-swinging stance to match. In the aftermath of World War I, in the twenties, there was a reversion to irresponsible, almost sexless, childhood and an awkward, gangling, leggy stance to go with this frame of mind. In the dark days of the thirties a more-sober and less-opulent atmosphere prevailed. The dresses seemed to droop along with the dampened spirits. The first stunned response to the explosion of the atomic bomb at the end of World War II (the single most shattering event in a century of shocks) was the adoption of the "New Look," which represented a subconscious return to the safety of the Victorian era, when females were sheltered, life was simple, and codes were clear-cut. The second reaction, appearing in the late fifties and early sixties, seemed to be an impulse to throw overboard all responsibility, look and act like children once more, and let somebody else worry about the H-bomb. In recent years, changes in styles have come faster and faster, and fashion designers have drawn inspiration from all corners of the world.

This study presents illustrations and written descriptions of American costume from 1915 to 1970 and includes suggestions for their adaptation to stage use. The fashions are limited to clothing worn by members of the general public (men, women, and children) in the United States and come from everyday life rather than from costumes worn on stage. A few of the models shown have appeared in theatrical productions — for example, Jean Harlow's ostrich-trimmed negligee from the thirties and the vamp's harem skirt from a silent film of World War I. Although they were worn in America, many of the designs emanated from Paris couturier shops and London tailors.

As the twentieth century progressed and mass production of clothing advanced, the latest styles were no longer exclusive items but became available in less-expensive models in clothing shops across the country. An original dress design that struck the fancy of the buyers at a Paris opening used to take months to reach the American public, first being worn by the wealthy and then being adopted by middle- and lower-income women in cheaper copies. A Paris original may now appear on the market in mass-produced copies three weeks after its first showing, at a price within the range of the average working woman. This short-circuiting of the old-fashioned routes means that class distinctions in clothing, which visually used to separate the master from the servant and the rich from those on a limited budget, have largely disappeared. The general line and style of a garment may be the same for a President's wife and a suburban housewife. Distinctions between expensive originals and cheaper copies are subtle ones of quality of material, excellence of workmanship, and fineness or elegance of detail, trim, and finish.

The fashions selected for illustration and discussion in the text are those worn by "typical Americans," if there are such persons. Admittedly, styles vary from New York to California, and from the hills of Kentucky to the ranch country of Wyoming. Climate and occupation modify what people wear. Locale in earlier decades perhaps made more difference in clothing than it does now. With today's increased mobility, business or pleasure may take the New Yorker to Hollywood for the weekend, or bring the rancher to Washington, D. C. The fashions described in this study are probably "city fashions," drawn from the pages of the *Ladies' Home Journal*, *Vogue*, *Vanity Fair*, *Esquire*, and *The New Yorker*. These styles do reflect the general fashionable silhouette and spirit of their times, however; and similar garments were available from coast to coast through mail-order houses and published paper patterns for making clothing at home. Since 1950, television has made the general public more aware of the latest fashions as they appear. (Many occupations have their own distinctive uniforms: the overalls of the farmer; the white cap and uniform of the nurse; the black dress suit of the butler and headwaiter. No attempt has been made to cover all these special areas of costume styles in this volume.)

A great many plays are timeless — "time, the present" — and may be updated perennially. The costuming will reflect the current mode whenever feasible and possible. However, some scripts are topical and timely and need to be set in the period they were written to reflect. Tales of a historic nature, plots centered on some particular episode, will under ordinary circumstances be costumed in the era when these historic events took place — the sinking of the *Titanic*, the stock market crash of 1929, or the early career of Franklin D. Roosevelt. Upon occasion, the director may elect to transfer a script forward or backward in time, although upon first inspection it would logically call for a particular period in costume. Sometimes this "tampering with time" may traverse several centuries, and when that is done, critics will be quick to comment on the shift.

"Modern dress" is frequently utilized for a period play to illustrate the timelessness and universality of the theme. Two notable examples of radical departure from period costuming, both productions of Shakespeare, were the Orson Welles staging of *Julius Caesar* in modern dress (wherein Welles was trying to draw an analogy between ancient Roman history and the fascist movement of the late 1930s) and the 1961 Stratford, Connecticut, version of *Troilus and Cressida*, in which the fall of Troy was forcibly and fancifully wrenched from its usual Greek setting and costumed in crinoline petticoats and Civil War uniforms amidst Conestoga wagons and cannon fire (presumably to do homage to the 100th anniversary of the American Civil War).

One must take into account the fact that a play is seen through "the glass of the present." Any audience brings to the enjoyment of a production a current point of view and a sense of what is right and proper. It is impossible to divorce oneself completely from the present era; hence the presentation of a historic period is always colored and influenced by contemporary modes, tastes, and fashions in style and design. That may be seen by comparing the treatment of some leading lady, such as Cleopatra, through successive decades. Since she must be beautiful, she is costumed to conform to what is "beautiful" at a given time — and the styles change drastically. In the 1890s she had a wasp waist and the suggestion of a bustle; in the early 1900s she had a full, curvaceous bosom; in the 1920s she was straight and flat-chested. In each case the Egyptian motif was an overlay on the popular silhouette of the era. The costume designer will be influenced, consciously or subconsciously, by the current fashion and spirit of the time and will strive to make the heroine attractive to the audience in terms of what is considered beautiful.

Many plays written and set at any time in the twentieth century may be brought up to date and staged in the current mode. The catalogs of play scripts generally list costume requirements as "modern" for any play later than 1910 or 1920. For scripts that are tied to a specific decade or era in the century, some further definition of "modern dress" may be helpful. Twentieth-century styles seem to fall into seven definite periods between 1915 and 1970. These divisions have been set in relation to distinct changes in women's styles (in terms of general silhouette, waist position, and hem length) rather than with regard to shifts in men's wear. Women's fashions have been much more subject to fluctuation than men's throughout these years. Since changes are gradual and are accepted at varying times in different locales and communities, the exact date of a shift in fashions is difficult to determine. Therefore the cut-off dates of the chapters have been subjectively and arbitrarily set by the author. The decade of the sixties was so diversified and eclectic in its styles that it almost defied classification and categorization.

Some of the photographs included are representative of garments worn by an elite segment of the population. They are models from the costume collections of The Metropolitan Museum of Art, the Museum of the City of New York, and the Smithsonian Institution. Many of them were worn by fashionable members of society who had considerable wealth and were able to buy their clothing in Paris or London. The designers are for the most part leading Paris couturiers, and the models are outstanding examples of the mode of the day, considered worthy of preservation in museum collections. Except for a limited number of fashion illustrations from *Vogue* and *Esquire*, the line drawings are my own.

The actual writing of this study took several years, during which time I received invaluable assistance from many institutions and persons. I am tempted to extend the list backward in time to include everyone who has exerted an influence on the formulation of design theories, production methods, and concepts of what constitutes good theatre.

Perhaps the first acknowledgment should be to Lucy Barton, whose phenomenal work, *Historic Costume for the Stage*, has served as my guide and inspiration through many years of costume designing. It was my privilege to receive her counsel on the initial planning and later revision of this study. The unfailing encouragement, sympathetic understanding, and sound advice of

Paul Kozelka of Teachers College, Columbia University, was a constant source of comfort and motivation to continue on a seemingly endless project. I am also indebted to Carl Thomas of the University of California at Sacramento for his willingness to adjust my teaching schedule to permit advancement of this study. For material assistance and moral support I should like to thank members of my family — Ashley S. Miles, Preston H. Miles, Jr., Russell L. Wise, Ruth M. Wise, and Margaret Birnie — and my friend Norma E. Berke. I wish to express my gratitude to Homer Abbeglen, Don Fibiger, Charles Horine, and Rudolph Pugliese for their critiques of my compiled lists of plays to be produced in each era. For help in assembling photographs, I am most grateful to Paul Ettesvold, Assistant Curator, and Gordon Stone, Librarian, of The Costume Institute of The Metropolitan Museum of Art; Mary Warlick in the Photograph and Slide Library at The Metropolitan Museum of Art; JoAnne Olian, Curator of the Costume Collection of the Museum of the City of New York; and Claudia Kidwell, Curator of the Division of Costume, The Smithsonian Institution.

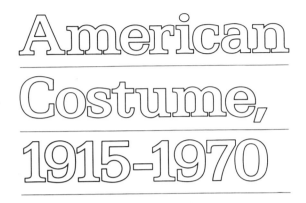

American Costume, 1915-1970

I

The First World War
(1915–1919)

IN TRACING THE SHIFTS of styles in apparel through the twentieth century, it is interesting to observe how the outward appearance of the American people has revealed their inner states of mind or attitudes. During these years new inventions, new materials, and faster modes of travel have come thick and fast and have meant a change in the way of living and a consequent change in the fashions and flavor of each era. As the straitlaced Victorian morality of the first decade of the century gradually gave way to a more-relaxed and carefree approach to life, the clothes people wore reflected these psychic changes. Quite literally, when women abandoned boned corsets about 1912, and soon thereafter some men discarded stiff, starched shirt collars, the entire country began to breathe and move more freely. The trend toward emancipation from nineteenth-century conservatism and restrictions had started on many fronts before the United States entered World War I.

CONCERNING THE PERIOD

In 1915 the United States was trying desperately to keep from getting involved in the bloody conflict in Europe. President Wilson was reelected in 1916 on the slogan "He kept us out of war." However, the temper of the times changed swiftly to a war psychology in 1917. As one historian noted, "Before the war, the people had been singing the pacifist song, 'I Didn't Raise My Boy to Be a Soldier,' and six months later they were singing George M. Cohan's rousing martial tune, 'Over There.'"[1] A tremendous upsurge of the movement for equality of the sexes, augmented immeasurably by the needs of the war effort and the war economy, swept women into public life, into jobs they had never held before, into positions of authority and responsibility. Small wonder that they achieved the goals they had set themselves during this era of upheaval (while their men were otherwise occupied in Europe) — the passing of the prohibition and women's suffrage amendments to the Constitution.

In the arts, the break from the old traditional, romantic, and representational style of painting continued. The public taste had been jolted by the exhibit of the "Ashcan school" of painters in New York in 1908, which portrayed the seamy side of life with stark realism. A further furore, amounting almost to hysteria, had been created by the first showing in America of works by modern Parisian artists, in abstract and cubist styles, which was held at the Armory in New York in 1913. In the realm of music, Paul Whiteman launched his first "jazz band" in 1915. A Russian flavor was imported with the first tour of the United States by the Ballet Russe, brought by Diaghilev. Theatre-goers were enthralled in 1916 with the dancing of the great Nijinsky, and that same year saw Anna Pavlova dancing at the Hippodrome in *The Big Show*. The Oriental note that had already crept into European design through the influence of Diaghilev (the designs of Léon Bakst for the Ballet Russe) and the creations of Paul Poiret in the Paris fashion world during the years just preceding World War I now found its way into American costume and interior decoration. Designer "Erté" (Russian-born Romain de Tirtoff) delighted the sophisticated world with the great theatrical flair of his costumes for the *Folies Bergère* and his cover designs for *Harper's Bazaar*.

Exemplifying this exotic splendor was fashion-setter Gaby Deslys, the English actress who bought her clothes in Paris and came to New York in 1915 to appear in the *Ziegfeld Follies* and several early silent films. In the same vein and exerting even stronger influence on tastes in American dress among the more-daring women, were the "vampires," who were rocketing to stardom in motion pictures during this era. Theda Bara (née Theodosia Goodman of Brooklyn) became the symbol of the sultry, heartless home-wrecker, wearing a series of clinging, trailing, bare-shouldered gowns (or divided "harem skirts"), dripping with beads, and garnished with a spray of feathers in her hair or a jeweled headband (Figure 51).

A very different image was introduced by the equally influential Irene Castle, whose innate fashion sense made her the idol of women aspiring to be well dressed. In direct opposition to the sticky, cluttered "vampire" style, the Castle silhouette was clean, graceful, lithe, and boyish. With her vigorous dancer's movement and her bobbed hair, she was a prophetic figure — a forerunner of the boyish ideal of the twenties. The Castles, Vernon and Irene, were a very popular husband-and-wife dance team appearing in night clubs and motion pictures. Their daring experiments with "animal dances" caught the public fancy, and many a ballroom was enlivened by the spectacle of well-dressed couples attempting the fox-trot, the turkey trot, and the grizzly bear.

The complete breakaway from the straitlaced morality of the Victorian era, which erupted in the 1920s, did not happen overnight. It had been brewing during the previous decade. The growing interest in syncopation and jazz patterns in music and dancing was one manifestation of the new order. The conservative elders were horrified at such goings-on; in New Jersey a young woman was jailed for fifty days for doing the turkey trot, and in Philadelphia fifteen girls were fired by their employer for turkey-trotting during their lunch hour.[2]

The first hints of the acceleration in the speed of living that has characterized this century were in the air. The sounds of the early twentieth century were still fairly quiet, but noise was on the way. For the most part, people still made their own music. One could hear the tinkle of a piano along with the close harmony of family song fests, and in summer there was the plunk of a ukelele being played on the porch swing, in the canoe, or beside the campfire. Horse-drawn buggies were being replaced by Henry Ford's "Tin Lizzie." Motoring was a rattling, bouncing, windblown adventure, as these new creations traveled at a reckless 25 miles per hour over dirt roads. In its early stages, such travel necessitated veils to protect the women's hats and faces, and goggles and visored caps for the men. Some variety of motoring coat was customarily worn; at first it was an all-enveloping "duster" (Figure 1), later some sort of belted jacket. Since breakdowns were frequent, a fashion writer in 1916 suggested that "an enthusiastic motorist should provide a doughty little cover-all suit of substantial dark denim, which may be drawn out from under the seat and slipped on for first aid to the injured car."[3] In the air, experiments with weird and wonderful flying machines had advanced to a point where the United States could send an air force to France in the spring of 1918. These planes were "notoriously unreliable, . . . more colorful than effective,"[4] but they gave a new dimension to warfare in this century.

GENERAL CHARACTERISTICS OF COSTUME

The war years were bound to give a military flavor to costume as the populace turned its attention to sending soldiers overseas. Those who remained at home adopted a great variety of civilian uniforms to provide a measure of comfort and freedom as they went about their tasks. Perhaps the cause of democracy was served more effectively by the liberating forces that were at work in all walks of life than by the slaughter at the front. Certainly women came closer to equality with men than ever before. They donned mannish jackets and plain skirts or breeches as they took over such jobs as driving automobiles and running elevators. By the time the war ended, the escape from the shackles of binding clothing was fairly well accomplished. Men had discarded long woolen underwear, had begun to rescue their necks and chins from the unyielding vise of the two-and-a-half inch stiff collar, were frequently leaving off their vests, and were generally more comfortable and casual as they became ever more interested in active sports — golf, tennis, and motoring. The female silhouette, which had been characterized by an S-curve since the 1870s (or "bustle period") — the bosom thrust out in front and the derrière thrust out behind — now reversed itself and became an opposite curve. As the murderously restricting corsets of the Victorian era were discarded and the lines of the figure relaxed and straightened, the prevailing stance became the "debutante slouch," with the shoulders sloping, the chest dropped, the hips slung forward, and the knees (in more pronounced cases) slightly bent.

MEN'S FASHIONS

Generally speaking, men's clothing in this era was characterized by broad shoulders, a princesse line or fitted waistline (even in sack coats), a close fit at the armhole, slender trousers, and ankle-high boots or spats. The neckline early in the period was still marked by a stiff high collar, often with rounded tabs. The vest was in evidence, and the coat buttoned rather high. Lapels might be braid-trimmed.

Hair Styles and Grooming

Men's hair was close-cropped, short over the ears, and shingled at the neckline. A few men wore middle parts, but the majority wore side parts (frequently brushed straight across the forehead) or pompadours. Men in general were clean-shaven. The well-groomed young man slicked his hair down with Vaseline or Wildroot Cream Oil until it resembled patent leather (à la Rudolph Valentino). The more-dapper male wore a small mustache, with carefully waxed ends. An elderly gentleman might still wear a brush or walrus mustache or a full beard or, rarely, muttonchop sideburns.

Hat Styles

The fedora, or felt hat, with rolled brim and fairly wide hatband was standard for daytime or business wear. The more-conservative or elegant man might wear a derby, with fairly high crown before 1917, a lower crown late in the period. The high silk hat was worn for formal occasions, church, and weddings. The straw hat, or "boater," was popular for summer, with a vivid band (often in college or club colors). For sports and college wear, cloth caps with visors were in vogue. These caps were popular in checks, plaid, or tweed. A fashion note from 1917 comments, "The top is made very full and almost covers the visor."[5]

Another innovation in caps for sports wear, which came out of World War I and was popular with both men and women, was a dark blue felt beret, which had been worn by some units of the French army.

Underwear, Loungewear, and Sleepwear

Long knitted underwear, wool for winter (often a dark red) and cotton for summer, had been worn for many years. Now it began to be replaced by lightweight one-piece cotton union suits (Figure 2) or by sleeveless jersey vests and cotton shorts ending above the knee. Pajamas were worn for sleeping, although older men might wear nightshirts. Flannel bathrobes in stripes or plaid were standard for lounging. For more-elegant evenings at home, a velvet smoking jacket or a silk smoking suit might be worn (Figure 3).

Neckwear

Men's shirts still had high, tight, white collars of starched linen, paper, or celluloid for dress and business wear. They might have wing tips, but more frequently had pointed or rounded tips, and were at least two inches wide (and three-eighths inch higher in back). The collar extended above the coat collar in back (and the shirt cuffs extended an inch or so beyond the coat sleeves). These stiff detachable collars were fastened to the neckband of the shirt with collar buttons. Soft shirts with attached turnover collars (often worn open) and attached cuffs were adopted increasingly for informal wear, sports, and manual labor. Ties in fashion were the cotton or string tie, the four-in-hand (wide with a large knot), or the bow tie. A fashion page in 1917 recommends a bow tie "with ends 1-7/8 inches wide."[6]

Day Wear

The Prince Albert, or frock, coat was still correct for formal day wear (Figures 4, 5), although it was fast being replaced by the cutaway (Figure 6). Frequently the lapels were faced with satin. Either coat might be worn with a pearl-gray or white vest, gray-and-black striped trousers, spats or cloth-topped boots, a wing collar and ascot or wide four-in-hand, and a silk top hat. A picture of President Theodore Roosevelt shows this typical frock coat attire, with striped trousers, but his vest is a festive polka-dot affair.[7] A black jacket might be worn with black-and-white trousers for a fairly formal day affair (Figure 7).

The sack coat was gaining popularity for informal and business wear (Figures 8, 9, 10, 11, 12). It was usually worn with matching vest and trousers. The majority of coats were single-breasted and could have from one to four buttons. The three- and four-button coats buttoned higher than present-day models, but frequently were worn open. The effect was fitted, at a rather high waistline. Vests were double- or single-breasted and often had lapels. Trousers might be cuffed or not; cuffs were quite wide and shortened the trouser legs to the ankle.

Evening Wear   Tailcoats of black worsted were worn for formal evening dress (Figure 13). They were high-waisted and had low lapels, often satin-faced. (The tailcoat pattern resembled that of the cutaway, but the lower fronts were set back at the waistline, and the evening tails were two inches longer at the center back.) The complete formal outfit consisted of black trousers with black silk braid stripes down the sides; a white piqué, faille, or satin waistcoat cut quite low; a stiff-bosomed shirt with a high standing collar or wing collar; a white bow tie; black patent leather pumps with bows; a black silk top hat; and white kid gloves. Increasingly popular was the more-informal "tuxedo" dinner jacket without tails, which had first appeared in the 1880s. Its name was acquired from Tuxedo Park, the "millionaire's retreat" about 40 miles north of Manhattan. This jacket was straighter, looser, and more comfortable than the tailcoat; it might have satin-faced peaked lapels or a shawl collar. Worn with the tuxedo jacket were black trousers with braid stripes down the side, a black waistcoat, a black bow tie, and patent leather pumps with bows or patent leather oxfords.

Sportswear   Standard dress for active sports was a rough tweed Norfolk jacket, with a belt stitched in at the waistline both back and front or only in back. The jacket was typically worn with knickers that were not too full and fastened just below the knee; a vest; a soft shirt with turnover collar, worn open or with a four-in-hand; ribbed golf socks with deep turnover cuffs; oxfords; and a cloth cap with visor (Figure 14).

Another popular jacket for vigorous activity (such as the new fast dances) was the "pinch-back coat," which also had a set-in belt in back and an inverted box pleat in the center back.

For informal wear sweaters were more and more in vogue, including cardigans and turtlenecks; pullovers with V-necks were worn in place of vests, particularly on campus. A dashing photograph of movie star William Garwood in 1916 shows him wearing a bulky knit white sweater-jacket with a roll collar, white flannel trousers, white oxfords, a soft shirt, and a full patterned four-in-hand.[8]

Still popular for sports wear was the lightweight unlined flannel sports jacket or "blazer." The original model of this garment, which appeared in the 1880s, was navy blue with a white braid trim, but more often it was now a bold, bright stripe. This striped blazer, worn with white flannel trousers and a straw hat, has become the traditional costume of the collegiate chorus boy in musicals from this period.

Swimming suits were of knitted wool jersey, with a short attached skirt (Figures 15, 16). Quite often they were in a bold stripe. Canvas bathing shoes were worn with them.

For hard manual labor, men might wear blue chambray work shirts (Figure 17) and denim overalls (Figure 18).

Overcoats might be of heavy dark wool and fairly long, slightly below the knee; or they might be lighter in weight and a little above the knee. The Chesterfield, in black or dark blue, usually with a velvet collar, was worn with formal evening attire (Figure 19). Topcoats might be single- or double-breasted, fitted at the waistline (Figures 20, 21) or straight and boxy (Figure 19). During this period a heavy wool overcoat, fleece-lined and with a fur collar, was popular (Figure 22). For sports or knockabout wear, the belted raglan coat was in order. It had sloping shoulders, with the sleeves set into the neckline. Shorter, belted jackets were also worn, about mid-thigh in length.

The United States Army uniform of World War I was of wool or cotton in khaki with a greenish cast, with all outer garments and accessories in matching color. Buttons and metal ornaments were of dull bronze. The jacket was single-breasted with five buttons, buttoned high at the neckline, and had a standing band collar (Figure 23); early styles might have a high turnover collar (Figure 24). The breeches were wide in the hip and fitted at the knee, similar to riding pants, and closed with lacings below the knee. Officers wore brown leather riding boots or leather puttees, and enlisted men wore canvas gaiters or puttees of khaki cloth strips bound round the leg (as in the Marine uniform shown in Figure 25). The typical soldier, or "doughboy," of World War I early in the war wore a "campaign hat," or "Montana peak," a broad-brimmed felt hat with quartered indentations in the crown, encircled by a cord (Figure 23); in the European field he wore a cloth "overseas cap" (Figure 25); in the trenches and in battle he wore a round-crowned shallow steel helmet with a chin strap (Figure 24). The service cap worn by officers differed from that worn in World War II by having a somewhat smaller bell crown, a slightly wider headband, and a smaller visor (as in the naval uniform, Figure 28). Officers wore the Sam Browne belt, a wide belt of brown leather with a narrower supporting strap passing over the right shoulder. It provided a convenient way of carrying a pistol (Figures 24, 25). The use of this belt was discontinued in the late thirties, before World War II. In cold weather the soldier might wear a double-breasted greatcoat of heavy wool or a shorter coat of waterproof canvas with a fleece collar and lining as in the coat shown in Figure 22.

The olive-drab service uniform was much the same for the infantry, Air Force, and Marines. The Air Force was not a separate division, but aviators flew under both Army and Navy jurisdiction. The naval aviator's working uniform shown in Figure 26 was khaki, with a leather jacket. The Marine might wear "day blues" — a navy blue tunic and visored cap, French blue trousers with a red stripe, white canvas belt, and black shoes. The Navy uniform remained the same as it had been for the previous 100 years: dark blue trousers with a thirteen-button fall front, a gusset laced in back, and bell bottoms; a dark blue middy blouse with a large collar (V-neck in front and square in back), trimmed with three rows of white braid, and slightly full sleeves gathered on a cuff, also trimmed with white braid; a dark blue flat cap (Figure 27); black silk neckerchief; and black shoes. The Navy summer uniform was white, in the same style, worn with a white washable round cap with turned-up brim, black neckerchief, and black shoes. Navy officers wore dark blue double-breasted jackets and dark blue trousers in winter, and white single-breasted jackets with standing collar and white trousers in summer (Figure 28).

Full-dress uniforms for both the Army and the Navy were dark blue. They had modified frock coats or tailcoats, and the collars, cuffs, and trousers were trimmed with gold braid. For special dress occasions a general or an admiral might wear a cocked hat, gold epaulettes, and a dress sword (Figure 29). However, full dress was discontinued soon after the war started and not reinstated until after World War II. Colonel Robert H. Rankin comments:

> World War I marked the end of uniforms in the old tradition in all countries. After the first few months of that bloody conflict, the profession of arms no longer was romantic. In the first of the modern technical wars, uniforms which blended into the background became a necessity. The Germans adopted a gray-green uniform, the French a "horizon blue," the British and Americans an olive drab. Dress uniforms were laid away in mothballs.[9]

Footwear

During World War I, men wore ankle-high laced shoes or oxfords that laced high on the instep; both styles had rather pointed toes. For evening wear black patent leather pumps were proper. For formal day dress, gray or fawn-colored spats were worn with black low-cut shoes; or ankle-high shoes of black calf with light uppers, giving the effect of spats, might be worn. Spats or cloth-topped boots also appeared frequently for business and street wear. Two-toned oxfords in white and brown, white and black, or white and tan were popular for sports wear. Ankle-high laced boots of heavy leather with rounded toes were worn for work and for Army service.

Accessories

Older men might carry a sober black umbrella with a crooked handle. The practice of carrying a cane was diminishing, although a cane was still part of formal dress. Sturdy sticks of Malacca with crooked handles were replacing the earlier style of canes in rare woods with gold or silver heads. Gloves were very generally worn, in both winter and summer — white kid for formal wear, and chamois, calfskin, and pigskin for day wear. The pocket watch was still in evidence, hung on a fob or carried in a vest pocket. The watch chain was sometimes linked across the vest front, and a pearl-handled knife might be suspended from it. The wristwatch had appeared about 1910 and was gaining in popularity. The war demonstrated its utility and greatly accelerated its general adoption. Cigarettes had also arrived on the scene and were supplanting pipes. Along with this change in smoking habits came the cigarette case, made of leather or metal, as a standard men's accessory. The wallet or billfold was taking the place of the pocket purse with a snap catch. Trousers were held up by belts or suspenders. Socks were frequently held up by garters. Jewelry might include a tie pin, a signet ring, a fraternity pin, cuff links, and, for evening wear, waistcoat buttons and shirt studs of gold, jade, or onyx. Daytime handkerchiefs might be colored or bordered, but fine white linen was preferred for evening and dress wear.

WOMEN'S FASHIONS

With the abandoning of the boned corset about 1912 or so, the female silhouette became straighter, softer, and more relaxed. The "pouter pigeon" breast (Figures 30, 31) returned to a more-normal line, and hips slimmed down a bit. The very restricting "hobble skirt" of 1910–1914 had vanished, but the "peg-top" silhouette of 1914 (full at the hip and narrow at the hem) still lingered in some models (Figure 34). Hemlines, which had hovered at ankle length for a few years ahead of the war period, began to creep up. During the years from 1915 to 1919 they stood at six to eight inches above the floor.

Hair Styles and Makeup

Most women had long hair early in the period, styled softly in waves over the ears and frequently done up in a Psyche knot low on the back of the head or higher (Figures 44, 47). After the war, bobbed hair was adopted swiftly, particularly by younger women. At first, it was flaunted only by the "fast" or daring woman. The marcel wave had been invented by a French hairdresser in 1907. Soon women were discarding curl papers and curling irons to sit under formidable electric machines that produced a "permanent wave." Beauty shops sprang up after the war and became a permanent and necessary part of American culture. The henna rinse, which imparted an auburn tone, was a favorite improvement on natural hair color. Cosmetics — rouge, powder, and lipstick — began to be used openly, in contrast to the long-standing Victorian concept that no lady would paint her face.

Hat Styles

Small hats were popular during this period, particularly the cloche and the toque, often with a feather trim (Figures 41, 58, 61). In 1915 there was a brief fad for the tricorne, or three-cornered hat (Figures 62, 66). Cockades used as trim were good in 1916 and 1917 (Figure 43). Big-brimmed hats were still popular, in straw or fabric (Figures 36, 38, 39, 46, 48, 54), and might be trimmed with plumes, bird wings, flowers, artificial fruit, or ribbons. Late in the period there was a fad for the "bellboy hat," high-crowned with a small visor and a bow or a plume in front (Figure 60). For sports, a close-fitting cap, a brimmed felt or panama hat, a straw sailor, or a beret might be worn (Figure 55). The evening headdress could be a simple band of silk or a more-elaborate concoction of flowers or feathers (Figures 49, 51).

Underwear, Loungewear, and Sleepwear

Older women still wore knitted underwear, long for winter and short for summer. The camisole, or corset cover, was being replaced by a semifitted waist-length brassiere. A combination garment had appeared, a straight, sheathlike affair with divided legs (called "camibockers" in England and "teddy-bears" or "teddies" in the United States) made of batiste, crepe de Chine, or silk. The petticoat was straight, slightly full, sometimes accordion-pleated, gathered with a ribbon at the waistline. All lingerie was dainty and feminine, trimmed with lace and ribbons.

For lounge wear, a kimono-style negligee was popular, with straight, full sleeves. The "tea gown" was also worn informally, for dinner at home; this negligee-like garment was soft and fluttery, often made of chiffon or crepe de Chine (Figure 53). Nightgowns were floor-length or trailing, sleeveless or with a short raglan sleeve, and frequently trimmed with lace and ribbon insertion. An exotic touch for the boudoir was a lacy or ruffled cap to match the gown (Figure 32). Pajamas for sleeping had appeared about 1912. They were plain and mannish in style, of soft cotton or silk. Another new addition to the boudoir scene were high-heeled slippers with toes but no backs, called "mules."

Day Wear

Skirts were above the ankle, reaching their shortest length of eight inches from the floor in 1918 (Figures 33, 34). Waistlines were belted in, a little higher or lower than normal. Bodices were usually full rather than closely fitted. Skirts were suddenly fuller in 1916 than they had been for the preceding several years (Figures 35, 36). Tailored suits and dresses were popular (Figures 37, 38, 39, 40). The jackets were long and frequently had flaring hiplines, and the skirts were full and often flared (Figures 41, 42, 43). During the war, materials were restricted and hard to get. Colors became more subdued with the embargo on imported fabrics; American dyes were poor and not equal to those of European manufacture. The sailor dress was popular for women and children, with braid-trimmed collar and cuffs (Figures 44, 74). The chemise dress appeared about 1916. At first it was a straight slip, over which was worn a straight tunic or overblouse with long sleeves (Figures 45, 46). Then the tunic lengthened and took on a belt placed low at the hips, and the underslip disappeared (Figure 47). Variations on this chemise-and-tunic style were the "apron tunic," with a draped front but no drape in back, and the "handkerchief tunic," with four corners hanging to the hem of the chemise. Another fashion that was gaining in popularity was the ensemble, or suit with three-quarter-length matching topcoat (Figure 48).

The prevailing style in evening dresses during this period was a softly *Evening Wear* draped ankle- or floor-length skirt with a train (Figures 49, 50, 51). The train might be square, or it might have a single "serpent" point or a double "fishtail" point. Large tassels were a popular finishing touch, on floating sleeve drapery or on the ends of sashes and loose panel drapes. Draped flounces and panels are seen in the dance gowns worn by Irene Castle in Figures 49 and 50. (The extended hoop skirt would probably be used only for exhibition dancing.) Several layers of pastel sheers might be used, in varying colors. The following descriptions accompany a page of "tea gowns" or "dinner gowns" for the hostess to wear at home:

> This year [1915] Fashion is smiling on the trained dinner gown. Handsome flowered silks, brocades, chiffon velvets and satins make the most beautiful house gowns, . . . which can be combined with chiffon, georgette crepe, tulle or lace.

> Rich brocaded satin in gray, with poppy designs, forms the trailing skirt . . . extending also into the surpliced pointed sections of the draped bodice. Delicately transparent is the chiffon yoke in a warm rose, with pointed sleeve openings . . . edged with smoked-pearl beads. From the yoke falls the rippling cape diminishing to a point just above the hem [in back] with a dull silver tassel.

> Japanese sleeves . . . and delicate coral-pink chiffon over-dress hung over a white satin skirt. Garlands of tiny flat marquisette flowers like embroidery are appliquéd to the waist, and larger ones weight the pleated overskirt [hemline]. Atop of the white satin girdle a band of sable squirrel gives a dark tone of contrast.

> A straight Greek neckline ends in back with a graceful hood drapery. Of transparent mauve chiffon are the bishop sleeves, and beads and stones adorn the girdle. The gown itself is made of two layers of chiffon, mauve over azure blue, giving a delightful opalescent effect.[10]

The gown illustrated in Figure 53 is described on the same fashion page as follows:

Through the delicate sleeveless chiffon coat of the home dinner gown . . . is revealed the pale-blue taffeta foundation dress with . . . quaintly plain bodice. In three pieces is the skirt, repeating at its hem the filmy texture of the coat and gathered ever so slightly round the waist. Of circular fullness is the fluttering ruffle of the coat, all one-toned in pale wisteria, meeting at the neck the pointed collar of the coat, which is made of silk.[11]

Formal evening dress was curtailed while the war was in progress, but reappeared quickly in 1919. A fashion commentator in the early spring of that year comments on the gown presented in Figure 54:

It is nice to be able to wear an evening gown once more without feeling apologetic, especially now that there are so many lovely styles in such beautiful glistening silks, luxurious brocades and glittering gold-and-silver tissues to tempt one. . . . In this [gown], American beauty charmeuse, forming the skirt and one-sided bodice ending in a strap over the right shoulder, is brilliantly contrasted with the black-and-gold broché of the straight bodice. Worn over this was a scarf cape of black satin, with a lining of pale biscuit-color crepe de Chine, and around the cape is a band of kolinsky.[12]

The "harem skirt," with divided legs and full bloused bloomer hemline, was worn by models and movie stars, but did not gain general acceptance.

Sportswear

Skirts, blouses, and jackets were adopted for active sports such as boating, golfing, and tennis (Figure 55). A close-fitting cap or a brimmed straw hat usually completed the outfit. Shoes might be low oxfords or ankle-high laced boots.

Swimming suits were still skirted, sleeved, and fairly decorous. The bathing ensemble included a "hat to match," stockings, and canvas bathing shoes (Figures 56, 57). In 1916 movie star Annette Kellerman introduced the one-piece knitted bathing suit, which eventually gained universal acceptance. The Mack Sennett bathing beauties helped to popularize a sleeveless model, progressively brief. Sennett stars Gloria Swanson, Marie Prevost, and Phyllis Haver were the pinup girls of World War I.

Striped blazers and sweaters were popular for women, as well as for men, in sports activities.

Coats and Wraps

The cape was popular in the daytime with tailored dresses or suits and in more-luxurious materials with evening dress (Figures 54, 58). A favorite style for coats was full and flared, with back free-swinging (Figures 59, 60) or belted (Figures 61, 62). Short bolero jackets were in vogue early in the period. A loose jacket or wrap with large sleeves was popular for day or evening wear (Figures 63, 64). The tubular silhouette is illustrated in two elegant daytime coats designed by Poiret (Figure 65). A straight boxy coat or jacket, or one with raglan sleeves, belted or unbelted, was worn for sports. Fur coats and capes and various fur-trimmed garments were much in evidence. A fur coat might have collar and cuffs or trim of a contrasting fur. Cloth suits might be trimmed in horizontal fur bands, or a chiffon evening gown might have a furred hemline. In summer, fur scarves and stoles were worn with light dresses. In winter, muffs were carried to complete the furred costume; they were of various sizes and shapes—small and round or large and pillow-shaped (Figures 40, 60).

Women served in several military departments during World War I. In general their uniforms consisted of ankle-length skirts and jackets similar to those worn by the men in service. The YWCA overseas uniform, designed by Worth (Figure 66), shows the prevailing silhouette. The Army nurse's jacket had a turnover collar and small lapels and was worn with a blouse and tie (Figure 67). The American Red Cross nurse wore an Oxford-gray uniform, white blouse, red scarf, white cotton gloves, gray overseas cap, and high-laced black shoes. A nurse on duty might also wear a white uniform, white cap or draped head-piece with a Red Cross insignia on it, and a navy blue cape with a red lining (Figures 68, 69). The "Marinettes," or Women Marines, and members of the Woman's Motor Corps wore khaki uniforms, with khaki blouses and ties, and wool overcoats to match (Figure 70). Those in the Army Nurse Corps, the Navy Nurse Corps, and the "Yeomanettes" wore navy blue uniforms, white blouses, blue ties, black shoes, and blue straw sailor hats with brims or overseas caps. Working outfits such as the one shown in Figure 71 came in a variety of styles, designed for freedom and comfort, and might well be made at home. Service uniforms were a part of the daily picture. Among them was the "Hoover apron," a wraparound uniform worn by women working in the Food Administration (Figure 72). The lap front proved so practical that this garment became a perennial for home and kitchen wear, and was also adopted as a uniform by many waitresses, beauticians, and nurses. It is still a standard style for "dirty work." For domestic service, the typical maid's uniform was a plain black dress worn with a frilled, starched white cap and apron (Figure 73).

Uniforms

High boots were still worn throughout the period, although they were disappearing by 1919. They came halfway up the lower leg, had soft tops of leather or fabric, and might lace or button up the front or outer side. Often the tops were gray, white, or tan, contrasting with a black

Footwear

vamp. The same effect was achieved by wearing high, buttoned spats with black pumps. Oxfords were worn for sports, and might be buttoned or laced; some were two-toned, white with black or brown. Low slippers were worn for evening or afternoon dress with less-tailored outfits. There was a fad for high tongues and buckles on pumps late in the period. All boots and shoes had long pointed toes and French or "Baby Louis" heels.

Stockings were neutral in color and usually matched the tops of the shoes—gray, sand, or beige. White stockings were worn in summer. Black stockings were worn for swimming. Early in the period stockings were of cotton or lisle. Silk stockings were an expensive luxury; they were worn with evening dress and might have fancy clocks or lace inserts.

Accessories   Jewelry during this period included short pearl necklaces worn with pearl button earrings as well as dangling strings of beads and pendant earrings. Costume jewelry (brightly colored brooches, rings, earrings, and necklaces made of imitation stones) was coming into vogue to be worn with the plain, simply designed chemise and tunic frocks. During the war the wristwatch gained general acceptance. It might be on a leather or grosgrain ribbon band or attached to a bracelet.

A long, slender "pencil umbrella" often completed a street costume. It would appear from the fashion illustrations, both English and American, that canes of a slender and dainty variety were also carried by well-dressed women in tailored outfits (Figure 61). In the summer, an ever-present accessory was a parasol, of typical Japanese design (Figure 47) or perhaps of flowered silk, possibly ruffled. It was still considered desirable to preserve a fair complexion and to protect one's face from the summer sun. The caption accompanying the bathing suit sketched in Figure 57 says: "Outwitting Old Sol's rays, the mermaid of this summer has a snug little brimmed hat."[13]

Handbags were of fabric, usually gathered on a cord or on a large ring that could be looped over the wrist, or they might be fastened with a snap catch and have a hinged opening. Very often they were finished off with a large tassel (Figure 43). Evening bags were of gold or silver mesh, velvet, or brocade. Compacts for face powder were carried, and cigarette cases began to appear among women's accessories. Ostrich plume fans were popular for evening dress. Folding fans might be carried in the daytime as well, during summer heat, since air conditioning was still nonexistent. In church, palm-leaf fans shared the rack with hymn books. Gloves were buttoned at the wrist with two or three buttons. Evening gloves were long, of white kid. They were removed while dancing more frequently than in the preceding decade.

Very little children, both boys and girls, wore "rompers," a one-piece suit with short sleeves and short legs, straight or bloomer style, gathered on a straight band or on elastic. Waistlines for both girls and boys were a little lower than normal and usually belted. Little girls often wore middy blouses with sailor collars and pleated skirts (Figure 74). Skirts for girls were full, gathered, pleated, or flared. All little girls wore a big hair ribbon high on the back of the head; usually it was of black taffeta, sometimes of plaid or flowered ribbon. A young girl might wear a brimmed hat with a ribbon or a voluminous tam-o'-shanter.

The "Buster Brown" suit for boys had a tunic blouse, double-breasted, with a detachable stiff-starched white Peter Pan collar, a big bow tie, and short bloomer pants. The "blouse suit," or "Russian suit," for little boys had a bloused tunic top and straight short pants (Figure 74). Small boys might also wear a Norfolk jacket, combined with knickers that fastened just above the knee. Children's shoes were more often than not high-buttoned or laced. The traditional Mary Jane shoe with a single strap was also worn.

TYPICAL MATERIALS, COLORS, MOTIFS, AND TRIMMINGS

Probably the most-typical color and material during a war period is khaki, and the most-prevalent motif is the military. As has been mentioned, materials were restricted and wool fabrics in particular were conserved in the war years. Colors were more subdued because American dyes were inferior.

Men's suits for formal wear were made of black broadcloth, with tailcoat or frock coat lapels of dull silk or satin. Sack suits were made of serge, worsted, or tweed. Summer suits were made of light flannel, duck, linen, or seersucker. Usually trousers of sack suits matched the coats, although they were sometimes lighter in color. In the summer, trousers of duck, linen, or white flannel were worn with coats of blue serge or pinstriped fabric. A fashion note in 1917 says: "Striped white flannel trousers with 1/8-inch stripes one inch apart will be very good this summer, but many all white will be worn too."[14] Suit colors were generally dark — blue, brown, gray, or black. Checks and plaids were also good for sack suits, vests, and overcoats. A trimming of contrasting braid on suit jackets gave a colorful touch — white on navy blue, or dark sienna brown on light beige or cream. Shirts were of linen or cotton, sometimes of silk for formal wear. Shirts for less-formal wear might be pastel or striped, but they were still combined with a stiff white collar. Wide four-in-hand ties were made of silk, crepe, or foulard, with diagonal satin-figured stripes, or they might be knitted.

Socks were often brightly colored, sometimes heavily clocked and sometimes polka-dotted.

Lingerie was made of fine soft cottons—such as batiste, cambric, nainsook, and dimity—and were trimmed with ribbons and embroidery. Early in the era, silk underwear was considered not quite respectable for ladies. Petticoats might be made of crepe de Chine. Raw silks were popular—pongee, shantung, tussah. A soft and supple variety of satin called "charmeuse" was much used for better dresses. Taffeta was a perennial favorite. Daytime dresses were made of serge, foulard, duvetyn, broadcloth, gabardine, or crepe de Chine. Evening gowns might be made of satin, chiffon, silk crepe or georgette, lamé, or metal brocade.

Rayon, the first of the synthetic fibers, had been discovered in the late nineteenth century and was originally placed on the market in 1890. This man-made material and the closely related acetate were derived from cellulose, or wood pulp. In these early days, fabrics made from "artificial silk" were still expensive and of inferior quality, and most silk fabrics were still products of the silkworm. The phenomenal growth of the synthetic fiber industry did not get under way until the end of World War I.

Just before the war, there had been a new liking for brilliant colors in women's costumes—bright pink, orange, jade, cerise or "American beauty," and peacock blue. This trend was epitomized in splashy batik prints on china silk and bold, multicolored embroidered trims, often Persian or Oriental in motif. During the war years this passion for color was toned down or subdued, but it recurred when the fighting ended and the victory celebration was in order. Wartime dresses were often navy blue or black.

Trimmings included ribbons (particularly picot-edged and grosgrain), lace, beadwork and passementerie (patterned networks of braid and cord), gold and silver fringe, ostrich fringe and marabou, tassels, imitation flowers (sometimes of fabric or ribbon), rows of buttons, fur edgings on almost anything, and hand embroidery.

SUGGESTIONS FOR COSTUMING PLAYS IN THE PERIOD

Men may be given the look of the period by removing a soft collar from a modern shirt and adding a stiff starched model at least two inches high, with rounded corners or wing tips. Vests buttoned rather high might help to give the period flavor, or an extra button might be added at the top of a modern coat closing to shorten the lapel. The waistline of the coat might be pinched in a little, and a braid trim might be applied. Derby hats for winter and straw hats for summer are good. If the outfit is sporty, trouser cuffs may be deepened and the legs may be shortened to ankle-length. Trouser legs should be fairly slender. A Norfolk jacket with knickers or a striped blazer with white flannels will help to give a sporty air.

For women, the look should be soft and feminine. Select fabrics that drape well. The cheaper varieties of satins and taffetas, with the least body, will capture the soft quality of "charmeuse." A fitted skirt pattern with four or six gores, or pleats set on a yoke, might serve as a start for a tailored suit. Jackets should be semifitted or even slightly bloused. An added hip-length cape, with slits for the arms, and a pencil umbrella would help to create the proper effect; or try a fur stole and an ample muff, "pillow" or "barrel" in shape. The draped skirt of an evening dress was often of rather intricate cut, but it could be simplified to a series of pleats or gathers on a low waistline. The train could be a panel hung from the waistline in back.

The effect of high boots for both men and women can be achieved by carefully tailored spats worn over pumps or oxfords — white or gray over black shoes and biege over brown. Toes of shoes should be pointed.

REPRESENTATIVE PLAYS AND MUSICALS SET IN THE PERIOD 1915-1919
("M" denotes musical)

TITLE	AUTHOR	PERIOD
All the Way Home	Tad Mosel	1915
Daddy Long-Legs	Jean Webster	1914
Dear Brutus	J. M. Barrie	1890s, 1917
Fiorello! (M)	Jerome Weidman, George Abbott	Pre-WW I, 1920s
Funny Girl (M)	Jule Styne, Bob Merrill, Isobel Lennert	Pre- and Post-WW I
George M! (M)	George M. Cohan, Michael Stewart, John & Fran Pascal	1878, 1900–19, 1937
Getting Married	George Bernard Shaw	1916
The Good Soldier Schweik	Erwin Piscator, Robert Kalfin	WW I
The Great White Hope	Howard Sackler	WW I
He Who Gets Slapped	Leonid Andreyev	1919
Heartbreak House	George Bernard Shaw	WW I
Irene (M)	Harry Tierney, Joseph McCarthy	1919
Johnny Johnson (M)	Paul Green, Kurt Weill	WW I
Journey's End	R. C. Sheriff	WW I
Justice	John Galsworthy	1916
A Kiss for Cinderella	J. M. Barrie	1916
Leave It to Jane (M)	Guy Bolton, P. G. Wodehouse, Jerome Kern	1917
Look Homeward, Angel	Ketti Frings	1916
Major Barbara	George Bernard Shaw	1915
A Night at an Inn	Lord Dunsany	1916
Oh, Boy! (M)	Guy Bolton, P. G. Wodehouse, Jerome Kern	1917
Oh! What a Lovely War (M)	Charles Chilton	WW I
The Old Lady Shows Her Medals	J. M. Barrie	WW I
Our Betters	Somerset Maugham	1917
The Plough and the Stars	Sean O'Casey	1916
Red Roses for Me	Sean O'Casey	1917
Ross	Terence Rattigan	1916–18, 1922
Ruggles of Red Gap	Harrison Rhodes, Harry Leon Wilson	1915
Seven Keys to Baldpate	George M. Cohan	1914
Seventeen	H. S. Stange, Stannard Mears, Booth Tarkington	1918
Seventh Heaven	Austin Strong	WW I
Summer and Smoke	Tennessee Williams	1916
Time and the Conways	J. B. Priestley	1919, 1939
Up in Mabel's Room	Wilson Collison, Otto Hauerbach	1919
Very Good, Eddie (M)	Guy Bolton, Philip Bartholomew, Jerome Kern	1915
What Price Glory?	Lawrence Stallings, Maxwell Anderson	WW I

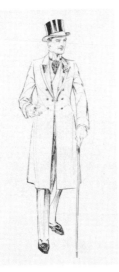

1. Linen duster and motoring cap. American, 1910. (The Costume Institute of The Metropolitan Museum of Art. Gift of Mrs. James S. Hedges.)

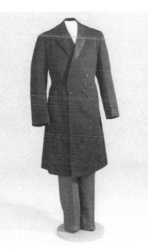

2. "BVD's": lightweight cotton union suit. 1916.

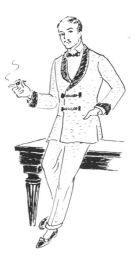

3. Smoking suit of black patterned silk, black silk collar and cuffs. 1918.

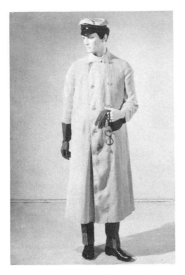

4. Black frock coat. Black cashmere trousers, with fine white line. Black varnished boots. Double-breasted white waistcoat and black ascot worn with wing collar. *Vanity Fair*, March 1918.

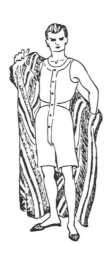

5. Suit with frock coat: black wool coat with silk satin-faced lapels; gray striped vest; gray-and-black striped wool trousers. About 1910. (Division of Costume, Smithsonian Institution.)

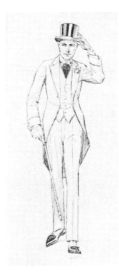

6. Oxford cutaway suit of undressed worsted. The coat has very narrow binding. Black calfskin boots with top cloth buttoned uppers. Throw-over scarf; wing collar. *Vanity Fair*, March 1918.

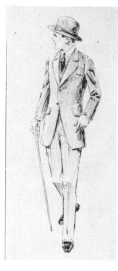

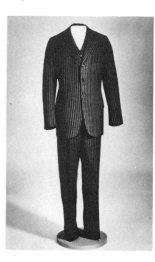

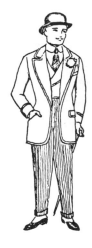

7. Black jacket worn with black-and-white striped trousers. Calfskin buttoned boots, waistcoat with white facing, colored shirt, white cuffs, black felt homburg. *Vanity Fair*, March 1918.

8. Three-piece suit in blue-black worsted with white pinstripe. Hart, Schaffner and Marx. About 1915. (Division of Costume, Smithsonian Institution.)

9. Sack suit for business wear, braid trim, vest with lapels. 1915.

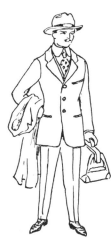

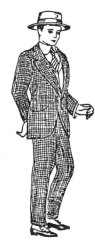

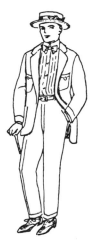

10. Business suit with single-breasted sack coat, fine check. 1918.

11. Sack suit with vest, small check. 1916.

12. Sack suit with patch pockets, straw hat, bow tie. 1916.

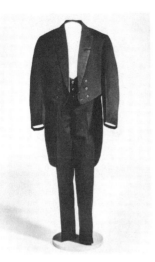

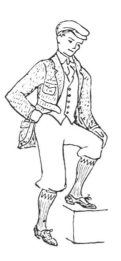

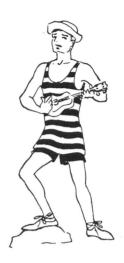

13. Three-piece full dress suit of black wool, formal tailcoat. Charleston, S. C., about 1910. (Division of Costume, Smithsonian Institution.)

14. Sport attire: Norfolk jacket with set-in belt, knickers, billed cap. 1918.

15. Striped wool bathing suit. 1917.

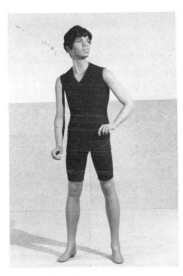

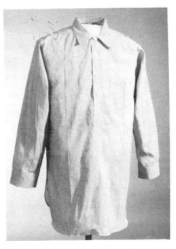

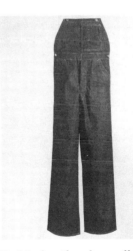

16. Wool bathing suit. American, 1918. (The Costume Institute of The Metropolitan Museum of Art. Gift of Gantner of California.)

17. Man's work shirt in blue chambray with white topstitching, front button placket, shoulder yoke. About 1915. (Division of Costume, Smithsonian Institution.)

18. Man's railroad overalls of blue denim. About 1915. (Division of Costume, Smithsonian Institution.)

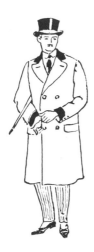

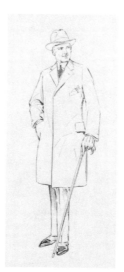

MEN'S UNIFORMS, WORLD WAR I

19. Black wool overcoat with velvet collar and cuffs; top hat. 1919.

20. Topcoat of dark oxford cut to follow easily the lines of the figure, lapels faced with dull silk. Three buttons. The coat is about knee-length and has three pockets. *Vanity Fair*, March 1918.

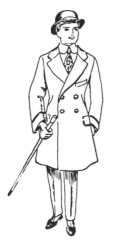

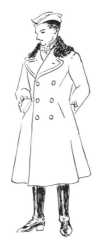

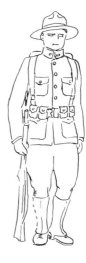

21. Double-breasted overcoat; bowler hat. 1915.

22. British military-style overcoat with fur collar; field boots. 1918.

23. Army officers' olive drab service dress with campaign hat and gaiters.

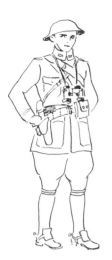

24. Army officers' olive drab service dress with steel helmet and boots.

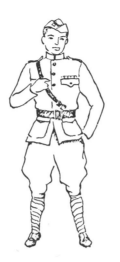

25. Marine field dress, forest green; wrapped puttees; overseas cap.

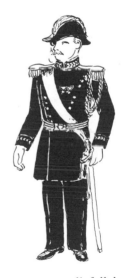

26. Naval aviator's khaki working dress; leather jacket.

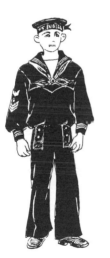

27. Navy enlisted man's blue dress; blue flat cap; black tie and shoes.

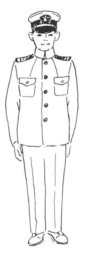

28. Naval officer's white service dress; white cap and shoes.

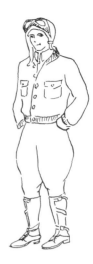

29. Army general's full dress; dark blue coat and trousers; cocked hat.

The "pouter pigeon" silhouette of the early prewar era.

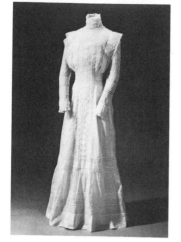

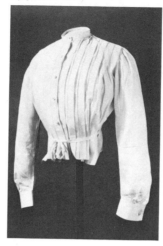

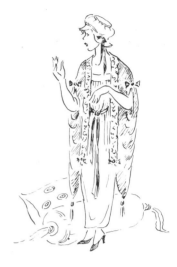

30. "Lingerie" dress: sheer white linen with machine-made lace insertions, high stand-up collar. About 1911. (Division of Costume, Smithsonian Institution.)

31. Woman's waist of white linen: long sleeves, pleated front, worn with detachable collar. Providence, R. I., about 1911. (Division of Costume, Smithsonian Institution.)

32. Negligee: peach satin slip; blue chiffon coat; boudoir cap. 1918.

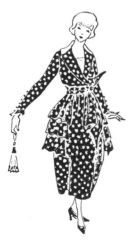

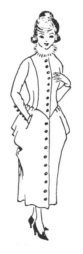

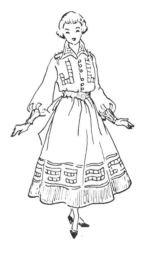

33. Navy foulard dress with white polka dots; white satin vest. 1918.

34. Wool dress with fur collar, draped bustle, fitted basque. 1917.

35. Sheer frock trimmed in hemstitching; taffeta cuffs, hem, and girdle. 1916.

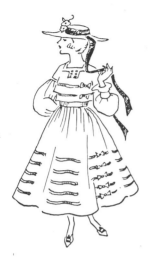

36. Dressy frock of organdy trimmed with inserted ribbons. 1916.

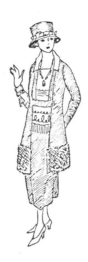

37. Semifitted coat dress; embroidered waistcoat. 1918.

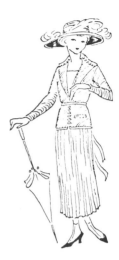

38. Dress of navy blue serge: pleated skirt, white satin vest. 1919.

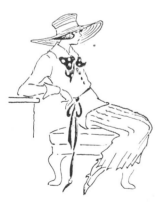

39. Matching pink silk jersey blouse and silk poplin pleated skirt; pink-dotted black tie. 1919.

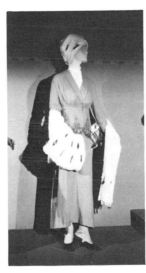

40. Afternoon suit of magenta cashmere twill: high-waisted jacket and softly flared skirt, trimmed with applied purple velvet and silk embroidery. By Poiret, 1919. (Museum of the City of New York. Gift of Mrs. Henry Clews.)

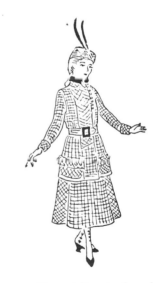

41. College girl's suit of wool plaid, with black velvet collar. 1915.

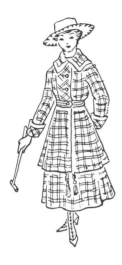

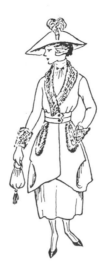

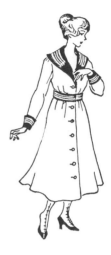

42. Sport suit of rose silk tussah. 1916.

43. Maroon satin suit trimmed in squirrel fur. 1917.

44. Sailor dress, braid trim. 1917.

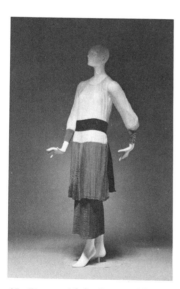

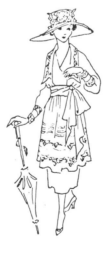

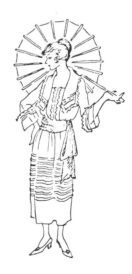

45. Dress with bodice and long sleeves of finely pleated white lawn; two-tiered skirt of finely pleated rose silk linen; sash of black ribbed silk. By Léon Bakst, 1915. (The Costume Institute of The Metropolitan Museum of Art. The Estate of Marcia Sand Fund.)

46. Net frock trimmed with tucks and embroidery, satin girdle. 1918.

47. Summer frock of organdy with satin girdle. 1918.

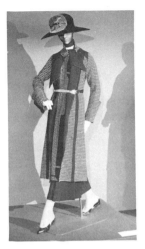

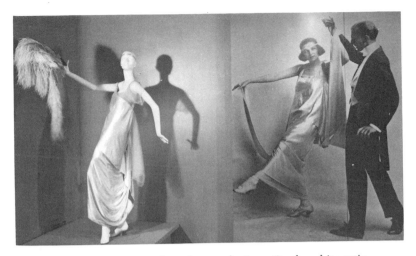

48. Tailored promenade ensemble of wool: long tunic dress in black-and-white woven checked pattern over plain black wool skirt; three-quarter-length coat woven in a larger black-and-white checked pattern with scarf tie at neck. By Poiret, 1919. (Museum of the City of New York. Gift of Mrs. Henry Clews).

49. Evening dresses of a style worn by Irene Castle: white satin trimmed with floating panels of silk net and ropes of pearls. By Callot Soeurs, 1913 – 14. (The Costume Institute of The Metropolitan Museum of Art. Purchase, Irene Lewisohn Bequest.)

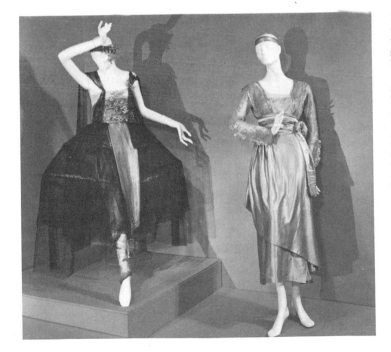

50. Left, dance dress with bodice of turquoise and gold lamé with tight trousers of gold tissue, shadowed by hooped skirt of black embroidered net. About 1914. Right, evening dress of a style worn by Irene Castle: bodice and sleeves of silver lace, skirt of chartreuse satin, sleeve tabs and waistband of mauve, pink, and blue satin. By Lucile, Ltd., 1914 – 16. (The Costume Institute of the Metropolitan Museum of Art. Gifts of Irene Castle and Isabel Shults.)

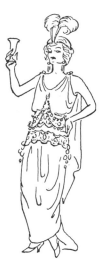

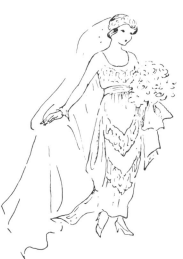

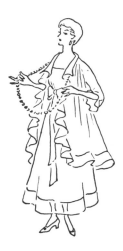

51. "Vamp" style evening gown, made popular by movie sirens; chiffon with beaded girdle. 1917.

52. Wedding gown of satin with overbodice and apron tunic of beaded tulle, bandeau of beaded lace, tulle veil. 1919.

53. Informal dinner gown of taffeta and chiffon. 1915.

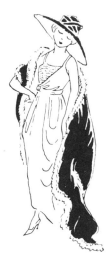

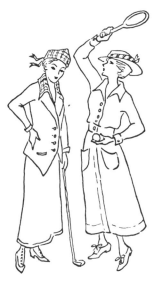

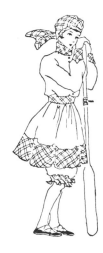

54. Evening gown of rose satin with bodice of black-and-gold brocade. black satin cape, fur-trimmed. 1919.

55. Left, plaid shirt and cap worn with jacket suit for golf. Right, shirtwaist and skirt for tennis. 1915.

56. Bathing suit of taffeta with plaid trim. 1918.

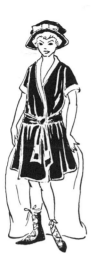

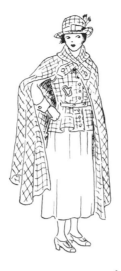

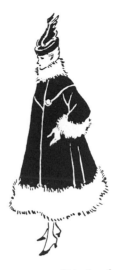

57. Bathing suit and hat of black taffeta. 1916.

58. Burberry cape coat and matching hat of checked Scotch tweed. 1917.

59. Winter coat of black velvet with fox fur trim. 1915.

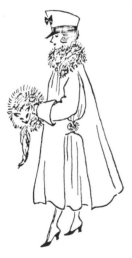

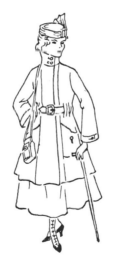

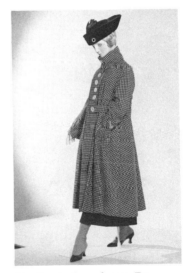

60. Wool coat; "bellboy hat" with visor; fox fur muff with head and tail. 1917.

61. Belted velveteen coat for sport or dress. 1916.

62. Checked wool coat. By Bergdorf Goodman, 1919. (The Costume Institute of The Metropolitan Museum of Art. Gift of Mr. Chisholm Beach.)

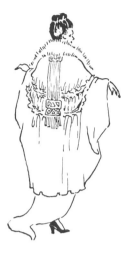

63. Velvet evening wrap worn over evening gown with train. 1915.

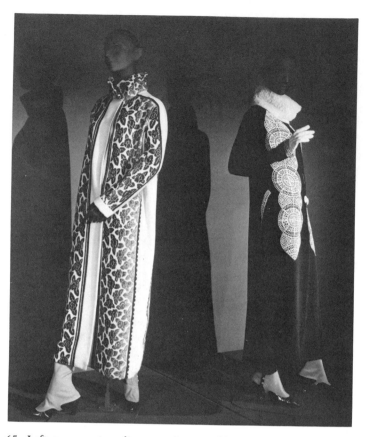

65. Left, summer traveling coat: ivory and brown cashmere twill; tubular silhouette with no fastening. By Poiret, late teens or early twenties. Right, daytime coat: black ribbed silk and wool, trimmed with applied bands of white leather cutwork; standing chin collar of white fur. By Poiret, 1919. (The Costume Institute of The Metropolitan Museum of Art. Gift of Mrs. David J. Colton.)

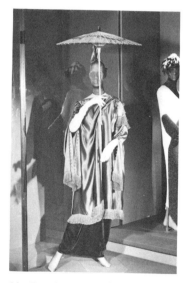

64. Evening wrap of purple satin lined with emerald green, trimmed with purple silk fringe, borders, and tassels. By Poiret, 1917. (Museum of the City of New York. Gift of Miss Matilda E. Frelinghuysen.)

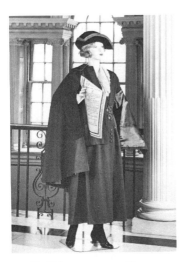

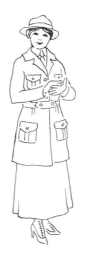

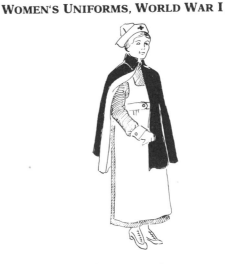

66. YWCA overseas uniform. Made in Paris by the House of Worth, 1918 – 19. Felt tricorne hat made in Paris by Georgette. About 1916 – 18. (Museum of the City of New York. Gifts of Margaret Merle-Smith and Mrs. Henry Clews.)

67. Army nurse's dark blue street dress; dark blue hat; black shoes.

68. Red Cross nurse's overseas uniform: gray dress; white apron; blue cape.

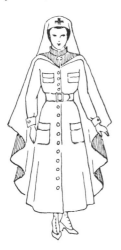

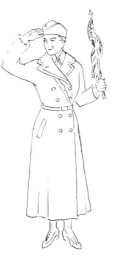

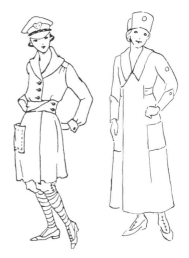

69. Red Cross nurse's white uniform; navy blue cape, red lining.

70. Woman's Motor Corps: khaki uniform; overcoat; garrison cap.

71, 72. Service uniform for war work: smock; breeches; puttees. "Hoover apron" (Food Administration uniform): light blue with white trim.

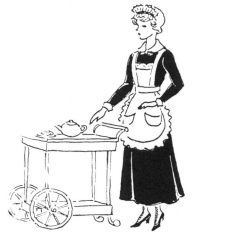

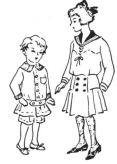

73. Maid's uniform: white organdy apron and frilled cap. 1919.

74. Boy's Russian suit; girl's sailor dress. 1916.

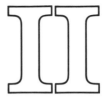

The Flaming Twenties
(1920–1929)

"TURNED-UP NOSE, turned-down hose — flapper, yes sir, one of those — has anybody seen my gal?" So went a popular song of this colorful era, when a girl's skirts flapped around her knees as she swung into the rumble seat of a Stutz Bearcat or danced the Charleston. Her unbuckled galoshes flapped as she strode across the campus in her yellow slicker. It was an age of unheard-of freedom for women, hard-won in World War I. Women had proved they could take the place of men on countless fronts when the latter went off to war and could work beside them in the uniforms of nurses, motor corps chauffeurs, or canteen hostesses. One might almost say that the idea of equality with the male had gone to a girl's head as she bobbed her hair to look like his; borrowed his shirt, tie, and felt hat to appear on the golf links; and flattened her curves with a bandeau that reduced her to subteen straightness.

CONCERNING THE PERIOD

The United States, in revulsion against the horrors of the conflict that had cost over 100,000 American lives on the battlefields of Europe, turned its back on the newly constituted League of Nations and returned to an isolationism that negated the elusive dream of world democracy. It was an age of feverish *laissez-faire*, of high tariffs, and of reparations demands that could never be met by impoverished and defeated nations. And while the United States went on a ten-year binge of partying, new problems were brewing in Europe; Mussolini marched into Rome and seized power in 1922, and Hitler published *Mein Kampf* two years later. In America there was an all-pervading "get-rich-quick" psychology, as paper fortunes were built on an inflationary economy. It was an era of speed and jazz and petting parties for a wild and reckless younger generation bent on forgetting the unpleasantness of the war. "The bawl of the saxophone was as characteristic of the period as the blare of the automobile horn."[1]

Prohibition of the drinking of alcoholic beverages, on the law books from 1920 to 1933 but not enforced, added its own peculiar quality of wildness. Gangsterism arose in the big cities, built on the illegal traffic in liquor; and café society supported the bootleggers by nocturnal trips to illicit "speak-easies," which flourished in dark alleys and side streets, behind doors that opened at a magic password. President Wilson had finished his second term in office with difficulty, in fast-failing health. In 1921 Warren G. Harding became the President, but after two years of political intrigue and scandal, he died suddenly of a heart attack. Calvin Coolidge succeeded him, and was elected to the office of President in 1924. He completed his full term but declined to run again. In 1929 Herbert Hoover took office. Thus the country had four presidents during this one decade.

The momentum of science was ever-increasing. The great upsurge of discovery and invention that had marked the end of the nineteenth century was now coming into full application, affecting all facets of life. Mass production of motor cars by Henry Ford and Will Durant was swiftly putting the nation on wheels. Mechanical appliances were appearing to lighten household chores and emancipate the housewife. The early models were not "streamlined." The refrigerator had its mechanism in a coil on top, and the washer had a wringer attachment and portable tubs. At the beginning of the decade, the Victrola in the parlor was still cranked by hand, and the radio was a crystal set with headphones. By the end of the twenties the dial telephone was replacing the wall-box model.

A succession of popular heroes caught the public fancy — "Babe" Ruth in baseball, Helen Wills and Bill Tilden in tennis, Gertrude Ederle swimming the English Channel, and Charles A. Lindbergh, who made the first solo flight across the Atlantic in May 1927. Milder excitement was generated by a succession of fads — flagpole sitting, marathon dancing, Ping-Pong, Ouija boards, Mah-Jongg, contract bridge, and crossword puzzles.

In the arts, the abstract painters were in their heyday. Picasso, Braque, Miró, and Kandinsky were experimenting with cubist techniques and rainbow-hued splashes, several steps removed from reality. Brancusi's abstract sculpture in bronze, *Bird in Space*, made headlines when it became "conspicuous as the center of a dispute between the United States Customs, who wanted to tax it as bric-a-brac, and its owner, who wanted it to enter the country duty-free as a work of art."[2] Piet Mondrian, working in straight-line arrangements and squares, has been given credit for being a major influence on the breakaway from traditional architectural patterns that was occurring in this decade. Major exponents of the new "form follows function" theories, utilizing freely arranged masses of steel, concrete, and glass, were Walter Gropius and Mies van der Rohe at the Bauhaus in Germany and Frank Lloyd Wright at Taliesin in Wisconsin. The masses paid little attention to the new architecture and continued to live in Edwardian ginger-bread, fake Tudor, or fake Spanish mission houses. Interior decoration took up the idea of abstraction and free form in an Art Moderne style, with results that were sometimes garish and not always functional. "The modern-minded let skyscraper furniture zag its way up walls, the zig provided by cacti."[3] Most living rooms were furnished with matched sets of overstuffed chairs and sofas covered in cretonne with cabbage-sized floral patterns.

The National and Columbia Broadcasting companies were both formed during the mid-twenties and were soon providing entertainment of increasing merit to the owners of new electric radio sets, which had appeared in 1925 — programs such as the N.B.C. Symphony Orchestra under Walter Damrosch, the Mormon Tabernacle Choir, newscasts by Lowell Thomas, and the popular comedy team of "Amos 'n Andy."

Jazz had come north from Dixieland (specifically New Orleans), and its syncopated rhythms pervaded the entire era, even getting into automobile horns. It was fast and staccato, and vocal numbers were punctuated with refrains like "boop-boop-a-doop" and "vo-do-de-oh," sung in an enchanting baby voice by popular singers like Helen Kane. The Charleston and the Black Bottom were athletic, vigorous dances requiring considerable muscle tone and coordination for the proper counterswivel of knee and ankle; they were definitely for the young or the very well preserved. It became fashionable for café society to make expeditions to Harlem night spots, seeking authentic jazz rhythms at their source.

Motion picture production had become a million-dollar business. Theatres became more and more luxurious, decorated in red plush and gilt. Some top-ranking stars were Pola Negri, Lillian and Dorothy Gish, Norma Talmadge, Mary Pickford, Gloria Swanson, and Marion Davies. Greta Garbo made her first film in 1926 and by the end of the decade was a leading star (her major impact on fashions belongs to the 1930s, however). Wallace Reid, John Gilbert, John Barrymore, and Douglas Fairbanks played male leads. Rudolph Valentino was perhaps the most sensationally popular male star of the era, specializing in exotic foreign types. In *Blood and Sand* he played a toreador dressed in a gorgeous red velvet outfit with gold embroidery. In *The Sheik* he wore the flowing robes of the Arabian desert. His untimely death in

1926 left a trail of feminine heartbreak across the continent. Comedy was raised to the heights of art with the antics of Charlie Chaplin, Harold Lloyd, and the Marx brothers. Clara Bow made a picture called *It* in 1927, and "it" became a synonym for "sex appeal." She certainly embodied the look of the period, with a cap of short marcelled curls and bangs, a baby face, and a rosebud mouth. Her figure was remarkably flat-chested for a sex symbol — but so went the twenties. Unfortunately, her voice was not of a caliber to survive the transition from silent films to talking pictures at the end of the decade; other casualties were John Gilbert and Norma Talmadge. Al Jolson appeared in the first "talkie," *The Jazz Singer*, in 1927. The metamorphosis was swift and complete — 85 percent of the movie theatres were equipped for sound by 1931.

The Broadway stage was experiencing a parallel surge of glorious activity. The musical theatre was developing as a new and distinctively American art form during the twenties, and a collection of giants — Jerome Kern, George and Ira Gershwin, Richard Rodgers and Lorenz Hart, Vincent Youmans, and Cole Porter — was producing successful shows packed with hit tunes, not just now and then, but season after season. Beatrice Lillie, Gertrude Lawrence, and Fanny Brice contributed to the hilarity of the decade. Florenz Ziegfeld in his *Follies* "glorified the American girl" with breathtaking spectacles, outdoing Hollywood in their lavishness and extravagance; George White's *Scandals* and Earl Carroll's *Vanities* were close rivals. Eugene O'Neill came to the fore as a playwright with *The Emperor Jones, Desire Under the Elms*, and *Strange Interlude* (which started at four in the afternoon and allowed time out for dinner).

It is seldom possible to fix an exact date for the end of a historic period, but the decade of the 1920s stopped with catastrophic suddenness on the day the Wall Street stock market crashed — October 24, 1929. The party was over.

GENERAL CHARACTERISTICS OF COSTUME

For the men, the twenties silhouette was a much looser, broader, baggier effect than the one that had prevailed in the first two decades of the century. The sack suits were straighter, having lost the "pinched-in" look at the waistline, and the shoulders were wide and padded. Lapels were wide, and the double-breasted jacket was popular. Trousers were full, pleated at the waistband, and in the middle of the decade the legs were wide to the point of floppiness. Vests were frequently discarded or replaced by pullover sweaters. Wide pinstripes and bold checks were popular with more-dashing personalities — such as gangsters and members of the theatrical profession. Knickers in a full "plus-fours" style were the prevailing outfit for active sports, particularly golf. A jaunty beret, a sleeveless pullover sweater in a wild pattern, and knee-high argyle socks completed the picture. Shirts had been converted to the soft turnover collar for the most part; ties were either an ample bow-tie or a wide four-in-hand and came in bold colors and patterns. Stiff collars (usually wing-tip) and cuffs were still worn for formal occasions. The raccoon coat, the hip flask, and the foot-long cigarette holder were hallmarks of the period.

Women's fashions were straight and simple, boyish and flat-chested, with a waistline at the hip and a hemline at the knee. In studying the illustrations and photographs from this decade, one wonders how women managed to defy nature and achieve this chestless, waistless, hipless look — a perfect 30–30–30. There seemed to be a movement afoot to erase the distinction between the sexes. One popular song complained:

Boys now wear pants that are wider than skirts;
Girlies wear ties and their big brothers' shirts.

Chanel, a leading designer of this era, came forth with styles that accented simplicity and comfort. A *Vogue* editor gives the following picturesque description of the "flapper":

In the 20's, after groping through the post-war wasteland of mahjong, disillusion and Dr. Coué, she finds herself. Rather, she finds that Chanel has given her back to herself with a dress that throws everything to the winds but chic, and exactly expresses the utter, unutterable freedom and blasé wisdom she feels is hers. Its essense is chemise, its silhouette is flat; in 1927 its waistline reaches an all-time low, its hem an all-time high. . . . She shingles her hair; affects a long cigarette holder, a debutante slouch, a rope of pearls, an ostrich feather fan, and pins an orchid on her shoulder; likes rooms that look like country club lounges; wears silk pyjamas on the beach; sits in dark cellars through the nights (it is mid-prohibition). Jazz is her music, gin her drink, "inhibitions" her scapegoat, divorce her burning question, and F. Scott Fitzgerald her biographer. After allowing herself a brief old-fashioned thrill when Lindbergh flies the Atlantic, she packs her Vuittons for Biarritz, and so long as she's on this side of paradise doesn't care what's on the other.[4]

The close-fitting cloche hat, which came down over the eyebrows, was most typical of the period. Long strings of beads, dangling earrings, and multiple bracelets from wrist to elbow were in vogue. Shoes had rather clubby-looking heels and often had a fairly wide strap across the instep.

MEN'S FASHIONS

A note of casual comfort and a loose fit characterized the men's fashions during this period. There was, however, an interest in good grooming and sleekness. As Cecil Beaton comments,

> All sorts of men suddenly wanted to look like Noel Coward — sleek and satiny, clipped and well groomed, with a cigarette, a telephone, or a cocktail at hand.[5]

London set the styles for the well-dressed male, as it had done since the beginning of the nineteenth century.

Hair Styles and Grooming

Men's hair styles continued to be short. Hair might be parted in the middle or on either side, or combed back in a pompadour; sometimes there was a combination of part and pompadour. Generally, the hair was clipped fairly high over the ears and shingled in back. A liberal amount of hair oil or Vaseline was used to keep the hair slicked down and in place, which frequently gave a "patent leather" look to a man's head. The vast majority of men were clean-shaven, but a few wore a small dapper mustache, neat and close-clipped. In some cases the "sleek" look was carried to the extreme of plucking and pencilling the eyebrows (Wallace Reid, Rudolph Valentino, Noel Coward).

Hat Styles

Hats in fashion were still the homburg, the low-crowned derby, and the silk top hat for formal wear. A fashion note in 1922 describes the current mode in top hats as having "a bell crown that is six inches high and a brim that is two inches wide at front and back."[6] The straw hat, the visored cap, and the beret were worn for informal and sports wear; and the soft felt fedora was a perennial favorite for business and informal occasions. About the middle of the decade the sportier models of felt hats acquired a snap-brim, i.e., it could be turned down over the eyes in front. The Panama hat of soft cream-colored straw, with a wide brim, was worn in summer, and a new silk shantung sport hat appeared (it resembled a fedora in shape and had rows of parallel stitching on the brim and crown). A new import was the "planter's punch," which arrived from Jamaica in 1923. It was of firm natural-colored straw and shaped like a fedora, with a creased crown and a wide pleated ornamental band.

Underwear, Loungewear, and Sleepwear

Some die-hards, mostly older men or dwellers in rural and small-town areas, still wore long knitted underwear of wool or cotton. The union suits of the preceding decade were being supplanted by knitted lisle undershirts (sleeveless or with short sleeves) and cotton shorts. The earlier models of undershorts were white; later they came in stripes, plaids, or prints. Pajamas and lounging robes were sometimes quite elegant. A smoking jacket for relaxing at home might be of velvet (Figure 1). The dressing gown illustrated in Figure 2 was shown in a heavy silk crepe in a striking print, lined with silk of contrasting color. Pajamas were also available in bold-patterned silks as well as in quieter cottons.

Neckwear

The majority of men wore stiff-bosomed white shirts with detachable stiff collars for formal day and evening wear. The semistiff pleated-front shirt, considered a little less formal, was usually worn with a dinner jacket. The preferred style of collar was the wing tip. Frequently seen was the "bat-wing" collar — "the wings are slightly rounded and it is intended that a wide bow tie, which also has rounded ends, should be worn with it."[7] For formal day dress, *Vanity Fair* recommended the wing collar with a flaring or narrow bow tie or a puff tie (ascot), or the turndown collar (stiff starched) with a sailor's knot as being equally correct. During the twenties, a detachable soft collar was developed, but many sport shirts had attached soft turndown collars. About 1924 men began to wear a collar pin, long and slender, which held the points of the collar down and passed under the knot of the tie. In the same season button-down tabs on sport shirts were occasionally seen. Colored shirts in pastel shades (light blue, green, or pink) were popular. These came in plain colors, small checks, or fine stripes and frequently had white collars and cuffs. Fabrics for dress shirts were fine cotton, linen, or piqué. Sport shirts were made of cotton — broadcloth, poplin, basketweave — flannel, or silk. The bow tie was correct for formal wear — white tie with tails, black tie with the dinner jacket or cutaway, possibly a quiet stripe or dot for formal day wear. With informal and sports outfits, the four-in-hand was universally worn. During this decade, its width was generous almost to ascot proportions. It might be quite lively in color and bold in pattern, in a polka dot, stripe, plaid, or upon occasion a daring Art Deco print.

Day Wear

Formal day attire remained much the same as in the preceding decade. The Prince Albert coat was making its final appearance during the season of 1920 or so. The accepted attire for formal day weddings was that shown in Figure 3: black silk top hat, cutaway coat of black or dark Oxford gray, finely striped gray cashmere trousers without cuffs, waistcoat of the same material as the coat or of white piqué or linen (double-breasted or single-breasted), patent leather shoes with pearl gray or white linen spats, wing collar, ascot of black-and-white or gray-and-black striped silk, and gray suede or white kid gloves. Possible variations were a bow tie with a wing collar or a four-in-hand with a turndown collar and a waistcoat of pearl gray or fawn with spats to match. The complete outfit included a cane.

For informal occasions, the sack suit was generally worn (Figure 4). During the twenties this garment was broad-shouldered and loose-fitting. The jacket was liberally padded in the shoulders, and the lapels were wide. Trousers were full, pleated at the waistband, and for several seasons in mid-decade rose to a high waistline. The range of colors was expanded over that worn in the teens, particularly for sports wear, but also for street and business wear. Wide stripes were popular and so were combinations of striped or checked jackets with plain trousers. Coats might be single- or double-breasted, and might fasten with one, two, or three buttons. Typical combinations were a single-breasted style with notched lapels or a double-breasted one with peaked lapels. The following descriptions, taken from the fashion pages of *Vanity Fair* during the 1920s, give a more-complete picture of the outfits presented in the illustrations:

> [Figure 5] Single-breasted gray sack. Striped flannel, stripes of darker gray and blue. Single-breasted waistcoat, no collar. Trousers regular, pleats in front. Blue pleated shirt, self-figured; white collar and cuffs. Black tie, small double horseshoe pin of diamonds and sapphires. Black low shoes and gray socks.[8]

> [Figure 6] Single-breasted black and white shepherd's check suit. Single-breasted waistcoat, regular trousers. Small black and white check shirt, black tie, white collar and cuffs. Black shoes, black socks. The monotony may be relieved by wearing a solid color shirt, such as pink, blue or tan, with white collar and cuffs.[9]

> [Figure 7] "Drury Lane" is a double-breasted sack suit exactly copied from the creation of a well known London tailor. The shoulders are extremely broad, with a welted seam at the join of sleeve and shoulders, and the extra fullness about the armholes — a detail of importance in English clothes. It has . . . the latest feature in smartly cut clothes, which is an absence of flaps on the side pocket.[10]

> [Figure 8] Single-breasted, three-button sack suit in brown mixture. Double-breasted brown linen waistcoat, pink shirt and collar, brown and white polka-dotted tie, black shoes.[11]

In this era of affluence, there was a general exodus to "posh" resorts in the winter season. Fashion notes were full of suggestions for vacation wear at the French Riviera or at Florida beaches. Part of the travel equipment for a well-dressed gentleman was a valet to take care of his vacation wardrobe. Lightweight tropical fabrics were becoming more and more popular. A 1927 issue of *Vanity Fair* comments: "White has once more become fashion's favourite colour for men's summer attire. White suits of tropical materials, white flannel slacks, odd jackets of white gabardine, white sweaters and white bathing trunks will be worn."[12] The vacation outfit pictured in Figure 9 is described as follows:

> For the well-turned out man on the beach in Florida. Jacket and trousers of thin herringbone twillet in pale blue and brown mixture, soft white silk shirt, scarf of two shades of blue and white, shoes of light brown canvas, tipped in darker brown calf, and straw boater hat with club band. A white handkerchief and corn colored socks complete the accessories.[13]

The fad for wide-bottomed trousers reached its extreme during the years 1924 to 1926. At one time they attained a width of 24 inches at the cuff. This style is illustrated in Figure 16, and the original sketch was accompanied by these comments:

> Mr. Jack Hulburt, of "By the Way," does a few steps for us. He is wearing a tobacco brown coat and double-breasted waistcoat, with trousers of similar color striped with gray, a brown butterfly foulard tie, buff socks and tan shoes. [There is a side-view diagram showing how the full trousers are draped], the idea being to get an unbroken straight line from the hip down to the ankle. These drape well in action.[14]

The extra-wide trousers (called "Oxford bags") were particularly popular with college students, who strove to uphold the image set by the comic-strip character "Harold Teen" and by the Charleston-dancing, saxophone-playing lads of the John Held, Jr., cartoons.

Evening Wear

Formal wear varies little from one era to another. "White tie and tails" was still the correct ensemble for the most-formal evening affairs. Tail-coats had either notched or peaked lapels. For less-formal events, dinner jackets were generally worn. The cut of evening jackets varied, as one fashion writer noted:

> This year they are advocating a notched lapel. A short time ago they advocated the peaked lapel. Next season, perhaps, they will revert to the "shawl" collar, which, properly speaking, has no lapels at all. The very fact that there are only three types of lapel and collar treatment, and that each type is made "fashionable," in a sort of never-ending rotation, is proof that it doesn't really matter whether a man wears one type or another.[15]

This advice would seem to hold true across the decades. Certainly one sees examples of each variety in every season. About the middle of the twenties midnight blue dinner jackets for semiformal occasions were widely adopted as a relief from the perennial black. The following description of the complete outfit recommended for correct formal evening wear accompanied the tailcoat shown in Figure 10:

> Silk hat; dark Chesterfield topcoat; a dress suit, tailcoat with satin-faced lapels; a white piqué waistcoat with pearl buttons or pearl rimmed with platinum; stiff, plain-bosomed linen shirt, with studs to match the waistcoat buttons; a square-tabbed wing collar and a white piqué hand-tied bow. Accompanying all this, white kid gloves, black socks, patent leather shoes or pumps minus defined toe caps, and a knob-topped stick. Spats are not worn indoors with evening dress.[16]

An article on the proper wardrobe for a well-dressed college student in 1929 comments: "'White tie' having now become *de rigeur* at parties in town, the well-dressed college man finds his wardrobe no longer complete with only the dinner jacket. This, however, is still the correct thing for most campus occasions."[17] The less-formal outfits with their accessories were described in *Vanity Fair* as follows:

> [Figure 11] A dinner jacket with a shawl collar is equally as smart as one with a notch lapel. In this illustration the lapels are faced in black silk, or satin, and the waistcoat is made in the same material. It is worn with a plain stiff bosom shirt, open wing collar, black silk or satin bow tie, patent leather dancing shoes and a top hat.[18]

> [Figure 12] The double-breasted dinner jacket in midnight blue with square end bow tie. London tailors now face the lapels of the double-breasted dinner jacket with glossy silk, instead of the usual dull ribbed silk, in order to distinguish it from the jacket of the dark blue double-breasted lounge suit. Single-breasted dinner jackets and tail coats, however, still have lapels of dull silk.[19]

Sportswear   Clothing for sports wear was loose and comfortable and very colorful. The standard outfit for the golf links or strenuous outdoor activity was likely to include knickers of a full cut, bloused on a band that buckled or buttoned below the knee (Figures 14, 15). They were considerably more voluminous and longer in cut than the knickerbockers worn in the preceding decade; they were called "plus-fours" because when they were unbuckled they fell four inches below the knee. With knickers one might wear a Norfolk jacket or a variation called the "Skokie," with a set-in belt in back and pleats or gathers to give extra fullness for action (Figure 13). A similar jacket was also worn with slacks for informal dress (Figure 17). Brightly colored pullover sweaters with V-necks were frequently worn with knickers (Figure 18). Knee-high golf socks in geometric patterns and with wide cuffs went with this ensemble. Caps with visors or felt hats might be worn in cooler weather; in the summertime, straw hats or Panamas appeared. For spectator sports, mixing colors was in vogue. Light trousers were worn with darker jackets, or plain colors were combined with plaid or stripes. The striped blazer was still popular for sports wear. For horseback riding, correct attire was a tweed jacket, jodhpurs, and boots (Figure 19). If one were riding in a fashionable fox hunt in the South, the jacket would probably be red flannel for a man, black for a woman, and the jodhpurs black.

In this decade, beach wear for men was briefer than formerly (as it was for women). The one-piece knitted suit was still worn (Figure 20), but it had been replaced in many locales by trunks and sleeveless tops, usually in plain colors (Figure 21). A fashion note in *Vanity Fair* for 1927 remarks on beach propriety:

> It is not an unusual sight on the beaches abroad, such as the Lido and Biarritz, to see men wearing only a pair of trunks, but in conservative America the nearest approach to this custom is the sunburn coloured upper, with white flannel trunks. At a distance this gives the same effect.[20]

The beach outfit shown in Figure 21 consisted of a bright orange knitted top, gray-green slacks, and a beach robe in a green and orange polka-dotted print with white terry cloth lining.

Sweaters were popular. Cardigans continued to be worn, and pullover styles — V-necks, crew necks, or turtlenecks — were coming into more general use for sports wear.

Coats and Wraps

The Chesterfield overcoat in black, dark gray, or dark blue was still the correct coat for formal wear in daytime or evening (Figure 22). There were several models of straight overcoats, usually in gray or tan, for street or business wear. They came in both single- and double-breasted styles, with the prevailing wide lapels, and were approximately knee-length or a little longer. The tan polo coat of camel's hair was very popular for casual wear (Figure 23). The belted raglan coat was worn for traveling or knockabout purposes (Figure 24). There was also a half-belted raglan coat of straighter cut, as well as a loose, flaring model with raglan sleeves called the "balmacaan," which often came in herringbone tweed or Glen plaid. War styles that carried over into peacetime fashions were the short overcoat with a fur collar and the long double-breasted military overcoat. The all-enveloping, shaggy raccoon coat was most typical of the era (Figure 25). It was a great favorite for campus wear (for both boys and girls) and a "must" for football games. Another college necessity was the yellow oilcloth raincoat, or "slicker" (Figure 26). This garment was also worn by both sexes, often accompanied by flapping, unbuckled galoshes.

A new sport item was the Lindbergh jacket of heavy wool or leather with elastic fitted waist and wrist bands.

Footwear

Shoes for formal evening wear were black patent leather, either oxfords or dancing pumps with bows. For formal day wear shoes might be black patent leather or calfskin, and were usually combined with spats of white linen, pearl gray, or fawn. In the early years of the decade ankle-high boots were still being worn, particularly by older or more-conservative men. Boots with light cloth tops gave much the same appearance as oxfords with spats. For informal wear, oxfords were most generally worn, in plain black, brown, or tan. Probably the most-popular style for sports wear was the two-tone saddle shoe in black and white or brown and white. They were all the rage and were considered much the smartest footwear with a natty sport outfit. Also favored were taupe and gray buckskin, or white shoes with black varnished soles. Sport oxfords might have fringed tongues (Figure 13).

Accessories

Jewelry for men included signet rings, fraternity pins, and tie clasps or stick pins. Formal shirts required studs and cuff links, which might be of pearl, gold, onyx, jade, or other stones. Dress waistcoat buttons might match the studs. Less-formal shirts frequently had French cuffs, single or double, and required cuff links. A narrow tie pin was worn beneath the knot of the four-in-hand to secure the tabs of the shirt collar. Pocket watches were still carried and might have ornamental watch chains and fobs. Wristwatches were very generally worn in this decade. Pipes and tobacco pouches might be carried, but cigarettes were smoked universally, and cigarette cases and pocket lighters were among the accessories carried by many men. Cigarette holders were considered very debonair by the smart set. Fountain pens and automatic pencils were part of the equipment of a man's vest pocket (or inside coat pocket). Trouser pockets were reserved for a wallet or a billfold and perhaps a jackknife. The well-dressed man wore gloves — white kid for formal evening wear; light gray or white for formal day wear; black, brown, gray, or tan calf or pigskin for street wear. White silk mufflers were worn with formal topcoats. Canes were still part of the well-turned-out attire — straight with a gold knob for more-formal occasions, Malacca with a crook handle for less-formal wear. An ever-present accessory of the twenties was the hip flask, to help the thirsty wayfarer bridge the gaps between forbidden oases during the dry days of Prohibition. The sober style for men's umbrellas, plain black with a crook handle, never varied through the years. In cold weather, earmuffs might be worn.

WOMEN'S FASHIONS

Within this decade, women's styles remained essentially straight and slim, with a low-slung waistline, but the hemline rose and fell from year to year. The general trend was upward, with the shortest skirts at knee level or just above in late 1925 through 1927. The brevity of women's garments caused panic in the textile industries. In 1928, manufacturers were dismayed at the small amount of material sold and influenced designers to create outfits that would require more fabric. At first, small pendants several inches long were attached to the hem in order to lengthen the above-the-knee costume. By 1930 hemlines were definitely lower, though uneven, and the waistline had crept back up to a normal position.

Hair Styles and Makeup

Permanent waving had come into general use by 1920. The early permanents were produced by baking under a complicated cluster of electric clamp-on curlers suspended overhead, with the victim immobilized during the process. The resulting spiral curls were kinky, frizzy, and somewhat hard to tame. In the first years of the decade, long hair was still styled softly over the ears and arranged in a knot at the back of the head. However, the vogue for bobbed hair was sweeping the country, and by 1924 most women were wearing their hair short. The coiffures frequently resembled close-fitting caps, sleek and neatly waved. The marcel wave was a regular arrangement of parallel undulations. Boyish bobs were popular, clipped over the ears and shingled in back. A straight Dutch bob with bangs was also prevalent. In 1929 some women were permitting their hair to grow again, and bobs were a little longer, curling softly on the back of the neck.

The twenties were frankly dedicated to conspicuous makeup. Mouths were painted a brilliant red and etched in a sharp line; a full pout or a cupid's bow was the ideal shape one tried to attain. The size of the mouth was often diminished by painting "bee-sting" lips in the center and ignoring the outer corners. Eyebrows were plucked, arched, and pencilled; lashes were loaded with mascara; cheeks were reddened with rouge; and noses were liberally powdered. Beauty parlors did a lively business in facials and rinses, and a great variety of creams, astringents, and beauty preparations appeared on the market. As more women went into the business world, increased emphasis was placed on careful grooming.

Hat Styles

Early in the twenties wide-brimmed hats were worn (Figures 35, 67). They might be trimmed with large bows, pom-poms, ostrich plumes, flowers, or artificial fruit. The typical hat of the period, however, was the small, close-fitting cloche, a bell-shaped hat with a narrow brim coming well down over the eyes (Figures 34, 40). Other models were turbans, toques, tam-o'-shanters, and berets. A brimmed hat of felt or velour might be worn for sports (Figures 61, 62). Evening headdresses were simpler than in the previous decade and might consist of a narrow silk headband or an ornamental comb.

Underwear, Loungewear, and Sleepwear

For those whom nature had blessed with straight and willowy figures, very little in the way of underclothing was required. They managed to discard everything except brief panties and short petticoats worn under the slim chemise gowns. Brassieres were very straight and flat in cut. For ampler figures, to assist women who had to fast and pray for boyish lines, there was a combination corset and brassiere made of silk jersey and elastic with vertical boning to erase the curves of the bosom and hip (Figure 27). A popular undergarment was the "teddy," or "teddy-bear," a one-piece combination consisting of a loose brassiere and panties, or a straight shift with a wide strap separating the skirt into two separate legs. Pajamas were gaining increasing popularity for sleepwear and were beginning to be seen on the beach and even in the drawing room (Figure 28). The following description accompanied the elegant pajama suit illustrated in Figure 29 and another of similar design by Molyneux:

> On the sands of the Lido, last summer, pajama suits first came into prominence as all-day attire. Of exotic and gorgeous materials, Molyneux is now heralding them as tea gowns of the perfect type, and they are the sensation of Paris. Modest they are, of a surety, with their demure little plaited-in trousers, straight jumper, and loose, high-collared coat of some sheer fabric that gives a very feminine gracefulness. One of the suits . . . is of gold cloth, printed in black, with a coat of black lace, banded at hem and cuffs with gold cloth; the other is of jade-green satin with a coat of printed black and white chiffon, and wide bands of black fox fur.[21]

Negligees continued to be made in a loose kimono style. There was a vogue for a wraparound model with wide sleeves and a shawl collar, which lapped across the front and tied low on the left hip (Figure 30).

Day Wear

The twenties featured the chemise. The silhouette was straight, slim, and simple; the effect was youthful and boyish — whether the wearer was eight, 28, or 80. A chart of the variations in the hemline through the decade would show that it started at about eight inches from the floor in 1920, rose another inch or two in 1921, went down again in 1922 and 1923 almost to the ankle (Figure 31), then began to rise sharply in 1924 to about ten inches off the floor (Figure 32). From 1925 to 1928 skirts were at knee level, just below or just above (Figures 33, 34). In 1928 hemlines were uneven, with the addition of draped panels or flounces, or perhaps were cut longer in back than in front. By 1929 hems were on a downward trend, though they were still uneven; the basic skirt line hovered about three inches below the knee. The natural waistline was almost completely lost or ignored during this period. At the beginning and end of the decade, a low natural waistline was the mode (Figure 35). Through most of the era, however, belts were worn at hip level, and draped girdle effects were placed at the same position (Figure 36).

The following descriptions were given for dressy afternoon outfits in 1921:

> [Figure 37] This frock of blue serge is bound with inch-wide black silk braid, and finished with a vest of black satin or cream lace. Black satin makes the underdress. The graceful side panels fall in points a few inches below the hem, giving the popular uneven line.

> [Figure 38] A circular tunic with a slightly circular underskirt and points falling below the hem proclaim this frock very much in the mode. Black serge or tricotine may be used, with an embroidered vest and fancy two-inch braid edging the tunic in both front and back.[22]

The Chanel suit appeared (one of its earliest forms is illustrated in Figure 39). Revised along simpler lines, the severely straight skirt and jacket became almost the uniform of the era. It has survived through all the years and was still in good style in the late fifties and sixties. For afternoon and spectator sports wear, a two-piece outfit of matching skirt and blouse was favored (Figures 40, 41, 42). The new, popular ensemble suit was a three-piece outfit of skirt, jacket, and matching topcoat, or tailored dress with matching coat in three-quarter or seven-eighths-length (Figures 43, 44, 45, 46).

Evening gowns were short. In the early twenties they might have an added train, a draped overskirt, or a length of sheer fabric hanging below the regular hemline or trailing on the floor (Figures 47, 48). In mid-decade formal evening gowns were knee-length, just as short as daytime dresses. Sheaths with an allover trim of beads, spangles, or sequins were popular (Figures 49, 50, 51, 54). Floating streamers (Figure 52) or cascades of long silk fringe were much admired. The "robe de style," with its long-waisted bodice and full gathered skirt, was a departure from the straight silhouette (Figures 53, 55). The Italian designer Fortuny created elegant accordion-pleated silk gowns, resembling classic Greek chitons (Figure 56), which continued in fashion through several decades. Tiers of ruffles for late evening appeared in the model by Poiret (Figure 54).

Evening Wear

Late in the decade, the lines of evening wear followed those of daytime garments, but in more exaggerated fashion. An evening gown might have a swooping drape on one side (Figure 57), or it might come just below the knee in front and descend to the floor in back. Much jewelry was worn with these outfits, a favorite mode being multiple bangle bracelets all the way up the arm. The cocoon-shaped wraps in velvet and satin from the preceding decade were still in vogue. Spanish shawls were rediscovered and worn as evening wraps (Figure 58). Ostrich plume fans (Figure 51) and feather headdresses (Figure 59) were sometimes seen.

Sportswear   Loosely fitted blouses and skirts were worn for sports. The tennis outfit illustrated in Figure 60 was made in two shades of gray silk jersey trimmed with navy blue taffeta bindings. Mannish shirtwaists and ties combined with tweed skirts were popular on the golf links (Figure 61). Simple shirtwaist dresses or straight chemise styles with full pleated skirts were also worn. In mid-decade a popular tennis dress was a sleeveless model of white crepe with a deep V-neck and a short skirt in wide box-pleats. A variety of sport jackets were in style—sweater-coats, silk jersey sweaters loosely belted, and sleeveless jackets of black velvet resembling long boleros. A typical three-piece sports outfit might consist of a long-sleeved jumper blouse and pleated skirt of beige crepe de Chine with a matching sleeveless cardigan of beige jersey. Sweaters were popular—cardigans and pullovers in V-neck, crew-neck, or turtleneck styles.

Bathing suits were shorter than in the preceding decade (Figures 63, 64). The one-piece maillot had come into use, although its wearers had been arrested for indecency when it first appeared on the beaches. Two-piece suits were also worn, consisting of short-skirted tunic tops over short bloomers. By this time stockings were omitted from the bathing costume.

Riding habits, across the years, consisted of neatly tailored jackets and jodhpurs (Figures 65, 66).

Coats and Wraps

Early in the period, coats tended to be voluminous wraparound models such as the one with full sleeves and shawl collar illustrated in Figure 67. The style with raglan sleeves shown in Figure 68 gave the same all-enveloping effect. The two Poiret coats from 1922 (Figures 69, 70) are dashing and dramatic. In the middle of the era, coats were straighter and slimmer and might have lavish fur collars and cuffs. At the end of the decade, the wraparound style was still good, but the line was slim and semifitted, as shown in the afternoon coat in Figure 71 and the evening coat in Figure 72. Capes, elbow-length or hem-length, were also worn throughout the period. There was also a cape coat — a straight, sleeveless coat with slit armholes and an attached wrist-length cape. For sports wear, one might appear in a belted double-breasted plaid tweed coat with patch pockets and raglan sleeves. Fur coats were popular and were frequently made in two different kinds of fur (for example, black sealskin with gray astrakhan trim).

Shoes in the twenties were rather heavy and "sturdy-looking," even in the high-heeled styles. Pumps were worn for dress, but the great majority of shoe styles had a strap over the instep or around the ankle, sometimes even two or three straps. Pumps often had high tongues and buckles. Two-toned combinations were popular. The illustrations of shoe styles in *Vogue* in 1928 show how festive and elaborate footwear might be and how often the feet were clad in beige to match the prevailing trend in costume color (Figure 73).[23] Silk and rayon hose came into general use during this decade. The most-popular shades were beige, taupe, and gray.

Footwear

Costume jewelry came into general use to enhance the very simple gowns. It was made of jewels of little intrinsic value, synthetic stones rather than real gems, but they were bright, attractive, and colorful. Matched sets of beads and earrings or brooches and earrings appeared. Sets of rings might match strings of beads or the jeweled trim on a bodice. Pearl necklaces and eardrops were always popular, and rhinestones were worn increasingly. It was an era of exaggeration in ornament. Strings of beads were very long and dangling, perhaps to below waist level, or were worn in multiple strands. Earrings were long, large, and elaborate. Bracelets were combined in profusion and might be worn all the way up the arm. Ornamental clips and brooches added an accent of color to a plain gown. In 1929 there was a recurrence of interest in antique jewelry.

Accessories

Accessories in this period were wristwatches, cigarette cases, long cigarette holders, vanity cases or compacts for carrying powder, rouge, and lipstick. Women also carried fountain pens, automatic pencils, and key cases in their purses. Handbags in the first years of the decade were tassel-trimmed fabric pouches closed with a drawstring (Figure 37). The most-prevalent style in purses, however, throughout this era was the envelope purse, or clutch bag, carried in the hand. Some styles of leather purses were suspended on a strap. Early in the period Japanese parasols and pencil umbrellas were still carried. Later, a short, stubby umbrella was in fashion. Folding fans or ostrich plume fans were carried with evening dress. An ornamental tortoise-shell comb might be added to the evening coiffure.

CHILDREN'S FASHIONS

Fashions for children reflected those of their elders, with knickers for the boys and short, straight skirts for the girls. A very small boy might wear a one-piece romper suit with short bloused pants, or a two-piece suit with short straight pants buttoned onto a blouse top. A fashion writer commenting on a boy's school wardrobe remarks: "The Norfolk suit, Buster Brown or Eton collar and the Windsor tie have given way to the more comfortable and far more practical suit of tweeds worn with a soft-collared shirt."[24] An eight-year-old boy might wear a jacket suit with straight short pants (Figure 74) and a ten- or twelve-year-old a suit with knickerbocker pants. A billed cap was worn with these outfits, and golf socks with wide-cuffed tops went with the short pants or knickers. At about fourteen years of age, a young man graduated into long trousers.

Very little girls might wear short, rather full dresses with matching bloomer panties (Figure 75). Those a little older wore replicas of their mothers' chemise frocks—straight, low-waisted, and short-skirted. Pleats were very popular. Matching sweater sets, a pullover and cardigan combination, were worn with tweed skirts. Matching coats and hats were in fashion (for little boys as well as little girls). For winter these sets often included wool leggings buttoned up the sides and, for the girls, a muff to keep the hands warm. A very elegant summer ensemble for a young lady was a matching dress, coat, and hat (cloche style) in pink taffeta.[25]

Little girls wore socks that came halfway up the calf, and older girls wore long cotton or lisle stockings. Boys' shoes were oxfords; girls wore oxfords, flat-heeled pumps, or simple strap shoes.

TYPICAL MATERIALS, COLORS, MOTIFS, AND TRIMMINGS

Materials for men's wear were serge or worsted in black, brown, navy, gray, or tan. Stripes and plaids were popular. Summer suitings were seersucker, linen, or Palm Beach cloth. Odd jackets came in tweed, light flannel, or gabardine. Art Deco abstract patterns appeared on four-in-hands. Shirts might be of pastel colors, striped or checked, with white collars and cuffs. Colorful sports jackets were combined with white or light-colored trousers.

For women, soft and draping fabrics were popular—georgette, crepe de Chine, chiffon, and silk jersey. Early in the period, serge and soft woolens, duvetyne, and velour were much used. Taffeta, soft satin (charmeuse), and velvet were popular. Rayons were used increasingly and were beginning to replace the more-expensive silk fabrics. Beige was probably the most-popular color during the twenties. An entire outfit might be in tones of beige—dress, sweater, coat, hat, and shoes.

White was also much worn, or white combined with brilliant trims. Off-colors such as mustard, citron, jade green, and copper were fashionable. Metallic effects, woven-in brocade patterns, and ribbon trims appeared frequently. One might see a white georgette gown embroidered in gold thread, a black velvet gown combined with gold lace, or orange brocade draped over a silver lamé sheath. Bead-embroidered trim in an allover pattern was much used. A pink chiffon-velvet gown might be decorated in a surface trim of crystal beads, or a black crepe gown might be trimmed with a bright red bead motif. Fringe was popular; it might be used as a hemline finish on a wool sports tunic, or a silk or beaded fringe might be used on an evening gown hem or in tiers covering the entire gown. Silk and rayon fabrics came in bold and exotic floral patterns. Large checks or plaids were popular, frequently made up on the diagonal, and bold stripes were also worn, horizontally as well as vertically. Fur trim was much used, and in mid-decade there was a fad for leopard, panther, and tiger-skin trimmings.

SUGGESTIONS FOR COSTUMING PLAYS IN THE PERIOD

To put the era of the twenties on stage is not very difficult at present, since women's styles in the sixties reverted for several years to the general flavor of that earlier decade. For men's wear, one may still find in second-hand clothing stores or thrift shops old suits that have jackets with broad, well-padded shoulders and wide lapels. To separate the genuine twenties and thirties models from the wide-lapelled Bill Blass "gangster suits" of the sixties, one must inspect the fit of the jackets and the cut of trousers. Twenties jackets are loose and draped in front; sixties jackets are more closely fitted and pinched in at the waistline. Twenties trousers are 18 to 24 inches wide at the cuff, and are full and baggy; the fullness at the hips is pleated into the front of the waistband. Sixties trousers are narrower in the leg and well fitted at the hip, with no pleats at the waistline. Trousers reproducing the wide-bottomed effect of the twenties trousers will probably need to be made for the occasion. Blazer jackets in stripes or plaids can be made using a present-day man's jacket pattern but it will be necessary to widen the lapels and increase the shoulder width. Hatbands and ties in bright stripes or in a flashy abstract motif give the color of the period. A long cigarette holder and a hip flask contribute to the atmosphere of the twenties. A cane and a straw hat help to complete the picture. One might be able to simulate a raccoon coat in a shaggy synthetic fur cloth. Two-tone shoes in brown and white or black and white also set the period. One may convert a pair of plain oxfords to a two-tone combination with shoe makeup.

Patterns and dresses for women that resemble those of the twenties are still available in thrift shops. In the sixties and seventies chemises were even shorter and some of the printed fabrics even wilder than those of the twenties. Today's array of knitted fabrics — Banlon, Estrella, Qiana, and metallic jerseys — lend themselves admirably to the drapes and tubular sheaths of the twenties. The beaded trim may be more difficult to achieve. The original models of beaded sheaths, made of weighted silk and crepe de Chine, are, alas, disintegrating. Old beaded dresses preserved in attics and museums must be handled with extreme care. It is sometimes possible to repair these fragile originals by making a new basic garment of net and appliqué-ing the old fabric and beadwork to this base. An allover sequin sheath could readily be created with the new knitted sequin fabrics. Silk or rayon fringe is available in fabric shops and trimming departments. The long strings of beads and fabulous dangling earrings are back on the market, in even more startling and theatrical versions than the twenties produced. Silk (nylon) stockings rolled below the knee would give a period touch; they should have seams in back. If seamed hose are unavailable, the effect can be produced with a felt-tipped marking pen. It is usually preferable to draw the fake seam on the leg rather than on the stocking.

The short hair styles of the twenties are extremely important to the period flavor. Nothing wrecks the authentic look faster than long flowing hair on men or women. If the members of a present-day cast are unwilling to sacrifice their long locks, their hair should be hidden under a short-cropped wig. Any dedicated actor should be willing to give up a full beard or trim off a luxurious mustache in order to appear in a twenties production!

TITLE	AUTHOR	PERIOD
The Adding Machine	Elmer Rice	1923
Anastasia	Guy Bolton	1926
archy and mehitabel (M)	George Kleinsinger, Joe Darien	1927
Auntie Mame; Mame (M)	Jerome Lawrence, Robert E. Lee	1928 – 46
Beggar on Horseback	George Kaufman, Marc Connelly	1923
The Boy Friend (M)	Sandy Wilson	1926
The Butter and Egg Man	George Kaufman	1925
Chicago (M)	Bob Fosse, Fred Ebb	late 1920s
The Circle	Somerset Maugham	1921
The Constant Wife	Somerset Maugham	1927
Dark at the Top of the Stairs	William Inge	early 1920s
The Desert Song (M)	Harbach, Hammerstein, Mandel, Romberg	1926
The Disenchanted	Budd Schulberg, Harvey Breit	1920s
Dracula	Hamilton Dean, John L. Balderston	1920s
Dulcy	George Kaufman, Marc Connelly	1921
The Front Page	Charles MacArthur, Ben Hecht	1928
Gentlemen Prefer Blondes (M)	Robin, Styne, Loos, J. Fields	1926
Good News (M)	Laurence Schwab, B. G. DeSylva	1927
The Great Gatsby	F. Scott Fitzgerald, Owen Davis	1926
Gypsy (M)	Laurents, Styne, Sondheim	1920s – 30s
The Hairy Ape	Eugene O'Neill	1922
The Happy Time	Samuel Taylor	early 1920s
Hay Fever	Noel Coward	1925
Hit the Deck (M)	Youmans, H. Fields, Robin, Grey	1927
I Do! I Do!	Tom Jones, Harvey Schmidt	1890 – 1925
Inherit the Wind	Jerome Lawrence, Robert E. Lee	1925
Juno and the Paycock	Sean O'Casey	1924
Lady, Be Good (M)	Bolton, Thompson, G. and I. Gershwin	1924
Morning's at Seven	Paul Osborn	1922
The Most Happy Fella (M)	Frank Loesser	1927
No, No, Nanette (M)	Youmans, Caesar, Harbach, Mandel	1925
Oh, Kay! (M)	Bolton, Wodehouse, G. and I. Gershwin	1926
Once in a Lifetime	Moss Hart, George Kaufman	1928
Rain	John Colton, Clemence Randolph	1920
Rose Marie (M)	Friml, Stothart, Harbach, Hammerstein	1924
Show Boat (M)	Ferber, Hammerstein, Kern	1880s; 1927
The Show-off	George Kelly	1923
The Silver Cord	Sidney Howard	1926
A Slight Case of Murder	Damon Runyon, Howard Lindsay	1920s
Strictly Dishonorable	Preston Sturgis	1929
Sunrise at Campobello	Dore Schary	1921 – 24
They Knew What They Wanted	Sidney Howard	1924
Tovarich; also (M)	Jacques Deval, Robert E. Sherwood	late 1920s

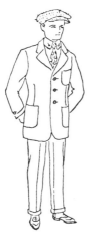

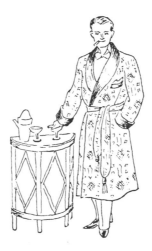

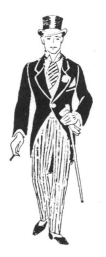

1. Velvet smoking jacket, braid trimmed, for lounging wear. 1929.

2. Dressing gown of heavy silk crepe, lined in silk of contrasting color. 1926.

3. Formal wedding attire: black cutaway; gray waistcoat; gray spats; striped trousers; striped ascot. 1925.

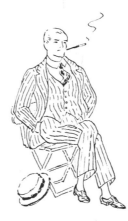

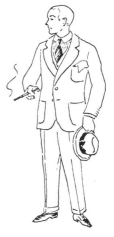

4. Sport suit: three-button sack coat with back vent; billed cap. 1921.

5. Single-breasted sack suit of striped gray flannel; matching vest. 1920.

6. Single-breasted suit with vest; striped shirt. 1920.

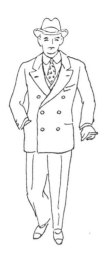

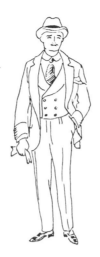

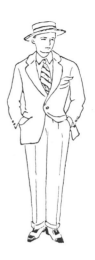

7. Double-breasted sack suit with broad shoulders and full trousers. 1924.

8. Single-breasted brown sack suit; brown waistcoat; pink shirt. 1921.

9. Lightweight summer suit; silk shirt; two-tone shoes; straw hat. 1923.

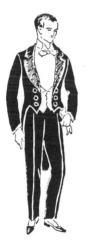

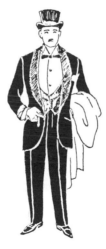

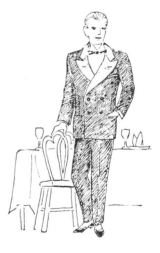

10. Black tailcoat with satin lapels; white tie and waistcoat. 1921.

11. Dinner jacket with shawl collar and satin lapels; satin waistcoat. 1922.

12. Double-breasted dinner jacket in midnight blue; black bow tie. 1928.

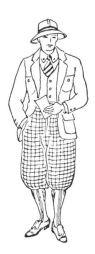

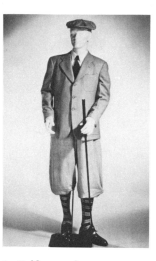

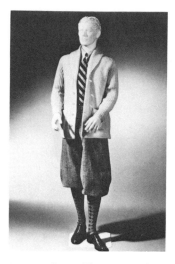

13. "Skokie" sports jacket, belted in back; vest; knickerbockers. 1924.

14. Golfing outfit: single-breasted tan wool jacket with three-button front; tan knickers with button fly and loops for belt at waistband. New Jersey, 1928 – 30. (Division of Costume, Smithsonian Institution.)

15. Knickers of brown wool tweed; cardigan sweater of tan ribbed knit wool, with shawl collar. New York City, by Cornell, 1928 – 29. (Division of Costume, Smithsonian Institution.)

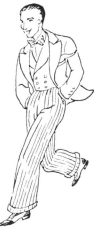

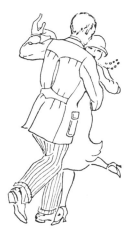

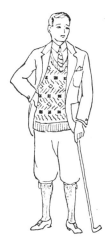

16. Brown coat and waistcoat; full, striped trousers with wide bottoms. 1926.

17. Gabardine sports coat, belted in back, set-in pleats. 1926.

18. For golf: plus-fours suit of gray flannel; bright pullover sweater. 1925.

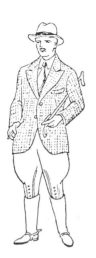

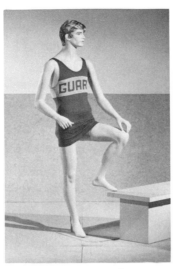

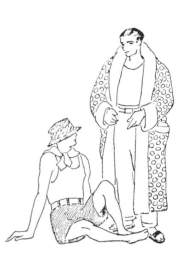

19. Riding outfit: tweed jacket; cord jodhpurs; boots. 1927.

20. Wool bathing suit for a lifeguard. San Francisco, by Gantner Company, 1923. (The Costume Institute of The Metropolitan Museum of Art. Gift of Gantner of California.)

21. Left, bathing shirt and trunks. Right, beach robe in flannel and terry cloth. 1929.

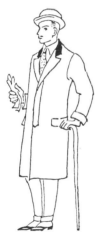

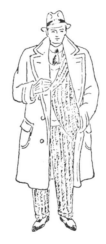

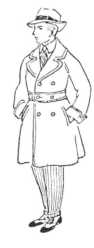

22. Chesterfield coat with velvet collar; bowler hat; spats; cane; gloves. 1923.

23. For motoring: tan polo coat; striped gray suit; yellow sweater. 1928.

24. Belted raglan coat of tan whipcord for traveling or motoring. 1923.

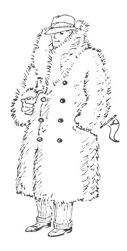

25. Raccoon coat, very popular with college boys. 1929.

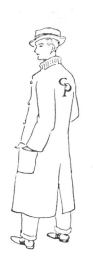

26. Yellow oilcloth slicker for rain and all-purpose campus wear. 1929.

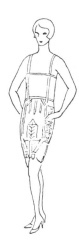

27. Combination corset and brassiere with vertical boning, to "create long straight lines." 1926.

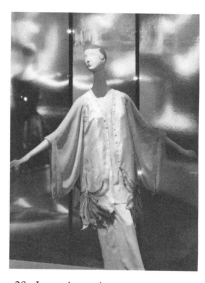

28. Lounging pajamas: yellow-chartreuse chiffon with sleeveless taffeta coat in peach and green with appliquéd tiger lilies. French, by Marie Nevitsky, 1925. (The Costume Institute of the Metropolitan Museum of Art. Gift of Mrs. Robert Lovett.)

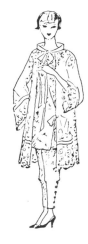

29. Molyneux pajama suit worn as tea gown: black-and-gold print, sheer coat of black lace. 1924.

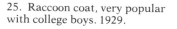

30. Poiret printed crepe gown with organdy collars and cuffs. 1923.

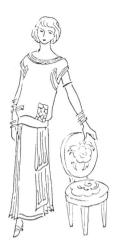

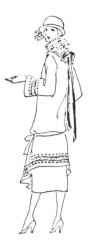

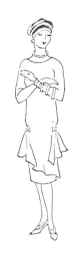

31. Patou white wool dress with pleated inserts in skirt, yellow-and-black embroidery. 1923.

32. Tunic dress of black wool embroidered in yellow and green silk; red beads; leopard collar. 1924.

33. Formal afternoon dress with long sleeves, of wine-red crepe. 1926.

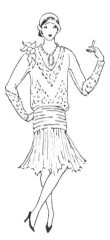

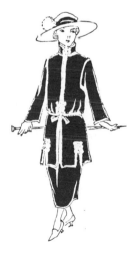

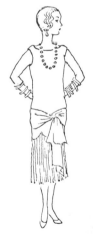

34. Spring frock of georgette and lace with accordion-pleated skirt. 1928.

35. Navy blue jersey suit in military style with edges bound in braid. 1921.

36. Afternoon frock of georgette, draped girdle on hip, silk fringe at hemline. 1924.

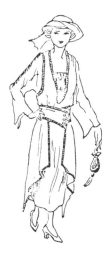

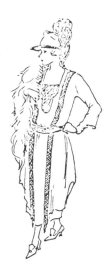

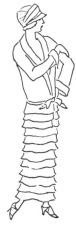

37. Frock of blue serge bound with black silk braid; underdress and vest of black satin. 1921.

38. Black jersey frock, circular over-tunic falling in points, two-inch braid trim. 1921.

39. Chanel suit of gray poplin; first three flounces are on jacket. 1923.

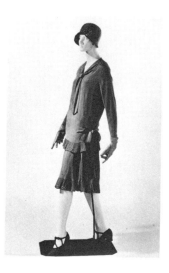

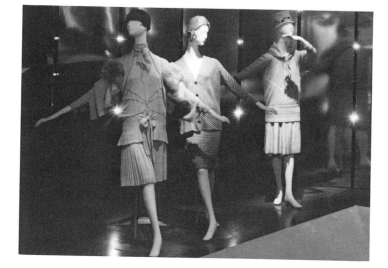

40. Two-piece dress of green silk crepe with long-sleeved overblouse. Knife-pleated ruffles border bottom edge of overblouse and hem of skirt. Cloche hat. 1924 – 28. (Division of Costume, Smithsonian Institution.)

41. Left, two-piece dress of rose-beige crepe trimmed with dyed fox fur. By Nellie Harrington of Corbeau et Cie, New York, 1928. Center, country tweed suit of coffee-and-beige houndstooth checked wool; bias-cut cardigan jacket and short skirt with loose back panels. By Molyneux, 1926 – 27. Right, two-piece sports dress with beige knit top and matching pleated silk crepe skirt and scarf trimmed with geranium silk crepe. By Nellie Harrington of Corbeau et Cie, New York, 1928. (The Costume Institute of the Metropolitan Museum of Art. Gifts of Mrs. Sidney Bernard and Mrs. Georges Gudefin.)

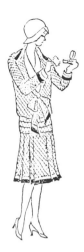

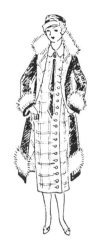

42. Spectator sports frock: checked blouse and box-pleated skirt; white vest. 1929.

43. Co-ed ensemble: jersey jacket over striped washable silk dress. 1928.

44. Jacket ensemble: fur-trimmed coat with plaid lining, over plaid dress. 1924.

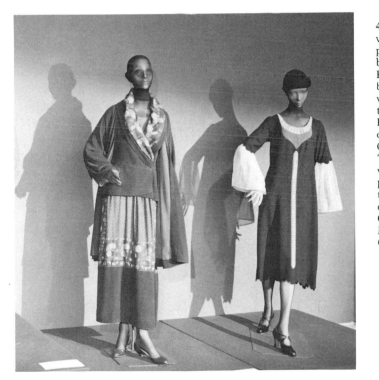

45. Left, afternoon ensemble in wine-red duvetyn and floral printed silk in shades of blue and beige on a wine-red ground. Printed silk dress with deep border of wool at hem; wool vest with shawl collar of printed silk; three-quarter length coat. By Poiret, 1920. (Museum of the City of New York. Gift of Mrs. Henry Clews.) Right, day frock, called "Bouclier": navy blue wool serge with accents of red and a band of printed buttons down the front, trumpet sleeves of cream-colored organdy. By Poiret, 1925. (The Costume Institute of The Metropolitan Museum of Art. Gift of Mrs. Alfred Rheinstein.)

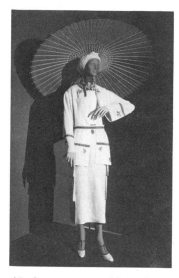

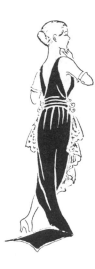

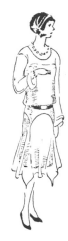

46. Summer ensemble: pale yellow linen dress and jacket trimmed with purple and green metallic bands and small floral sprays. Dress has inset vestee of pleated white linen. By Poiret, 1920. (Museum of the City of New York. Gift of Mrs. Henry Clews.)

47. Black satin evening gown with train and black lace flounces. 1920.

48. Dinner dress of black mousseline de soie. 1928.

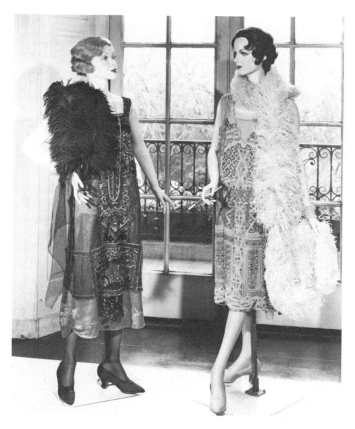

49. Evening dresses. Left, embroidered black net over magenta silk. By Callot Soeurs, early 1920s. Right, chiffon embroidered with metal thread and pearl beads. By Paquin, 1924–25. (Museum of the City of New York. Gift of Martha Lyon Slater.)

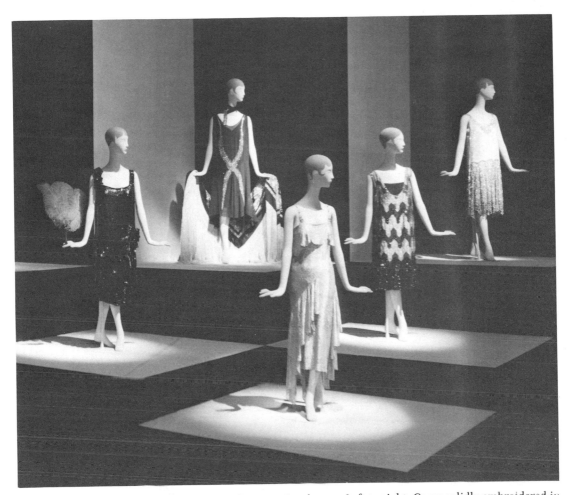

50. Short evening dresses. Left to right: Gown solidly embroidered in black sequins, with low-cut décolletage and tiered skirt. By Chanel, 1925. Black georgette studded with rhinestones in a lyre motif; worn with Spanish shawl of black silk, heavily embroidered and fringed in white. 1926. Pale gold lace with diagonal flounces and long uneven hemline. 1929. Dancing dress of black and gold metallic lace with flared flounce of black sequins. By Chanel, 1926–27. Beaded net encrusted with crystal bugle beads and gold sequined flowers, over silver lamé. 1926–27. (The Costume Institute of The Metropolitan Museum of Art.)

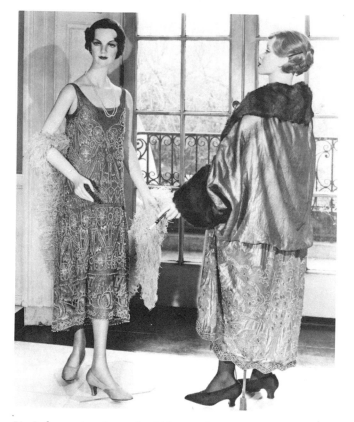

51. Left, evening dress of gold lace embroidered with rhinestones and pearls, over crepe de Chine slip. By Chanel, 1920s. Right, evening coat of gold lamé trimmed in mink and embroidered with pave bugle beads, rhinestones, and pearls. From Henri Bendel, Inc., 1920s. (Museum of the City of New York. Gift of Martha Lyon Slater.)

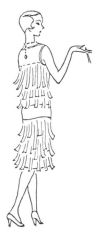

52. Evening dress of flesh-pink crepe with floating streamers. 1926.

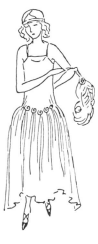

53. Evening dress with green moiré redingote, over gold cloth. 1923.

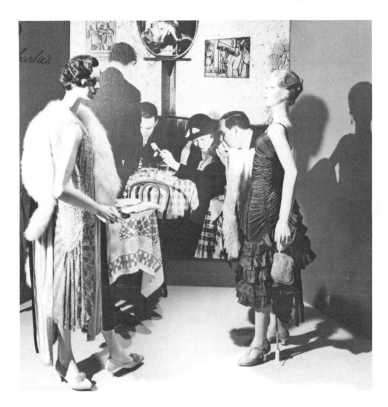

54. Left, gold sequined evening dress. Made in Shanghai, 1929. Right, evening dress of shirred black taffeta, called "La Poule." By Poiret, 1929. Background shot of "21" Club by Margaret Bourke White, lent by H. Jerome Berns. (Museum of the City of New York. Gift of Mrs. Theodore Roosevelt, Jr.)

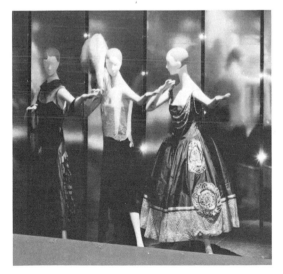

55. Left, dress for late evening: bias-cut black chiffon with rows of black satin ruffles; hipline defined by a wide satin sash. French, by Vionnet, 1929–30. Center, evening dress: petal-pink bugle-beaded bodice; black velvet skirt with descending side and back panels. French, by Worth, 1928. Right, "robe de style": long-waisted dress with full skirt of black silk taffeta trimmed with silver and green embroidered and beaded medallions. This silhouette was the exception to the prevailing unfitted line. French, by Lanvin, 1924. (The Costume Institute of the Metropolitan Museum of Art.)

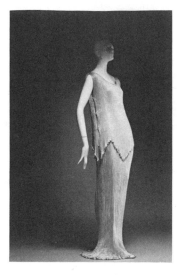

56. Evening gown of pale pink pleated silk, trimmed with matching cords and glass beads. Italian, by Fortuny, 1920s. (The Costume Institute of The Metropolitan Museum of Art. Gift of Claudia Lyon.)

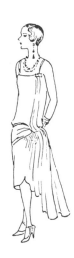

57. Evening dress of light blue stiff satin with elaborate drape. 1928.

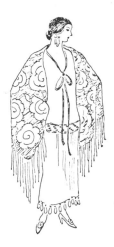

58. Spanish shawl worn over white crepe evening gown; crystal beads at waist and hemline. 1924.

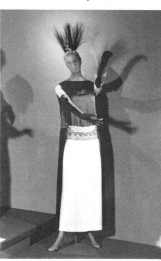

59. Evening dress: bodice and floating side panels of black satin over white satin skirt; waistline defined by a band of embroidery. By Poiret, 1922. (Museum of the City of New York. Gift of Mrs. Henry Clews.)

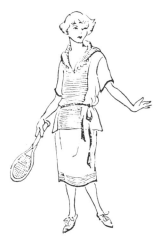

60. Sports dress of light and dark gray silk jersey with navy taffeta trim. 1921.

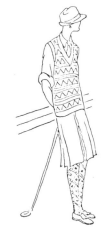

61. Borrowed masculine styles for sports: shirt, tie, sleeveless sweater, golf socks, felt hat. 1926.

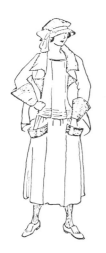

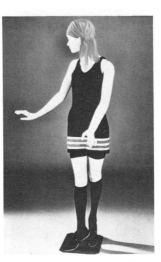

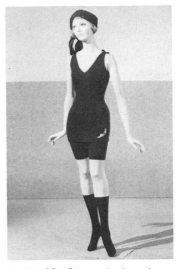

62. Sports ensemble; beige velour with brown leather trim. 1923.

63. One-piece black wool knit bathing suit. sleeveless, scoop-neck long top with white horizontal stripes at bottom; short trunks attached at waist. California, by Gantner and Mattern Company, 1925 – 27. (Division of Costume, Smithsonian Institution.)

64. Wool bathing suit. American, by Jantzen, 1920. (The Costume Institute of The Metropolitan Museum of Art. Gift of Vera Gawansky.)

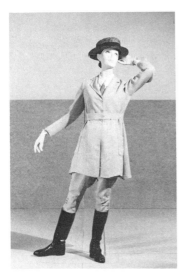

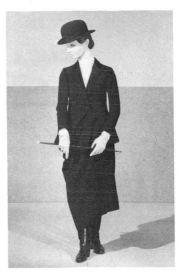

65. Linen riding habit. American, 1920. (The Costume Institute of The Metropolitan Museum of Art. Gift of Mrs. James Orme.)

66. Wool riding habit. English, London, by Arthur Cannon, 1920. (The Costume Institute of The Metropolitan Museum of Art. Gift of Mrs. Harrison Williams.)

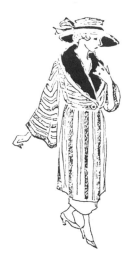

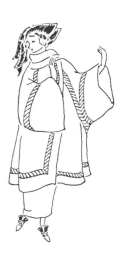

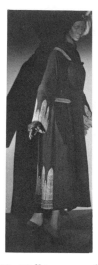

67. Black-and-red striped wool coat with Hudson seal collar. 1921.

68. Coat of navy wool rep with openwork trim. 1923.

69. Walking coat of dark blue wool with woven border pattern; coat wraps and buttons to one side. By Poiret, 1922. (Museum of the City of New York. Gift of Mrs. Henry Clews.)

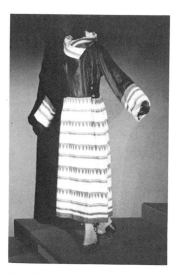

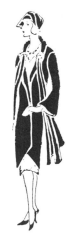

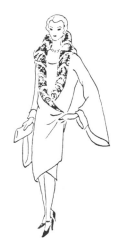

70. Afternoon coat: black satin top; cartridge pleated skirt of white wool with woven patterned bands in black; wool collar and cuffs. By Poiret, 1922. (Museum of the City of New York. Gift of Mrs. Henry Clews.)

71. Afternoon coat of dull black crepe satin. 1928.

72. Evening coat of beige velvet, lined with lighter satin; marten collar. 1926.

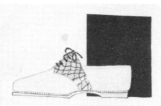

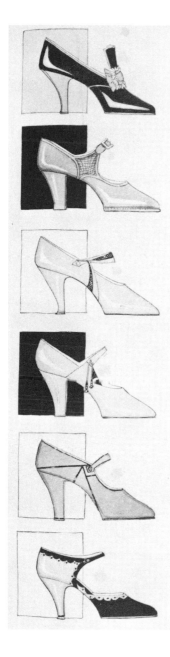

73. From lower left, clockwise: Evening shoe of sapphire-blue crepe de Chine combined with scalloped silver kid. Daytime shoe of dark beige antelope, with fine lines in brown patent leather. Beige kid shoe with insert of black patent leather. Daytime shoe of beige kid trimmed with sections of dark brown lizard. Morning shoe of heavy brown leather, edged with bands, trimmed with lizard. Black satin Louis XIV evening slipper with crimson satin heel and binding; large buckle. Sports shoe of white antelope and brown alligator; rubber sole. Evening slipper of black satin; band and heel of silver kid; trimmed with gold and silver roses. Silver kid evening slipper; heel and cutaway patterned trim in pomegranate-red suede. Afternoon shoe of gray lizard with straps of dark and light gray kid edged in silver. Sports shoe of white antelope and brown leather. Afternoon shoe of beige kid trimmed in brown patent leather. Evening shoe of green crepe de Chine with green satin inserts edged with gold. Page of 1920 shoe styles from *Vogue*, February 15, 1928.

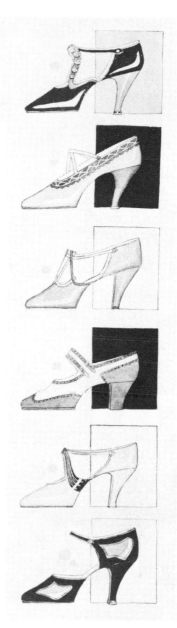

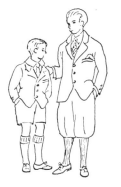 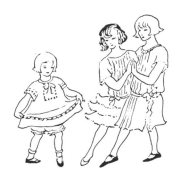

74. Boys' suits: 8-year-old in English shorts; 12-year-old in knickers. 1926.

75. Girls' dancing frocks of crepe de Chine; cross-stitched bloomers; tucks, ruffles, picoted edges. 1924.

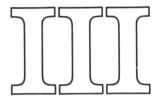

The Depressed Thirties
(1930–1939)

THE WOMAN'S COSTUME of the 1930s is characterized by the bias cut, bare back and bare midriff, and bobby socks. As the starch vanished from the national morale, the clothing sagged accordingly. As money disappeared from the scene, "fancy dress" became less fancy. A large section of the populace wore old clothes left over from an earlier era of affluence or made their own clothing. The term "banker" became an epithet, and, in the depths of the Depression, a high silk hat became an object of ridicule. This reaction is reminiscent of the days of the French Revolution, when it was dangerous for the nobility of Paris to appear on the streets in fine clothing; the mobs were highly sensitive to disparities in wealth between the upper and lower classes. That newly created American aristocracy of wealth, the big city gangsters, paid silent tribute to this frame of mind by replacing the top hat with a black felt fedora when they donned black tie and tuxedos for the evening. A cult of the sun developed as a population literally "on the beach" sought inexpensive diversion on the shores of lakes and oceans. Perhaps it is only a coincidence that the two-piece playsuits and bathing suits required less fabric than ever before.

CONCERNING THE PERIOD
The stock market crash late in 1929 ushered in a desperate era in America that prevailed throughout the following decade. The collapse of the economic system created an atmosphere much akin to that of war. After an unbelievable series of bank failures, bankruptcies, collapses of large corporations and small businesses, and mortgage foreclosures across the land, a black pall settled over the nation and a defeatist psychology prevailed — at the opposite pole from the high

spirits and optimism of the 1920s. Faced with this crisis when he came to office in 1933, President Franklin D. Roosevelt launched a drastic legislative program, setting new controls on banking and stock market speculation, repealing Prohibition, establishing many federal welfare agencies, and inaugurating a system of social security for the aged. Within one short decade America veered from a system of rugged individualism and private enterprise toward a welfare state with strong centralized responsibility and control of planning.

In the arts, Picasso was painting his two-faced *Girl with a Mirror*, and Dali was exploring the subconscious with his dreamlike deserts, while Ben Shahn was depicting the desperate situation of the unemployed and Grant Wood was caricaturing midwestern farmers. And across the nation, WPA artists were painting murals on the walls of public buildings, specializing in blocky representations of men and machines. In building and architecture, some courageous and daring souls were following the lead of Walter Gropius at the Bauhaus in Germany and Frank Lloyd Wright in America and experimenting with the new free forms of modern steel and concrete homes. Early in the thirties, these new styles began to appear on the West Coast in the work of Richard Neutra and in the East in industrial buildings designed by Lescaze. Rockefeller Center, built in 1931–1933, was the last word in "1930s modern."

The great majority still clung to Colonial-style in homes. Two international fairs helped to orient the public toward the new movement in architecture and interior decorating. At the Chicago World's Fair in 1933 an exhibit called "The House of the Future" featured new designs in furniture, including styles from Sweden and Denmark. The New York World's Fair in 1939 exemplified the new "modern" style in the design of its buildings, displays, and exhibits, and in the simple geometric shape of its symbol and trademark, the Trylon and Perisphere. With the curtailment of income during the thirties, most families were making do with furnishings from an earlier era; modernizing frequently meant a fresh coat of paint and new slipcovers. Where innovations could be afforded, they occurred first in the kitchen and bathroom, where the most-direct contributions were made to human comfort, in line with technological improvements.

The popular music of the thirties was produced by big bands, some of them "sweet" — those led by Wayne King, Guy Lombardo, Eddy Duchin, Paul Whiteman — and some of them "hot" — headed by Benny Goodman, Artie Shaw, Tommy Dorsey, and Glenn Miller. The latter breed developed a jazz rhythm labeled "swing," which led to a fast, syncopated dance called the Lindy Hop. This step emanated from the Savoy Ballroom in Harlem, a center featuring big-name bands. Embellishments on this dance included the Susie-Q, truckin', and peckin'. The Lindy, or Jitterbug, was an off-beat step that went into a breakaway, during which the man whirled his partner out at arm's length and then brought her in again, never missing a beat. The breakaway encouraged unlimited improvisation and creativity in new dance steps. The "Big Apple," a mass version of the Lindy, came out of South Carolina and was based on an old-fashioned square dance. A caller stood in the center of the dance floor and invited couples in turn to "rise and shine." Costume notes associated with the dances of the 1930s include the following:

> The girls quickly evolved their own uniforms — saddle shoes, full skirts, and sloppy sweaters — while all across the land at high school proms young ladies in "formals" began to jitterbug, presenting a happily incongruous spectacle.[1]

The "zoot suit" was an outfit developed in the late thirties by teen-age male "hep-cats" and "jitterbugs," particularly the blacks in Harlem and the Mexican-Americans in the Los Angeles area. This costume consisted of pegged pants and an absurdly exaggerated "draped-shape" jacket with broad shoulders and extreme length, almost to the knees; it was worn with out-sized accessories, a huge bow-tie, and an ankle-length key chain attached to a belt loop.

At the beginning of the thirties, the shift from silent to sound motion pictures was under way. Experiments were also being made in the use of Technicolor, and its quality gradually improved during this decade. The style in sirens was set by two seductive blondes, Mae West and Jean Harlow. Greta Garbo established her own particular style, a combination of aloofness and mystery costumed in a rather mannish simplicity and dash — slim and svelte with a slight air of slouch. This look became the ultimate in glamor for the thirties, and a devoted following strove to achieve the same careless assured elegance. At the opposite pole was the feminine softness and lushness of the Harlow — West brand of temptress — cotton-candy fluff achieved with slinky, bias-cut satin trimmed with ostrich feathers (Figure 27). Another variety of sophisticated high fashion, usually streamlined, draped, and clinging, often lavishly fur-trimmed, was exemplified by such figures as Norma Shearer and Kay Francis, who also ranked as fashion-setters.

In the Broadway theatre, some outstanding playwrights developed a social consciousness. Reflecting the universal concern with an economy gone wrong, such authors as Maxwell Anderson, Robert Emmett Sherwood, and Clifford Odets built stirring plays around such themes as the miscarriage of justice, the encroachments upon individual freedom by the all-powerful fascist state, and the rights of labor. In Manhattan the experimental Group Theatre produced several of these scripts and evolved the "method" school of acting. A unique development of the Depression era was the WPA venture into theatrical production, the Federal Theatre Project. Under the inspired guidance of Hallie Flanagan, who was the head of the Drama Department of Vassar College, the Federal Theatre gave work to thousands of unemployed actors and theatre workers and at the same time brought a variety of dramatic productions to cities across the nation. Among its experimental ventures were plays produced in a "living newspaper" style, usually with arena staging, minimal sets, an atmosphere of harsh realism under stark white lights, and projected images and film clips. The Federal Theatre Project lasted only four years, from 1935 to 1939. It might be considered a failure, since no outstanding plays or playwrights emerged. Yet it has doubtless been responsible for the sowing of seeds for a decentralized theatre across the country and for a network of vigorous community and college theatres built with WPA funds.

Against this background of social unrest and ferment, what were people wearing? In an era of experimentation, science was contributing more and more to costume, particularly synthetic fabrics. As the decade ended, in the Du Pont Exhibit at the great New York World's Fair, a beautiful model in a giant bird cage displayed a new product from the "Wonder World of Chemistry" — the first pair of nylon hose!

GENERAL CHARACTERISTICS OF COSTUME

In the Depression, fashions in men's clothing continued the trend of the late twenties. Suit jackets were predominantly double-breasted and broad-shouldered, with wide lapels (usually peaked) and a semi-fitted waistline. Trousers were still wide (about twenty inches at the cuff) and full at the waistline, with pleats on either side of the front seam, and they were long enough to break over the instep. A dark pinstripe was one of the most-popular models, in a dark gray or navy blue worsted with narrow white stripes spaced as much as two inches apart. Such suits became the uniform of the nattily dressed gangster portrayed in films by James Cagney and Humphrey Bogart. With this outfit he might wear a rather voluminous double-breasted polo coat or trench coat. Early in this decade, when men dressed for golf or other active sports, they shifted from knickerbockers to long trousers or slacks combined with a sport jacket or sweater. The same transition occurred in the younger set — grammar-school boys and young teenagers no longer wore knee pants, but converted to slacks.

Women's fashions during the thirties were for the most part slender and clinging. The French designer Madeleine Vionnet was credited with inaugurating the bias cut (or what the English call the "cut on the cross"), which became the hallmark of this era. Throughout the period, it was frequently used to produce an intricate network of zig-zag lines in a complicated and cut-up pattern (Figure 42). Diagonal seams in the new synthetic fabrics lent a much-desired soft drape to everything. Rayon-backed satin had a supple, spineless quality that made the negligees and evening gowns adhere to the wearer like a second skin.

Schiaparelli contributed her own exotic touch to the costume of the thirties. She was the most-extreme couturière of the era, noted or notorious for her startling effects. She promoted a violent shade of fuchsia, which she labeled "shocking pink"; and at one point in the late thirties she experimented with surrealist effects influenced by Salvadore Dali—hats trimmed with muttonchops, a suit decorated with closed bureau drawers. At the opposite extreme was Mainbocher's look of understated elegance. He created a starkly simple sculptured gown of blue-gray crepe for Wallis Warfield Simpson to wear at her wedding to the Duke of Windsor in 1937. At the outbreak of World War II, Mainbocher forsook Paris and set up shop in Manhattan. American designers were beginning to come to the fore in the fashion world during the thirties. New on the scene were Claire McCardell and Norman Norell, both of whom attained eminence in the 1940s. Working at Hattie Carnegie's establishment in New York during this decade, Norell designed for such theatre personalities as Constance Bennett, Katharine Hepburn, Grace Moore, Joan Crawford, and Gertrude Lawrence. The temperamental refugee Valentina contributed flamboyant color to the Manhattan fashion picture at this time and did some stage designing in addition to her work for a socialite clientele. The production of *Amphitryon 38*, starring Alfred Lunt and Lynn Fontanne, was enhanced by her beautifully draped costumes.

During the thirties the center of attention in women's fashions seemed to be the back and the hip area. Evening dresses were frequently very bare-backed, with necklines plunging to the waistline or lower, revealing shoulder blades and vertebrae. The hipline might be accented with a closely fitted yoke or with hip-flounces. Bustle effects were popular, with bows, drapery, or flounces at the rear. Lounging pajamas were more fashionable than they had been in the twenties and were worn for beach, boudoir, or formal evening affairs. Playsuits appeared in great variety, including a bare-midriff model that was worn on the street as well as on the beach.

MEN'S FASHIONS

The trend toward casual comfort in men's clothing, developed in the 1920s, continued in the thirties. Men strove for a look of carefree nonchalance—a loose drape across the chest, buttons unbuttoned, hands in pockets, full trousers flapping about the ankles. Innovations occurred in sportswear with the advent of knitted shirts and Bermuda shorts and a general tendency to bare more skin at the beach. Informal evening dress took on added color with the appearance of white evening jackets and bright cummerbunds.

Hair Styles and Grooming

Men's hair continued to be short, clipped over the ears, and shingled in back. Hair might be parted in the middle or on either side, with the left-hand part predominating. Some men still preferred the pompadour popular with the collegiate youth of the twenties. Photographs of movie stars in this era (such as Robert Montgomery, Robert Taylor, and George Raft) show the liberal use of hair oil to maintain neatly slicked-down hair with a precise part. Some went so far as to flaunt a marcel wave, lacquered in its every-hair-in-place perfection. The large majority of men were clean-shaven. A few sported small, neatly clipped mustaches (Ronald Colman, William Powell, Clark Gable). There was not a beard anywhere in sight.

Hat Styles

Although the high silk hat had fallen from favor, it was still required upon occasion to complete a formal evening outfit of "white tie and tails" or to be worn with a cutaway at a formal day wedding. Gangsters seemed to prefer black fedoras or derbies as a complement to their tuxedos. A wedding guest might wear a black homburg (or frequently went hatless). For town and business wear and for semiformal daytime occasions, the homburg or derby was worn by the more-conservative man. For general wear, the lightweight felt fedora was most popular. For a sporty flavor, it might have a porkpie shape (squared-off crown with a dishlike crease in the top, as shown in Figure 22) or a snap-brim pulled down in front (Figures 3, 11, 14). The billed cap was still sometimes worn for sports, often in checked tweed. Another style seen with sports outfits was the Alpine or Tyrolean hat with sloping crown, narrow brim, cord band, and a feather at the side (Figure 15). The straw boater, with a bright regimental band, was popular for summer and resort wear. It might even be worn with informal summer evening attire (Figure 9). Still appearing on the scene was the cream-toned Panama hat of fine handwoven straw (Figure 2). There was also a new variety of summer straw hat made of a darker tan coconut fiber with a gaily colored wide silk band.

Underwear, Loungewear, and Sleepwear

As more and more homes acquired central heating, the need for long knitted underwear in the wintertime diminished. Of course, there is a perennial need for "longies" in cold weather for such outdoor pursuits as farming, camping, and skiing. By this time, one-piece cotton union suits for summer wear had been replaced by cotton shorts and sleeveless knitted lisle undershirts. Many men wore only the boxer shorts and omitted the undershirt.

Lounging robes continued in a traditional style with a lapped front, shawl collar, and tie-belt. Bathrobes and beach robes in terry cloth were popular (Figure 19). Pajamas were the prevailing garment for sleepwear — printed or plain, of soft flannel or cotton, rayon, or silk. The tops might button up the front or slip over the head.

Neckwear

The stiff-bosomed dress shirt with wing collar was correct for formal evening wear with tails or formal day wear with a cutaway coat. Men were shifting more and more to dress shirts with attached turnover collars for semiformal occasions; a soft white silk shirt might be worn with an evening jacket. For day wear most shirts in the thirties had soft, attached, turnover collars. Early in the decade the collar ends might be blunt and rounded. Toward the end of the era collars were wider and more pointed, particularly in sport shirts. Shirts were colorful — pastels were used in the early thirties, brighter or deeper shades a few years later. Narrow stripes were also popular. Shirts came in tan, beige, light blue, pink, or gray, often with attached white collar and cuffs. Even at a formal daytime wedding, the best man and guests could (according to *Esquire Magazine*) properly wear blue or pink broadcloth shirts with starched white turnover collars. Collar tips were usually secured by fastening them with a long bar or collar pin that went under the knot of the four-in-hand. The button-down collar was also seen (i.e., with small buttons sewn to the shirt-front to which the collar tips were buttoned). About mid-decade a vogue for wearing dark shirts in shades of navy, wine, or brown with lighter suits came into fashion. The navy blue sport shirt shown in Figure 12 was included as a part of a "basic Southern wardrobe" for a well-dressed man in 1934. The caption says:

> White flannels, white shoes, white socks and belt, and a navy blue knitted sports shirt [are] excellent for deck tennis and other deck games, and for lawn tennis and golf ashore. The navy blue shirt, long popular in the south of France, is becoming popular here.[2]

Bolder and brighter patterns and colors were seen at resorts and beaches in the late thirties. Wide stripes, madras weaves, herringbone weaves in lightweight wool, plaids and checks — all were being made into sport shirts, with long sleeves for cool weather and short sleeves for summer. Collars were more often than not worn open. A variety of styles appeared for sports and lounging, such as the military shirt in Figure 18 and the tropical bush shirt in Figure 16. For added dash and color, the neckline might be filled in with a casually knotted scarf.

A white bow tie was worn with a formal evening tailcoat. Black bow ties were standard for informal wear with tuxedos or white jackets. A puff tie or ascot was worn with a cutaway. Early in the decade, bow ties were still being worn occasionally for daytime dress. By the end of the thirties, the four-in-hand was by far the most-popular style in ties. A bold diagonal stripe was the most-prevalent pattern; dots, plaids, and checks were also in favor. The fabric might be foulard or printed satin. The width was a lavish three or four inches.

Day Wear   The double-breasted lounge suit, often pin-striped, was perhaps the most-typical outfit of the thirties (Figures 1, 2). The shoulders were wide, the waistline was semifitted, and the lapels were very wide and peaked. The description accompanying the model in Figure 3 said:

> a striped flannel suit in blue-grey with a smoke-grey felt hat, white soft collar, blue shirt, dark blue tie, and brown-and-white shoes. Note the longer jacket. This suit is quite as appropriate in the country as an odd jacket and flannel trousers. However, such an outfit, while appropriate at resorts, is not the thing to wear in town, nor is it correct for traveling, except by motor.[3]

In another year or so the dark pinstripe was quite acceptable for town wear, though it might be combined with a double-breasted cotton waistcoat, a dark homburg hat, and black shoes. The broadly curving lapel line and a soft drape in the jacket front were designed to "give more apparent weight to the chest, and the suggested waistline, not actually tight or fitted, . . . to minimize the girth at that point."[4] Sack suits were popular in single-breasted two- or three-button models, with wide notched lapels (Figures 4, 5, 6). Usually only one button at the waistline was buttoned. Combinations of separate jackets and trousers were in high favor for town as well as country and sports wear.

Vanity Fair presented a fascinating page on a varied vacation wardrobe with a formula for mixing and matching ("4 suits plus 4 accessories equals 14 outfits"). The ingredients consisted of a plain gray flannel suit (double-breasted); one white suit (double-breasted) of linen, Palm Beach cloth, or tropical worsted; a checked tweed suit (single-breasted) with matching waistcoat; and a black or midnight blue evening outfit (preferably double-breasted dinner jacket), plus a white dinner coat with shawl collar and a white mess jacket. The fashion writer commented:

> Men who know how to dress know how to mix the colors and patterns in their outfits in order to achieve variety, just as an experienced cocktail mixer, given a few essential ingredients, can make a variety of drinks.[5]

The gray flannel jacket could be combined with the white trousers or the tweed trousers, the white suit jacket with the gray trousers or the tweed trousers, and the tweed jacket with the white trousers or the gray trousers; and the evening outfit could be varied with three different jackets. A dark blue jacket with lighter trousers was one of the favorite combinations of that era. "Perhaps the foremost exponent of mixed outfits (and certainly the best known)" observed *Vanity Fair*, "is the Prince of Wales. Even at public functions, during the day, the Prince has been seen wearing a dark lounge coat with light grey trousers."[6] Sack suits frequently had matching vests or waistcoats. The vests might be single-breasted or double-breasted with wide lapels (Figure 7). Trousers were generous in cut, high-waisted, pleated into the waistband, and full at the cuffs (20 inches). Now and then cuffs were omitted on suits for daytime wear (Figure 6).

It might be interesting to list the attire considered correct for a formal day wedding in the thirties. The following prescription appeared in the pages of *Esquire* in 1938:

A. The groom wears a one-button oxford grey morning coat [cutaway] with grey striped trousers, plain black calf shoes, double breasted waistcoat, white pleated shirt with wing collar, blue-grey ascot, pearl stickpin, white pocket handkerchief and lilies of the valley boutonnière.

B. An usher wears a one-button morning coat, striped trousers, double breasted white linen waistcoat, soft white shirt, white starched turn-over collar, grey Spitalfields tie [four-in-hand], white linen spats, plain black calf shoes, white handkerchief, white carnation boutonnière.

C. A page boy wears a black Eton jacket, single breasted waistcoat, striped trousers, plain black shoes, white shirt, white Eton collar, narrow black tie, silk hat [Figure 64].

D. The best man wears a morning coat, checked trousers, black shoes with button tops, fawn waistcoat, blue shirt with white cuffs and collar, checked tie, white pocket handkerchief, gardenia.

E. The bride's father wears a two-button morning coat, single-breasted waistcoat, striped trousers, black shoes with button tops, demi-bosom shirt with white cuffs, white wing collar, foulard bow tie, carnation.

F. A guest wears an oxford grey jacket [double-breasted], herringbone trousers, pink broadcloth shirt, white starched turn-over collar, black satin tie, pearl stickpin, pink carnation, white pocket handkerchief, plain black shoes, black Homburg, white mocha gloves.[7]

Another discussion of appropriate dress for the groom in wedding ceremonies under various circumstances (as illustrated in Figure 8) included the following:

Semi-formal town, daytime: Oxford gray single-breasted two-button jacket with peaked lapel, gray striped trousers, double-breasted waistcoat, white shirt, turn-over collar, black four-in-hand tie, black calf shoes.

Informal town, daytime: Medium gray flannel suit, double-breasted with peaked lapel, white shirt, turn-over collar, blue-and-white checked four-in-hand tie, black calf shoes, straw hat with black band.

Informal country, daytime: Navy blue double-breasted jacket, white trousers, white shirt, turn-over collar, light blue tie with white dots, black-and-white shoes.

Formal town or country, daytime: Oxford gray morning coat, striped trousers, white waistcoat, stiff-bosomed shirt, wing collar, blue-gray ascot, black calf shoes.

Formal town or country, evening: Full evening dress, tailcoat, white waistcoat, stiff-bosomed shirt, wing collar, white tie, black patent leather shoes.

Semi-formal town, evening: Single-breasted black tuxedo jacket, satin-faced peaked lapels, black trousers, stiff-bosomed white shirt, wing collar, black bow tie, black calf shoes.

Semi-formal country, evening: Double-breasted white dinner jacket, shawl collar, black trousers, white shirt, turn-over collar, black bow tie, black calf shoes.[8]

Evening Wear   Formal evening attire required a tailcoat, black or midnight blue (bottom, center, Figure 8). It followed the prevailing broad-shouldered contour of men's jackets for this era, with very wide, peaked, satin-faced lapels. The trousers were full, trimmed with braid on the side seams, pleated at the waistline, wide at the bottom, and uncuffed. Worn with them were a stiff-bosomed white shirt with wing collar and pearl studs, a white washable piqué single-breasted waistcoat, a white piqué bow tie, black or dark blue silk hose, and patent leather oxfords or dancing pumps. The full outfit included a black silk top hat or opera hat, a black or dark blue Chesterfield overcoat (single- or double-breasted), gloves of white buck or kid, and sometimes a cane.

For informal evening wear, the double-breasted dinner jacket with satin-faced collar and lapels was the most-popular style during the thirties (Figure 9). Variations were many — it might be black or midnight blue; it might have a shawl collar or peaked lapels. A single-breasted model in tuxedo jackets was also seen, with shawl collar or peaked lapels. A waistcoat, single- or double-breasted, of white piqué or black silk, or a black cummerbund completed the outfit. Popular for resort wear was the white dinner jacket, single- or double-breasted with shawl collar (Figure 8), or the shorter white mess jacket, which might be worn with a bright red cummerbund (Figure 10). Trousers were black or midnight blue, with braided side seams and wide uncuffed bottoms. Early in the thirties stiff wing collars were worn with tuxedo jackets, but toward the end of the decade the stiff collar and stiff-bosomed shirt were increasingly discarded in favor of the soft turnover collar for informal evening wear. Completing the ensemble were a black or midnight blue silk bow tie; hose of blue or black silk, plain or clocked; studs of pearl, gold, enamel, or colored stones; and gloves of white mocha, buck, or chamois. Dress shoes for evening were patent leather oxfords or pumps; low-cut pumps might be trimmed with black grosgrain ribbon bows. With their tuxedos, men might go hatless or wear black fedoras or homburgs, or on summer evenings they might wear a straw hat. One illustration for resort wear showed a dark coconut straw hat with white silk pleated band worn with a white dinner jacket. The proper overcoat for informal evenings was a single- or double-breasted Chesterfield, or a box coat, in black, Oxford gray, or midnight blue.

For active sports, knickerbockers (Figure 11) were still worn at the be- *Sportswear* ginning of the thirties. By the end of the decade, most men had converted to sport shirts and slacks for golf and other such pursuits. A dark knitted shirt with white flannel slacks was popular on the tennis courts (Figure 12). The Norfolk jacket in tweed and plaid was a perennial favorite (Figure 13). Mixing separate sports jackets and slacks in various combinations — patterned and plain, dark and light — continued to be a popular approach to casual sportswear throughout the decade (Figures 14, 15). With casual attire for country wear and spectator sports, pullover sweaters were frequently substituted for vests (Figures 11, 14). Beach and resort wear was colorful and comfortable. New styles appeared, such as the bush jacket (Figure 16), brightly striped or patterned short-sleeved cotton shirts, and shorts just above the knee (Figure 17). Bathing suits began to omit the tops and often consisted of a pair of brief trunks (Figure 18). Skiing required its own special cold-weather outfit (Figure 20).

Two-toned shoes for sports wear, brown and white or black and white, were still very popular in this decade, as they had been in the twenties. Headgear for sports or casual wear included lightweight felt hats (the porkpie was especially popular with college youth), straw hats in the usual boater style with regimental or club-striped band, darker coconut straws, and billed caps in tweed.

Coats and Wraps

The Chesterfield coat in black or midnight blue continued to be the appropriate wrap for evening wear. A popular dressy topcoat in this era was a double-breasted, peaked-lapel model with broad shoulders and a semifitted waistline, such as the coat illustrated in Figure 21, which was recommended as part of a college man's wardrobe. For campus and casual wear, the balmacaan coat was very popular; it was loose and wide, with raglan sleeves (Figure 22). Raccoon coats were still being worn in the early thirties, and a fur-lined coat was also favored for cold weather. The style illustrated in Figure 23, made of dark wool cloth with fur lining and collar, was advertised in 1932 for motoring, football games, and evening wear. The same page lists a less-expensive "good sports coat of wombat."[9] The voluminous polo coat of tan camel's hair was still around, worn loose or belted. A single-breasted fly-front raincoat of tan covert cloth, with notched or semipeaked lapels, large patch pockets, and raglan sleeves, was popular for stormy weather or all-purpose wear. The double-breasted trench coat of weatherproofed gabardine, styled with raglan sleeves and belted, was also worn for heavy weather.

Short jackets were increasingly popular, particularly with school boys and college youth. Among the styles in jackets were the Lindbergh jacket, with elastic cuffs and belt; the windbreaker of wool or leather, with set-on belt and zipper closing (Figure 24); and the sheep-lined jacket, which might have a fur collar. The parka, a heavy jacket with attached hood, first appeared for winter sports during this decade.

Footwear

For evening wear, black patent leather pumps (which might be bow-trimmed) or oxfords were proper. For formal day dress, plain black calf shoes were worn. Occasionally cloth-topped boots were seen. Spats were worn less frequently than in the previous decade. For daytime wear at business or dress occasions, dark oxfords of brown or black calf were the fashion. For country or sports wear, by far the most-popular style was the two-toned black-and-white or brown-and-white oxford (with dark toe-cap and heel). Another version was the saddle shoe, white with a black or brown section across the instep. In the summer or at the resorts, a "smart white buck with black rubber soles" was also favored. The Blucher shoe, originally named for a Prussian general, appeared in this decade; it was a half-boot laced or strapped over a tongue that came high on the instep. A new model for sports wear was the chukka boot, almost ankle-high, tied high on the instep, with heavy soles. At the end of the thirties a new Norwegian model in a low-cut slip-on moccasin style (later called the "loafer") appeared; in the next decade it became very popular. Shoes for the beach included canvas shoes with thick cork or rope soles and a variety of sandals. Heavy crepe rubber soles on sports shoes were seen frequently during these years. Galoshes graduated from the buckled fasteners of the twenties to the new zipper closings.

Accessories

Men's accessories did not change to any appreciable extent from the twenties to the thirties. Jewelry included cuff links, tie clasps, and shirt studs. Pearl studs and cuff links were worn with formal evening dress; studs and links with colored stones, enameled, or gold, might be worn with informal dress. A pearl stickpin was worn with an ascot tie. A college man might wear a class or fraternity ring, or a fraternity pin on his vest. A wristwatch was standard equipment for most men. An elderly man might still carry a pocket watch in his vest pocket, with a chain festooned across his waistcoat front. A wallet or billfold was carried in the hip pocket. Some sports jackets and topcoats had an extra "cash pocket," quite small, placed just above the usual lower right-hand pocket, designed to carry a change purse or theatre tickets. A neatly folded handkerchief with points showing out of the breast pocket of his jacket has been a part of any well-dressed man's ensemble for day or evening since early in the century. A fine white linen or batiste handkerchief was the choice for formal or dress occasions; one with a colored border or in plaid or a dark color (sometimes matching a dark shirt) might be worn with informal outfits. Other objects to be found in a man's pockets were a cigarette case, cigarette lighter, pipe, tobacco pouch of pigskin, key case, "little black book" for addresses, and sometimes a folding jackknife. A fountain pen and an automatic pencil were usually found in the vest pocket or inside coat pocket. With the repeal of Prohibition in 1933, the hip pocket flask, which had been ever-present in the twenties, was no longer part of the scene. Mufflers, fringed or not, were wrapped about the neck in cold weather; a white muffler was correct for evening wear. Gloves were worn for dress or for cold weather. White gloves were part of the evening costume and were made of fine leather, mocha, kid, or chamois. Gloves for daytime might be in shades of brown, gray, or tan, and were made of buckskin or pigskin. Earmuffs appeared in this decade, small ovals of fur or deep-piled wool attached to a springy strip of metal. Most men kept their trousers up with a belt, although some wore suspenders, particularly for formal dress. Elastic garters, fastened below the knee, were still used to support short socks. Canes were still in fashion for rather formal dress — black with gold heads, Malacca or white ash with crooked handles. Some men, usually of the older generation, carried black umbrellas with crooked handles, whether it was raining or not.

WOMEN'S FASHIONS

By the 1930s, the idea of wearing a particular outfit for a particular pursuit had taken hold; for many on a restricted budget, this practice may have been more an ideal than a reality. Those who could afford the wardrobe to support the notion owned different costumes for town and for country wear, for cocktail parties, for informal evenings at home, for formal evening dress, for active sports, and for spectator sports. Science was making its contribution to the costume arts. Synthetic fabrics — rayon and acetate — which were less expensive than silk, were becoming more prevalent on the market. Zipper fasteners were replacing buttons and snaps.

The female silhouette shifted considerably from the beginning to the end of the thirties. Early in the decade hemlines were uneven, often with flounces or drapery that dipped below the basic skirt line, or sometimes high in front and low in back (Figure 29). In reaction to the knee-high styles of the twenties, skirts went down almost to the ankles and then remained at about ten or twelve inches above ground during the first years of the 1930s. Gradually the hems went upward until they stood at fifteen to seventeen inches off the floor in 1939. Early in the decade shoulders were natural and sloping. About 1935, sleeves became fuller at the shoulder, puffed or gathered, or tailored in a squared, wide style filled out with shoulder pads. The square-shouldered line continued through the period of World War II. Waistlines were low or ignored at the beginning of the thirties (Figure 31), soon returned to a natural waist level, and went even higher at the end of the period in some models with a "princesse" cut (Figure 36).

Hair Styles and Makeup

The very short shingled haircut and boyish bob of the twenties was allowed to grow a bit longer in the thirties. Coiffures were still close to the head and likely to be precisely set. The typical style early in the decade was a short bob with a definite part, neatly waved on the top of the head and done up in small curls or rolls over the ears and at the back of the neck. The allover permanent wave, often frizzy, seen in the twenties had subsided into an end-curl. About mid-decade a pompadour style came into fashion, with the hair dressed higher over the forehead and on top of the head; clusters of curls or bangs on the forehead also appeared. A longer bob, worn rather plain around the face and with loose curls on the neck, was popularized by such movie stars as Marlene Dietrich and Carole Lombard. A long shoulder-length pageboy bob became popular toward the end of the era, particularly with teen-agers and younger women. The pageboy was worn with the ends turned under neatly in a loose roll on the shoulders; sometimes the hair was brushed back smoothly from the forehead, or it might be worn in bangs. The loose-flowing hair might be held back with a head-band running behind the ears and tied on top of the head (Figure 57). Jean Harlow's platinum blonde hair inspired many women to bleach their own locks. Hair dyeing became more general and more acceptable. A blue or lavender rinse for gray hair was popular.

The fashion in makeup was still the frankly painted look of the twenties. Lipsticks were bright and mouths were sharply defined. The flapper's preference for the small "bee-sting" mouth had passed, and lips were outlined more generously. The use of rouge diminished in this decade. The pink cheek patches of the twenties disappeared in favor of a softer tone, but often rouge was omitted. Eye shadow was used to darken the eyelids, and eyebrow pencils outlined the eyes. Eyebrows were tweezed, arched, and penciled (often to a fine line at the outer ends). During this decade, the interest in beaches and sun-bathing increased the desirability of the sun-tanned complexion, so that darker tones of face powder came into fashion. A new vogue developed for lacquering the fingernails (and toenails when they were exposed) in various shades of red, from pale pink to deep vermillion or fuchsia.

Hat Styles

At the beginning of the decade, the cloche hat continued to be worn, sometimes modified with a fold or drape at the side of the head or back of the neck (Figures 29, 31). In general, hats in the thirties tended to be small and close to the head. The Empress Eugénie style, a small black velvet hat with a rolled brim and miniature derby shape, appeared in 1931 and was worn tipped demurely forward over the eyes, usually with a black ostrich tip plume that swooped over the crown and downward, cupping the curls at the back of the wearer's head. Small hats, more often than not, were tipped forward at a rakish angle over one eye, or might be worn clinging to one side of the head. There was much variety in shape: the pillbox, the tricorne, the Tyrolean, the flat-crowned straw sailor with wide or narrow brim, the fez, the turban, the toque, the Russian Cossack cap, and the calotte (skull cap or "beanie"). In 1938 Schiaparelli introduced the "doll hat," a tiny confection of flowers and feathers attached to a velvet ribbon that tied under the chin. An off-the-face treatment was also favored, with the hat pushed back on the head. If the hat was small, it was frequently held on with a nose-veil. A large floppy brim might be folded back over the crown. A wide-brimmed hat worn well back on the head gave the effect of serving up the wearer's face on a platter. A great favorite of this era was the beret; it came in several sizes and treatments, from the small flat felt model to a full, luxurious, draped velvet. (The beret was rediscovered in 1968 with the advent of the film *Bonnie and Clyde*.) Late in the decade, when shoulder-length bobs were more prevalent, women began to go without hats. Velvet hairbows on combs might be added to the coiffure. The snood, of wide-meshed net, was worn over the loose back curls and was either secured with a ribbon tie or attached to a hat. The "babushka," a gaily printed kerchief covering the hair and tied under the chin, came into fashion about 1938 and continued through the war and into the fifties. Another novelty late in the thirties was the wimple, or jersey drape, attached to a hat; it went under the chin, covering the neck and resting on the shoulders.

Early in the decade, the simply dressed short bobs went unadorned with evening costumes. Later in the period, for evening one might wear a sequin cap, a velvet hairbow, a flower in the hair, a Spanish comb with a black lace mantilla, or a fancy snood.

Underwear, Loungewear, and Sleepwear

Foundation garments once more took into account the natural contours of the female figure. The flattened look of the twenties was modified to admit a rounded bosom, and, as the decade progressed, a sleek and rounded hipline was more and more prized. The boned corset was replaced by a girdle or brassiere-and-girdle combination made of Lastex, an elasticized material of interwoven rubber and fabric. The "two-way stretch" girdle signaled emancipation from the rigors of boning. Brassieres were redesigned to give an uplift contour to the bosom. Brief panties and a brassiere constituted standard underwear for most women. Slips and petticoats were as slim and clinging as the dresses worn over them. Made of a soft satin or rayon, the most-popular style in slips had a fitted brassierelike top and a princesse-line body cut on the bias, which draped beautifully.

The outstanding item in loungewear during this decade was the pajama. Pajamas were worn for daytime and evening, formally and informally, in private and in public. The following descriptions from a full page devoted to "pyjamas" (using the Continental spelling) in a *Vogue* issue of June 1931 (Figure 25) give some idea of the variety:

Boudoir:
The original meaning of pyjama had most to do with bedroom. Here is the bedroom pyjama, now and always something soft and feminine. Of peach satin, in two pieces, it is appliquéd with Alençon lace.

Beach:
When you come to the beach, pyjamas are something else again. These are of heavy denim, the colour of rust. The trousers are enormous and so make your hips look almost minute. A jacket with a semi-sailor collar goes gaily on top.

Lounging:
Black-and-white crepe pyjamas to lounge in. You can lounge with or without the coat.
In this pyjama with a long coat — kinder than a bolero — of orange crepe over a print, you have all the advantages and none of the disadvantages of an older woman.
A two-piece pyjama, with the blouse worn over the trousers, is in two shades of blue crepe — very cool.
Deep rose and pink crepe pyjama, with nice pipings and buttons. The coat comes off if you like.

Informal dinner:
You can go to a not-too-white-tie dinner in this pink-and-green printed crepe pyjama. It is more formal if you take off the bolero.
This black crepe pyjama has white pleats in the skirt that make you look vaguely medieval. The white pleats occur again in the sleeves — to give the covered-shoulder effect.
You could fool anybody with this dress-like pyjama. It is made of a green-and-white printed crepe and has a fichu scarf that disguises the very low décolletage.

Formal dinner:
The topmost pajama is of crepe roma, the colour of peach ice-cream. The pleats make you look tall and Greek.
Chartreuse crepe and a beaded baby-bolero make a pyjama that is formal as an evening dress.
An older woman would look divine in the black crepe pyjama with panels fore and aft.
When you wear this pyjama of dead-white lace, you look for all the world as if you were in a very swell evening dress.[10]

All the models shown were made of soft fabrics that drape in full folds around the ankles. The voluminous trouser legs give the effect of skirts. It will be noted that many of the outfits were ensembles with jackets in varying lengths, from a short bolero to a three-quarter-length coat. A bolero removed from the evening pajama revealed a back bare to the waist. These were indeed the "cats' pajamas"!

A floor-length nightgown was still in style for sleeping — usually slim, bias-cut, and lace-trimmed. A short and frilly bed jacket might be worn when one was indisposed or reading in bed. Housecoats and lounging robes came in a variety of styles, from the organdy model for summer (Figure 26) to the slinky satin negligee (as seen on Jean Harlow in *Dinner at Eight* and illustrated in Figure 27).

The fluctuation of the hemline for daytime wear is described above. *Day Wear*
The length that was most typical for the thirties was below mid-calf, about twelve inches off the floor. Some of the distinguishing touches of dresses worn early in the decade were the following: slim skirts (Figure 28), sloping shoulders (Figure 29), circular flounces, fluttering drapery at the shoulder or hip, intricately cut bias yokes and inset shapes fitted together in diagonal networks (bodice or hipline) (Figures 29, 30, 31, 32), large floral prints, decorative bows around the hip (centered, one-sided, front or back), draped cowl necklines, scarves or ties, detachable shoulder capes or bolero jackets (Figure 33), long fitted sleeves or dolman sleeves, and long slim tunics over slim skirts. About mid-decade shoulders became wider and squarer (Figures 34, 35) and

were held out with shoulder pads (the square, broad-shouldered look continued through World War II). Skirts began to flare a little and sleeves were fuller, particularly at the shoulder (Figure 36). Suits were popular throughout the period, at first with straight, rather long jackets (Figure 31) and later more tailored and fitted (Figures 35, 37). A formal dress suit might be very elegant, perhaps made of velvet with fur trim. A formal black wool suit with leopard trim is shown in Figure 38. The ensemble suit—a dress with matching jacket or coat (Figure 39)—was in high favor. The "little black dress" was perennially popular for afternoon and cocktail hours, although its silhouette changed to conform to the prevailing fashion (Figure 40). Blouse-and-skirt combinations came into vogue, and when made of fine fabrics might be worn for dress occasions. The "swing skirt," made of a full circle or with wide gores, was adopted by teen-agers for dancing to swing music. The dirndl skirt, a length of material gathered into a waistband, first appeared in 1937. The shirtwaist dress appeared in the thirties and has continued in the mode ever since in various versions—with straight, flaring, or pleated skirts, short sleeves or long. It is an eminently practical and comfortable style.

Evening Wear The most-popular styles in evening gowns for the early part of the decade were the slinking, bias, backless numbers (Figures 41, 42, 43, 44, 45, 46, 47). Bare shoulders might be covered, for at least part of the evening, by a chiffon scarf, a shoulder cape, a bolero, or a shrug jacket. Floral prints were favored, as in Figure 48 (particularly in England, where florals were the height of fashion for formal evening affairs and at the Ascot races). Another popular mode, with a little-girl or ingénue flavor, featured full skirts, fitted bodices, and frills. The organdy model illustrated in Figure 43 was recommended to "bring out the Jane Eyre in you."[11] Full overskirts of net might have an appliquéd trim, as seen in Figures 49 and 50. A blouse-and-skirt outfit for evening was versatile; one could "change it with vari-colored sashes and sandals"[12] (Figure 52). The dinner suit, a slim floor-length skirt with a tailored jacket or long-sleeved overblouse, was introduced by Schiaparelli late in the decade (Figures 41, 51). Variations in décolletage were the halter-neck bodice, backless with a strap around the neck to support the front, and a midriff style consisting of a skirt and brief top (sometimes with long sleeves) that bared the torso from waistline to bosom. In 1939 Alix introduced an evening gown with a strapless bodice, tightly fitted, and a tremendous flaring skirt that foreshadowed styles of the fifties. Wedding gowns followed the prevailing style and were often soft, bias-cut, and clinging (Figure 53).

In addition to the numerous kinds of short jackets worn over evening gowns, there were floor-length evening wraps, capes, and a hooded mantle. In the latter part of the decade evening coiffures were enhanced by ribbon bows, artificial flowers, jeweled hair clips, sequined caps or hats, combs and mantillas, or snoods.

Sportswear

For active sports in the winter, a sweater-and-skirt or blouse-and-skirt combination was popular; or one might wear a tweed suit or separate jacket and skirt. The Metropolitan Costume Institute has in its collection a five-piece sports ensemble designed by Claire McCardell in 1934; it includes a sunback halter, wide-legged slacks, culottes, a jacket, and a skirt made of black wool jersey (Figure 54). New styles in summer play clothes were the one-piece short suit (Figure 55), the slack suit in various styles (Figure 56), and the midriff outfit with button-on skirt (Figure 57). Beach wear was colorful; bright prints were popular in cotton, rayon, or silk. A smart wool bathing suit from Paris had a matching coat (Figure 58). There was more bare skin showing than in the previous decade, with an increasing number of two-piece styles — halter tops, bra tops, and midriff models (Figure 59). Beach pajamas also appeared in two-piece versions, with separate trousers and tops. The summer dresses of cotton or rayon were frequently bare-necked and bare-backed (Figures 60, 61). A sunback dress might be made more demure or proper with the addition of a bolero jacket. However, the bare-backed models were worn on the street as well. The midriff style shown in Figure 57 was recommended as part of a wardrobe to be worn to the New York World's Fair in 1939.

For spectator sports one might wear a tailored suit (Figures 35, 37) or a dress-and-coat ensemble (Figure 39). There was a vogue for black-and-white combinations in summer outfits (Figure 28). Two-toned black-and-white shoes were as popular with women as with men in this decade. A swagger coat was appropriate for sporty occasions (Figure 63).

Coats and Wraps

The fitted coat with a fur collar was typical of the early part of the thirties (Figure 62). The straight box coat and flaring swagger coat also appeared early in the decade in three-quarter- or seven-eighths-length (Figure 63). In the latter part of the era, both fitted and unfitted coats appeared with broader shoulders and fuller sleeves. A popular model was the double-breasted man-tailored tweed coat ("reefer"), with wide lapels and six or eight large buttons. The redingote was another style in favor; it was fitted and fastened at the waistline, and its flaring skirt swung open in front to show the dress beneath. Fur coats or jackets were a symbol of material success (perhaps they always have been). This was the era when the heroine of *Stage Door* held out against the Hollywood lure of "little ermine jackets up to here." The more-luxurious long fur coats were made of chinchilla, sable, mink, broadtail, baum marten, caracul, and Persian lamb. Silver fox was used for short coats and stoles. Less-expensive coats of muskrat, beaver, and nutria were also in fashion. Sports coats were made of leopard, lamb, or goat skins. Ermine and white broadtail were worn for evening. Small fur muffs were still carried upon occasion.

Evening wraps were very short jackets, or three-quarter-length or floor-length coats, usually fitted. Favorite fabrics were satin and velvet. A hooded mantle came into fashion for evening wear late in the decade; capes in varying lengths were also worn.

Footwear

Footwear in the first half of the thirties resembled that of the twenties. A sturdy or clubby look prevailed, and shoes had rounded toes and rather low, heavy heels of baby Louis or Cuban height. Fairly wide instep straps were still popular. Heels for day and evening wear grew higher and more slender as the decade progressed; the greatest height was probably about three inches and the narrowest width about one inch. Two-toned pumps were favorites for spectator sports wear, two-toned oxfords for active sports. The sling-back shoe came into vogue, often open-toed, with a strap at the back to hold it on the heel. The wedge sandal was another new style. Late in the decade, platform soles appeared; combined with high heels, they might elevate the wearer as much as three or four inches. Toes continued to be round throughout the period, and open-toed styles became more and more popular. Evening slippers attained a lighter, airier quality by the end of the thirties, as popular favor settled upon sandals with slim heels and a network of narrow straps.

Accessories

Costume jewelry continued to be popular. The bangle bracelets of the twenties were still worn, although fewer might be piled on an arm at one time. The long strings of beads that had given added color to the Jazz Age were now replaced by shorter necklaces of pearls or gold, silver, and set stones. Brooches, lapel pins, and clips gained in favor and were used in many ways, as simple adornment or to hold scarves and ties in place. Earrings began to be made with clip-fasteners instead of screws. Wristwatches were smaller and daintier in feminine styles. Artificial flowers were frequently added to a simple basic dress. Short pull-on gloves were popular. A loose medium-length glove, worn wrinkled, and a flared gauntlet style were also seen. Opera-length gloves for evening were rarely worn in this era; for evening, arms were almost universally bare. It was fashionable to wear black or dark gloves with a light costume and light gloves with a dark outfit. Gloves might be worn with a dinner suit. The folding fan had vanished as an evening accessory. Purses were of leather or fabric, in clutch or strap styles. In mid-decade a shoulder-strap bag appeared, at first on the beaches and then as a complement to street costumes; during the forties this style became very popular (Figure 59). Evening bags were small and ornamental; they might be made of velvet or brocade, trimmed with sequins or beaded. The contents of a woman's purse might include: a compact for powder, sometimes also containing rouge and lipstick; a comb; a cigarette case and lighter; possibly a cigarette holder; a key case; eyeglasses; fountain pen and automatic pencil; coin purse or wallet; and a handkerchief. Handkerchiefs with floral prints were popular. Scarves were much used, as neckties, sashes, head kerchiefs, shoulder capes, or possibly as ornamental drapery tied to the belt, wrist, or hat. Umbrellas were short and stubby and might be carried in a leather or fabric case, slung over the shoulder on a strap, or inserted in a pouch compartment of a large handbag. Women as well as men sometimes wore earmuffs in bitter weather. Muffs were carried in cold weather, for day or evening, frequently matching a short fur jacket or fur-trimmed coat or suit.

CHILDREN'S FASHIONS

It is generally true that the children's garments reflect the line and spirit of their parents' attire. The wardrobes of boys and girls of the thirties were no exception to this rule. In the early or mid-Depression years, when fathers abandoned the wearing of knickers on the golf links and changed to slacks and shirts, their sons gave up knee pants and graduated directly from short pants to long trousers at the age of about six or eight years. The knicker suit of the early thirties usually had a single-breasted jacket and matching vest and was worn with a cotton shirt, four-in-hand or bow tie, golf socks (which might be patterned), and oxfords. A billed cap completed the outfit. The jacket and vest were worn for Sunday School and dress occasions; for school and play, knickers were likely to be combined with a shirt, a tie, and a pullover sweater with a round or V-neck. Topcoats, raincoats, and short jackets for boys were similar in style to those worn by men, such as the leather windbreaker with zipper closing, which was new in this era (Figure 24). The following list of clothing suggested for the boy going away to school in 1937 seems more than ample:

> A complete wardrobe as recommended by schools and colleges: 3 sack suits; 1 dinner or evening suit; sports jacket and several pairs of flannel slacks; overcoat; sheep-lined coat; windbreaker; raincoat; 4 pairs of pajamas; 12 suits of underwear; 18 shirts for general and sports wear; 12 collars; 24 handkerchiefs; 12 pairs of socks; 2 pairs of gloves; bathrobe; 2 sweaters; 12 neckties; soft felt hat; cap; 3 pairs of shoes for general wear — 2 pairs of tan and one of black — in addition to sports shoes, galoshes, slippers; 2 belts.[13]

When, upon rare occasions, a small boy had to appear in formal dress, the Eton jacket and striped trousers shown in Figure 64 were worn.

Girls' dresses were straight and slim early in the decade, quite often bias-cut or made in many pieces joined on diagonal lines. Pleated skirts were popular; skirts were mid-thigh in length for the pre-school miss, just below the knee for the grammar-school girl, and at mid-calf for the teen-ager. Late in the decade a higher waistline and a flared or gathered skirt were adopted for girls of all sizes. Jumpers worn over blouses were popular in the later thirties. Tailored suits or dresses with bolero jackets were popular (Figure 65). A wider and fuller shoulder line came into fashion at the end of the period. Young teen-agers might wear a princesse style coat (Figure 66) or a dress similar to the one shown for an adult in Figure 36. For fast dancing the female "jitter-bug" wore a swing skirt cut with a circular flare and a shirtwaist, sporty blouse, or pullover sweater; anklets ("bobby socks"); and saddle shoes.

TYPICAL MATERIALS, COLORS, MOTIFS, AND TRIMMINGS

The traditional fabrics in cotton, wool, linen, and silk were all still in evidence. In addition, the textile industry had made great strides in the production of synthetic materials since the first appearance of rayon early in the century. A new man-made material on the market in this decade was acetate. During the thirties, crepe was perhaps the most-popular fabric of all — cotton, wool, silk, and rayon crepe, as well as crepe-backed satin and satin-backed crepe. Soft jerseys in wool, silk, and rayon also worked admirably for the bias-cut and draped models of this era. Soft, sheer fabrics such as chiffon and voile were popular, particularly in flowered prints. Early in the period, georgette and crepe de Chine were still much used. Some of the novelty fabrics were moleskin velvet and wrinkled velvet, matelassé (blistered silk), and crinkled crepe. For summer dresses, crisp fabrics such as piqué, linen, and gingham were popular. Summer evening dresses were made of sheer cottons — organdy, dotted Swiss, tissue gingham, and net — silk organza, or the new synthetics. Floral prints were popular for evening gowns, afternoon dresses, lounging pajamas, or beachwear. Polka dots, stripes, checks, and plaids were also in vogue. Playsuits were made of denim or sailcloth. Taffeta was available in stripes or plaid, sometimes with a metallic thread.

The decade of the thirties was relatively plain in regard to trimmings. The elaborate passementerie, beadwork, lace insertion, fringe, tassels, and embroideries of the two preceding decades had disappeared. Decoration was supplied by elaborate cut and contrasting values, added drapery and flounces, artificial flowers and clips, or ornamental buttons. Fur trim was popular; all kinds of fur were used for collars, cuffs, revers, or borders. Evening gowns or cocktail gowns might be trimmed with sequins or rhinestones.

Colors were often quite brilliant, sometimes even garish. High contrast was considered attractive; black-and-white or various light-and-dark combinations were frequently used. Schiaparelli's "shocking pink" combined with black was worn with matching fuchsia lipstick and nail polish. Some random examples of startling color combinations are: pink-and-green large floral printed crepe for formal evening pajamas with bolero jacket; blue, gray, and yellow evening gown with solid-color collar and sash, because "gargantuan prints are very chic at night";[14] ruby-red velvet bolero jacket worn over a white crepe evening dress; an evening gown by Valentina of striped gold lamé and black velvet (Figure 54); an evening gown by Claire McCardell of beige acetate jersey worn with a wide silver-studded red suede belt and a long coat of red wool tweed; and, for the daytime, a dress of raspberry-red and dull blue plaid wool worn with a boxy jacket of blue wool with plaid revers; a burnt-orange wool redingote over a black-and-orange floral print silk crepe dress. Other popular shades of this period were emerald green, chartreuse, wine or plum, rust, and brown.

Men's suits continued to be made of flannel, worsted, or cheviot. Herringbone tweeds were popular for sportswear or topcoats. Glen plaids were also in style for sports jackets or even for business suits. The widely spaced pinstripe was perhaps the most-prized suit fabric of the era. For summer, suits were made of linen, Palm Beach cloth, or seersucker. A new rayon gabardine came into favor for white dinner jackets or light sports jackets. Shirts were made of the traditional white cotton or linen as well as silk or rayon. Shirts worn with suits might be in pastels or deeper colors, or might be pinstriped. Sport shirts appeared in bright colors and might be patterned in bold stripes, checks, or plaid.

SUGGESTIONS FOR COSTUMING PLAYS IN THE PERIOD

To capture the flavor of men's wear in the thirties, the costumer should scour the thrift shops for broad-shouldered, double-breasted suits with wide lapels. Those in dark gray or navy blue with a white pinstripe are especially good. Trousers should be pleated at the waistband and wide at the cuffs. A double-breasted tan trench coat or voluminous, broad-lapeled polo coat would help to create the proper atmosphere. A natty sports ensemble might consist of a dark shirt and handkerchief combined with a white or light suit, or a dark blue double-breasted sports jacket worn with light gray or white flannel slacks. Shoes should be two-toned black-and-white oxfords or white with black soles. If the costume collection does not include shoes of this style, use a little shoe makeup on plain models. For evening wear, a double-breasted tuxedo jacket in midnight blue with wide, satin-faced lapels is especially good. The double-breasted white dinner jacket with shawl collar and the short white mess jacket are also appropriate for this period. A boater or coconut straw hat with white band could be worn with a summer informal evening outfit. For winter evenings, a black fedora or homburg would be preferable to a high silk hat. A stiff wing collar and a stiff-bosomed shirt would be worn for only the most-formal occasions. Four-in-hands should be a generous three inches wide. As in the twenties, men should have short hair styles and a clean-shaven look.

Dresses in thirties style should be made of soft fabrics cut on the bias. If the intricate jigsaw patterns take more time than the costumer can spare, the general effect can be achieved with simpler patterns by using set-on drapery in circular flounces or handkerchief squares. As was recommended for costuming the twenties, it is desirable to select fabrics of a cheaper variety — one might almost say "sleazy" — to give the spineless drape that was typical of the crepe-backed satins, the moleskin velvets, and some of the early rayon and acetate fabrics of the thirties. Some of the old bias-cut dresses may still be found in second-hand shops. The skirt length that is right for the period — almost down to the ankle — may have to be modified to conform to the shorter styles currently in fashion. (The *Bonnie and Clyde* recapitulation of Depression styles combined the thirties flavor with the knee-length skirts of the sixties.) An actress may be too hampered to perform well in a drooping skirt at mid-calf length, which she feels makes her look dowdy, awkward, and unattractive. A cloche is appropriate for the early part of the period. A broad-brimmed slouch felt hat might be worn by a sophisticated or Garbo type. A feminine style might call for a tiny doll hat tipped over one eye. A beret is very typical for the era.

TITLE	AUTHOR	PERIOD
All the King's Men	Robert Penn Warren	1935
Annie (M)	T. Meehan, C. Strouse, M. Charnin	1933
Anything Goes (M)	Bolton, Wodehouse, Lindsay, Crouse	1934
Awake and Sing	Clifford Odets	1935
Babes in Arms (M)	Richard Rodgers, Lorenz Hart	1937
Both Your Houses	Maxwell Anderson	1933
Cabaret (M)	J. Masteroff, J. Kander, F. Ebb	1930
The Children's Hour	Lillian Hellman	1934
The Cradle Will Rock (M)	Mark Blitzstein	1937
Dames at Sea (M)	G. Haimsohn, R. Miller, J. Wise	1930s
Dead End	Sidney Kingsley	1935
Death of Bessie Smith	Edward Albee	1937
Design for Living	Noel Coward	1932
Dinner at Eight	Noel Coward	1932
Fallen Angels	Noel Coward	1930
42nd Street (M)	Warren, Dubin, Stewart, Bramble	1933
The Glass Menagerie	Tennessee Williams	1930s; 1945
Golden Boy	Clifford Odets	1937
High Tor	Maxwell Anderson	1937
Idiot's Delight	Robert E. Sherwood	1936
The Late Christopher Bean	Sidney Howard	1932
The Man Who Came to Dinner	George Kaufman, Moss Hart	1939
Margin for Error	Clare Booth	1939
Music in the Air (M)	Jerome Kern, Oscar Hammerstein	1932
Night Must Fall	Emlyn Williams	1936
Of Mice and Men	John Steinbeck	1937
On the Twentieth Century (M)	B. Comden, A. Green, C. Coleman	early 1930s
The Petrified Forest	Robert E. Sherwood	1935
The Philadelphia Story	Philip Barry	1939
Point of No Return	Paul Osborn	1929; 1930s
Porgy and Bess	DuBose Heyward, G. and I. Gershwin	1935
Private Lives	Noel Coward	1931
Reunion in Vienna	Robert E. Sherwood	1931
Roberta (M)	Jerome Kern, Otto Harbach	1933
Room Service	John Murray and Allen Boretz	1937
She Loves Me (M)	J. Masteroff, J. Bock, S. Hernick	1933
The Sound of Music (M)	Rodgers, Hammerstein, Lindsay, Crouse	1938
Stage Door	Edna Ferber, George Kaufman	1936
Sugar (M)	Jule Styne, Bob Merrill	1931
Three Men on a Horse	John Cecil Holm, George Abbott	1935
The Time of Your Life	William Saroyan	1939
Tobacco Road	Erskine Caldwell	1933
Winterset	Maxwell Anderson	1935
The Women	Clare Booth	1936
You Can't Take It With You	George Kaufman, Moss Hart	1936

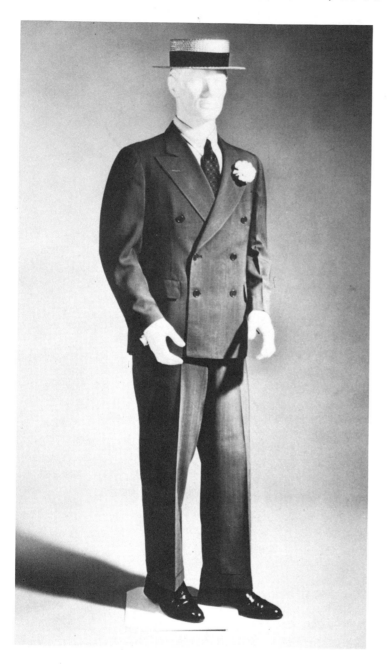

1. Two-piece suit: brown with gray and tan stripes; double-breasted, three-button jacket; cuffed trousers. Central Pennsylvania, 1930s. (Division of Costume, Smithsonian Institution.)

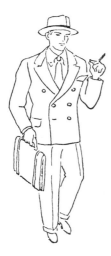

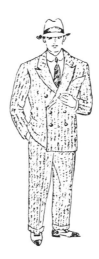

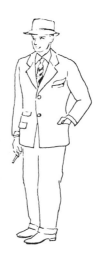

2. Summer suit of seersucker; shirt with button-down collar; Panama hat. 1934.

3. Double-breasted suit in striped gray flannel; brown-and-white shoes. 1930.

4. Semi-sports wear: square-front jacket with pin check and plaid overlay. 1939.

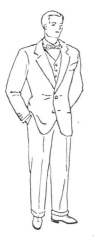

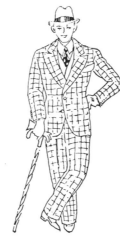

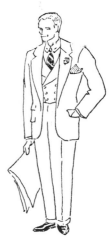

5. White Palm Beach suit, linen or gabardine. 1930.

6. Spring suit of gray sharkskin with cuffless trousers; homburg. 1937.

7. Business suit with double-breasted matching waistcoat with wide lapels. 1934.

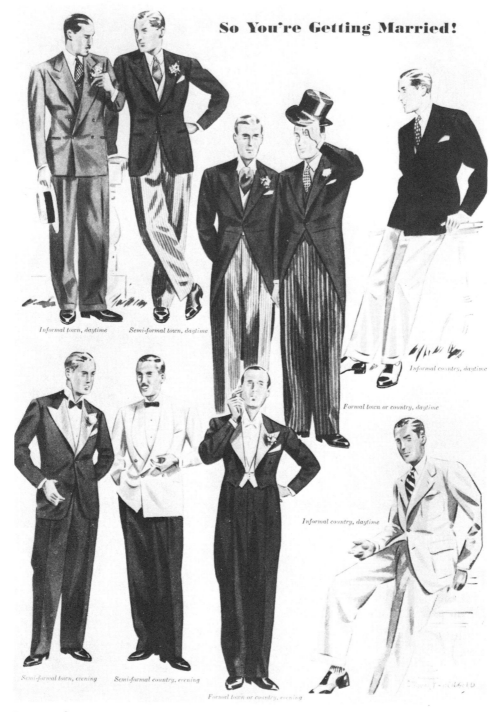

So You're Getting Married!

Informal town, daytime   *Semi-formal town, daytime*

Informal country, daytime

Formal town or country, daytime

Informal country, daytime

Semi-formal town, evening   *Semi-formal country, evening*

Formal town or country, evening

8. A page from *Esquire*, June 1937, showing correct attire for the groom.

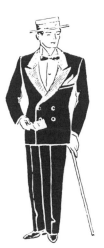

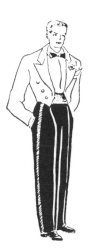

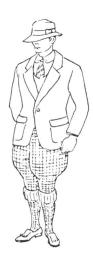

9. Resort wear: double-breasted dinner jacket; straw hat. 1930.

10. White mess jacket; black trousers; red cummerbund; black tie. 1934.

11. Country outfit: tweed jacket; checked knickers. 1931.

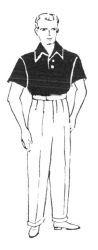

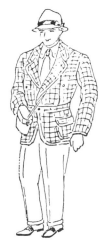

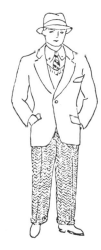

12. Sports outfit: white flannel slacks; navy blue knitted shirt. 1934.

13. Sports outfit: tan Norfolk jacket; white slacks; saddle shoes. 1934.

14. Country outfit: brown jacket; brown hat; gray flannel slacks; yellow sweater. 1931.

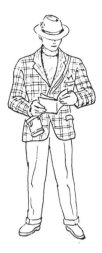

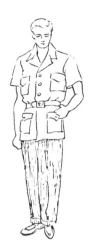

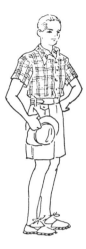

15. Country wear: tweed jacket; turtleneck sweater; Tyrolean hat. 1939.

16. For lounging or sports: tropical bush shirt; corduroy slacks. 1936.

17. Sports outfit: plaid cotton shirt; Bermuda shorts; canvas shoes. 1938.

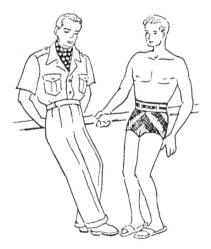

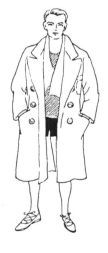

18. Beach wear. Left, lightweight military shirt and slacks. Right, herringbone knitted trunks. 1936.

19. Terry cloth beach coat; dark blue trunks; blue shirt. 1930.

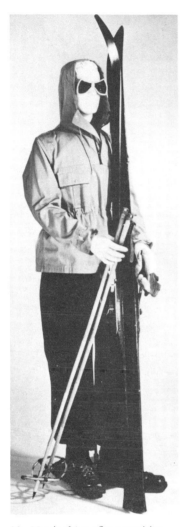

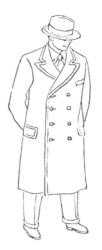

21. Double-breasted overcoat; felt hat. 1934.

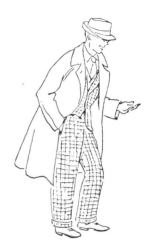

22. Reversible tweed balmacaan coat; checked suit; porkpie hat. 1935.

20. Man's ski outfit: navy blue wool trousers; brown cotton jacket with hood. New England, by Burton's, 1937 – 40. Ski accessories (goggles, gloves, boots, skis, and ski poles) original to outfit. (Division of Costume, Smithsonian Institution.)

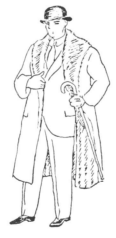

23. Cloth overcoat with fur collar and lining; derby. 1932.

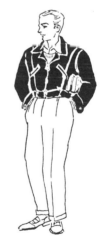

24. Windbreaker sports jacket of lined leather or wool with zipper closing. 1937.

25. "Pyjamas — When Are They Worn?" Page from *Vogue*, June 1, 1931.

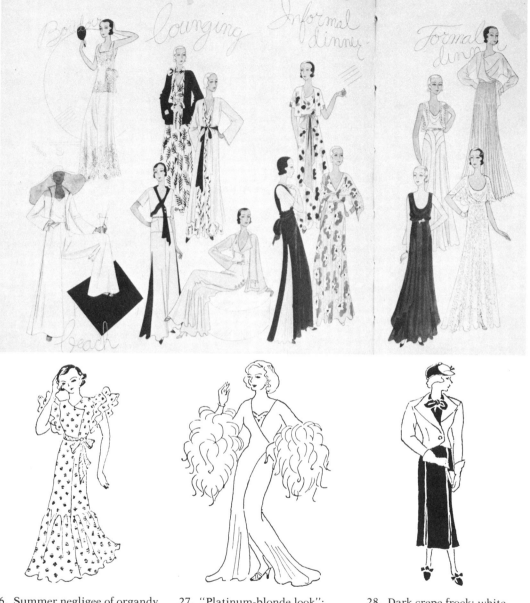

26. Summer negligee of organdy in coin-dot print with ruffled hem and sleeves. 1933.

27. "Platinum-blonde look": white-and-silver negligee with ostrich trim. 1933.

28. Dark crepe frock; white piqué jacket; matching hat. 1933.

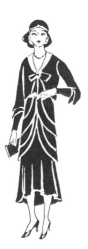

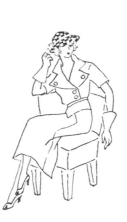

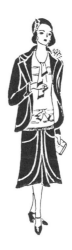

29. Afternoon frock of black crepe with white roll collar; bolero jacket. 1930.

30. Summer town frock of white linen. 1933.

31. Chanel suit: black tweed jacket and skirt; pink blouse and lining. 1930.

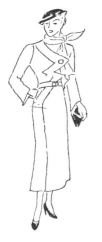

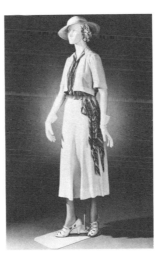

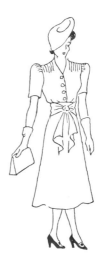

32. Maggy Rouf tailored street frock; scarf fastened with clip. 1932.

33. Afternoon dress: white skirt and false bolero jacket; multicolored striped bodice and sash. About 1934. (Division of Costume, Smithsonian Institution.)

34. Afternoon dress of crepe silk with soft blouse and sash. 1938.

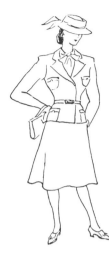

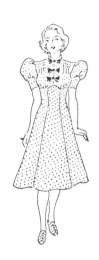

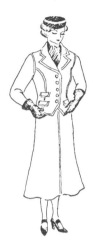

35. Chanel jersey suit: short fitted jacket; felt hat; oxfords. 1939.

36. "Princesse" dress in cotton print with puffed sleeves and flared skirt. 1939.

37. Suit with short fitted jacket and flared, four-gore skirt. 1936.

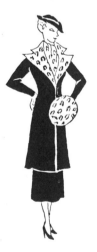

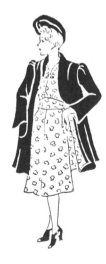

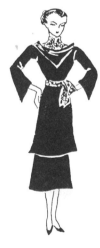

38. Formal suit of black wool with leopard revers, scarf, and muff. 1934.

39. Ensemble: plain coat, three-quarter length; print dress and lining. 1939.

40. "Little black dress": black crepe tunic with rose-red sequin trim. 1934.

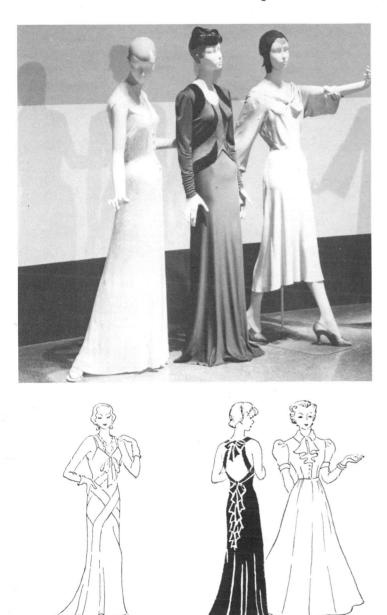

41. Left, after-dinner gown: clinging, backless dress with halter neckline of crystal and silver beaded chiffon. American, by Sophie Gimbel, 1936. Center, dinner suit of black silk jersey and black velvet; long-sleeved overblouse; bias-cut floor-length skirt. French, by Schiaparelli, 1939. Right, afternoon dress of silk crepe. By Vionnet, 1933. (The Costume Institute of The Metropolitan Museum of Art. Gifts of Mrs. Sophie Gimbel, Bettina Ballard, and Isabel Shults.)

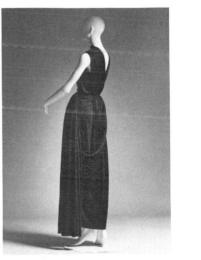

42. Molyneux evening gown: bias-cut white crepe in molded silhouette. 1931.

43. Evening gowns. Left, velvet, bow-trimmed, 1935. Right, full-gored skirt, fitted bodice, 1937.

44. Draped evening gown of black silk jersey. By Alix Grès, 1937 – 39. (The Costume Institute of The Metropolitan Museum of Art. Gift of Z. E. Marguerite Pick.)

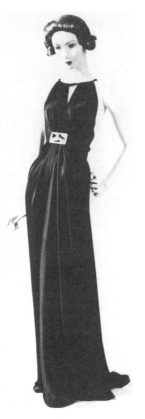

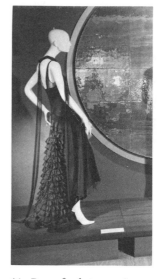

45. Evening gown of black satin: slim bias cut with deep décolletage; dress shaped by drawing folds together in front with large white buckle. By Vionnet, 1935. (The Costume Institute of The Metropolitan Museum of Art. Gift of Madame Madeleine Vionnet.)

46. Dress for late evening: bias-cut black chiffon, trimmed with tiers of black satin ruffles; hipline defined by wide black satin sash and bow. By Vionnet, 1929 – 30. (The Costume Institute of The Metropolitan Museum of Art. Gift of Madame Madeleine Vionnet.)

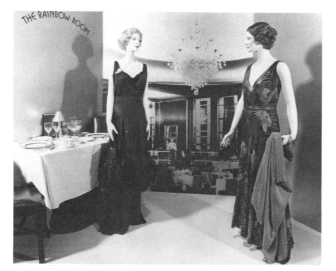

47. Left, tunic evening dress of black satin trimmed with monkey fur. By Mainbocher, 1930s. Right, evening dress of flowered lamé. By Alan Kramer, about 1933. Background photo of the Rainbow Room courtesy of Anthony May. (Museum of the City of New York. Gifts of Mrs. Frederick Childs, Jr., and Miss Louise B. Scott.)

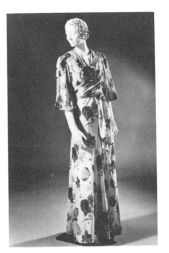

48. Evening dress with matching jacket in tan, brown, green, and gold printed georgette. Sleeveless, V-neck gown has large attached flower. Wraparound jacket has long sleeves, shirred at the shoulder. About 1936. (Division of Costume, Smithsonian Institution.)

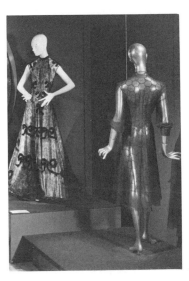

49. Left, dinner dress of black lace appliquéd with velvet bows, over a bias-cut silver-pink lamé underdress. By Vionnet, 1938. Right, cocktail dress of black silk voile, entirely hand-tucked in a graduated honeycomb pattern. By Vionnet, 1936. (The Costume Institute of The Metropolitan Museum of Art. Gifts of Countess de Martini and Mrs. John Chambers Hughes.)

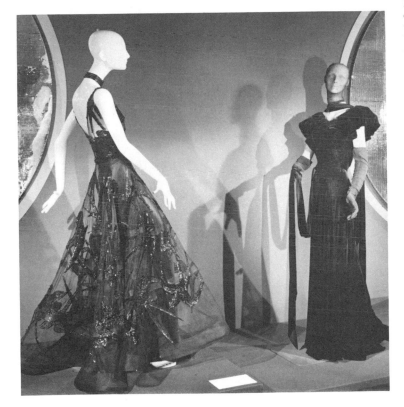

50. Left, ball gown with full circular skirt of black silk net embroidered with black sequins in a flying bird design; black satin underdress. By Vionnet, 1938. Right, dinner gown of black silk velvet, bias cut, with draped bodice and short puffed sleeves, soft skirt falling in folds. By Vionnet, 1932–33. (The Costume Institute of The Metropolitan Museum of Art. Gift of Countess de Martini, Lady Mendl, and Mrs. Ector Munn; velvet gown on loan from the Museum of the City of New York.)

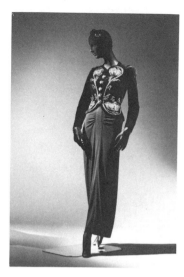

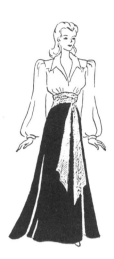

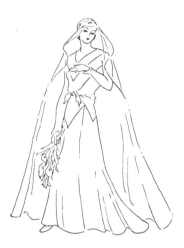

51. Theatre suit of dark green crepe satin, bias cut: jacket of dark green velvet, embroidered with gold tinsel and red stones. By Schiaparelli, 1937. (The Costume Institute of The Metropolitan Museum of Art. Gift of Julia B. Henry.)

52. Evening blouse and skirt, with cummerbund; sandals. 1939.

53. Bridal gown in white satin with train attached to bias-cut hip yoke. 1931.

54. Left, evening gown of striped gold lamé and black velvet, cut in flowing lines, with narrow pendant bands falling from shoulders. By Valentina, 1938. Center, tailored dinner suit of black broadcloth with white linen frills, made over during World War II from a man's tailsuit of 1929. American, 1943. Right, separates for sports: sunback halter and wide-legged slacks of black wool jersey; part of a five-piece matching set that includes culottes, jacket, and skirt — a capsule weekend wardrobe. By Claire McCardell, 1934. (The Costume Institute of The Metropolitan Museum of Art. Gifts of Mrs. Clarkson Runyon, Harper's Bazaar, and Claire McCardell.)

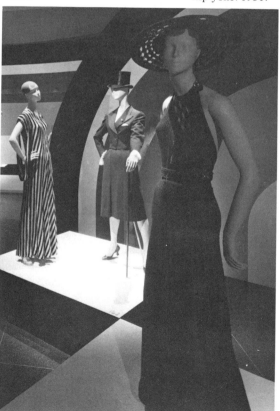

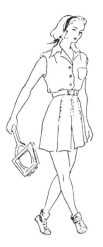

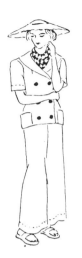

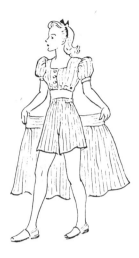

55. One-piece play suit of cotton or linen. 1936.

56. Jacket and slacks suit for lounging or beach wear. 1936.

57. Playsuit in striped cotton: shorts, bodice, and wraparound skirt. 1939.

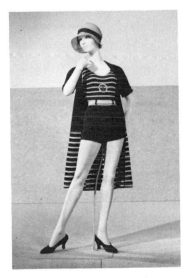

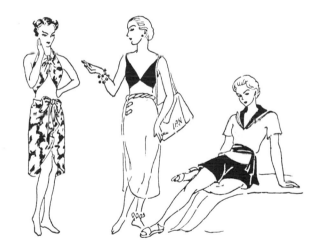

58. Wool bathing suit with matching coat. Paris, by Hermes, 1930. (The Costume Institute of The Metropolitan Museum of Art. Gift of Mrs. Sidney Bernard.)

59. Beach wear. Left, Tahitian paru with halter top of flowered silk print. 1934. Center, rough flax skirt with brown jersey top. Right, middy and shorts. 1934.

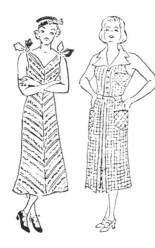

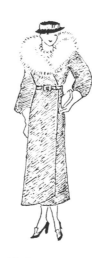

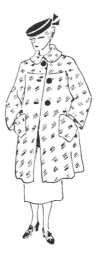

60, 61. Tennis dress of candy-striped cotton with V-neck back, buttoned to waist. 1933. Sunback dress of checked cotton; to be worn with bolero jacket. 1936.

62. Double-breasted coat with full sleeves and fur collar. By Mainbocher, 1932.

63. Swagger coat with full sleeves and box pleat in back. 1935.

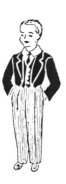

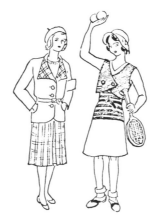

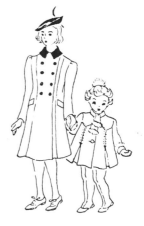

64. Formal wear for small boy: Eton jacket; striped trousers. 1935.

65. Left, girl's suit of green plaid tweed. Right, green-and-white linen dress. 1931.

66. Wool coat for girl; coat and leggings for 4-year-old. 1936.

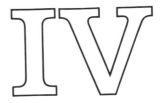

The Second World War
(1940–1946)

THE STYLES OF THE forties were modified to accommodate the needs of a country at war. Thousands of men and women were serving in the armed forces and were consequently wearing the uniforms of the Army, Navy, Marine Corps, and Air Force. Thousands more were working in service units such as the Red Cross and Civil Defense Corps, with their own characteristic service uniforms. The workers, male and female, on production lines at factories turning out products in support of the war were dressed in outfits designed for comfort, safety, and durability rather than for beauty. Eighteen million women were employed in war industries. Thousands more went into the female branches of the armed services: the WACs (Army), the WAVEs (Navy), the WASPs (Air Force), and the SPARs (Coast Guard). A soldiers' ditty of those years went:

> The WACs and the WAVEs are winning the war
> So what in the hell are we fighting for?

The women's uniforms were trim, short-skirted, and more functional than those worn in World War I. For this war the government drew upon the services of leading clothing designers: Philip Mangone helped design women's uniforms for the Army, Mainbocher for the Navy.

CONCERNING THE PERIOD

World War II started in mid-Europe, just as World War I had done, with another German thrust for power, this time under the leadership of the Nazi dictator, Adolf Hitler. And with the same reluctance to get embroiled in the conflict that she had shown in 1917, America stayed out of the war just as long as possible. But when Japan bombed the ships and planes of the United States Navy at Pearl Harbor on December 7, 1941, America was suddenly at war with Japan, and three days later with Germany and Italy. It then became imperative to convert the national economy from peacetime production to all-out war production. Civilians went to work on farms and in factories to help provide the necessary food and war materials to support the fighting men in Europe, North Africa, and the Pacific.

Although scientific development was focused on the war effort, some advancement occurred in the world of everyday living. The frequency modulation (FM) radio was being perfected, and the mechanics and techniques of television were being improved. In the laundry corner, old-style washing machines with tubs and wringers were being replaced by automatic washers that would wash, rinse, and spin the clothing, untouched by human hands. A new invention, the clothes dryer, was also on the market. During the war, however, production of many home appliances was suspended, and this improved equipment did not become available until the war ended. The New York World's Fair, which closed in the fall of 1940, had given new impetus to the public acceptance of modern styles in furniture and home decoration, including an increased awareness of the beauty and simplicity of Scandinavian designs — "Swedish modern" and "Danish modern." Good American designers of household objects during these years were Russel Wright, who produced simple, unadorned china and silverware; Charles Eames, who was experimenting with molded plastics and shaped plywood in his styling of chairs; and Raymond Loewy, who streamlined the contours of many items, from toasters to motor cars.

The arts in America profited from an influx of outstanding European refugees — Mondrian, Léger, Moholy-Nagy, and Lipchitz, to name a few. The art center of the Western world had shifted from Paris to New York. Mondrian absorbed the cadences of America, and now painted his geometric squares with a new syncopated rhythm in *Broadway Boogie Woogie*. Interest in abstract expressionism was growing and would come to full flower when the war ended. In the early forties first shows were held by Jackson Pollock, Hans Hofmann, Arshile Gorky, and Mark Rothko. John Marin was painting explosive, splashy seascapes, and Andrew Wyeth was working in a style of dreamlike realism. Alexander Calder was adding the factor of mobility to his abstract sculptures suspended on wires. The WPA Federal Art Project, which had sustained many talented painters through the latter days of the Depression, finally came to an end in 1941. Many artists recorded the story of the war on canvas. Jack Levine painted his own satiric view of the war in such paintings as *Welcome Home*. (Picasso had earlier expressed his response to the war in Spain with his horrifying *Guernica*, a huge fractured mural that until 1981 hung in the Museum of Modern Art. It had been painted in 1937, but in spirit surely belonged to this war era.)

Popular music and dancing during the war years continued in the style and spirit of the thirties. The favorite big bands were either sweet or hot, and at the USO centers the most-played jukebox records were the fast swing numbers to which the soldiers could jitterbug or dance the Lindy Hop. The syncopated rolling-bass beat was showing up in such numbers as "The Boogie Woogie Bugle Boy from Company B" (sung in close harmony by the Andrews Sisters). War songs were less fervent and a little more cynical than those sung in World War I. Kate Smith tugged at patriotic heartstrings with "God Bless America," but the general attitude toward this war for survival was more in the spirit of "Praise the Lord and Pass the Ammunition." Frank Sinatra became the bobby-soxers' idol with his sentimental crooning to the music of Harry James's orchestra. Another musical motif of this period was a Spanish or Latin American idiom, exemplified in the popular orchestra of Xavier Cugat; and for a while the tango, the rhumba, and the samba were vying with swing for popularity on the dance floor. As one popular song lamented: "Take back your conga, ay, your rhumba, ay, your samba, ay, ay, ay, . . . I've got a crack in the back of my sac-ro-iliac!" An exuberant crowd was quite likely to form a snake-dancing conga line, as everybody did in Times Square on the night of May 7, 1945 (V-E Day).

During the war the night-time blaze of Manhattan's Great White Way was dimmed, but the theatre went on as usual. Several light-hearted musical productions provided escape from the harsh realities of the war. Rodgers and Hart wrote *Pal Joey* before Hart's death, and then Richard Rodgers and Oscar Hammerstein formed a successful new team. Their first effort was *Oklahoma!*, which opened in 1943; it set a new style in Broadway shows, being the first to feature serious ballet and to use music as an organic part of the plot. Gertrude Lawrence and Danny Kaye starred in *Lady in the Dark*, which explored the world of the subconscious mind. The nostalgic comedy *Life with Father* ran for seven years. Thornton Wilder was represented on the New York stage by *The Skin of Our Teeth* and Eugene O'Neill by *The Iceman Cometh*. Comedies new in this era, which have since joined the repertory of American theatre classics, were *The Male Animal*, *Harvey*, and *Born Yesterday*. Tennessee Williams came to prominence as a playwright with his first Broadway production, *The Glass Menagerie*.

Many Hollywood stars had gone into the armed services — among them Clark Gable, James Stewart, Robert Montgomery, and Robert Taylor. Many more were serving overseas as entertainers at canteens and USO centers. Favorite pinup girls were Betty Grable, Hedy

Lamarr, and Rita Hayworth. The flowing shoulder-length bob and square-shouldered silhouette, the tailored suit and the mannish stride, were promoted by such reigning favorites as Katharine Hepburn, Marlene Dietrich, Carole Lombard, and Lauren Bacall. Veronica Lake furnished the model for an exotic hair style, parted on one side with a long swooping lock combed forward to hide one eye. Charlie Chaplin satirized Hitler in his film *The Great Dictator*. Humphrey Bogart portrayed international intrigue in *Casablanca*. Bing Crosby and Bob Hope went on *The Road to Singapore* and *The Road to Morocco*. In the stepped-up pace of a country working around the clock, where night and day were intermixed with swing shifts and graveyard shifts, movies were shown all night long.

GENERAL CHARACTERISTICS OF COSTUME

The clothing of this era expressed masculine strength, practicality, and common sense, with no frivolous details. Perhaps the broad, square shoulders that evolved in the garments of both sexes were a subconscious response to the heavy burdens that had to be borne by the entire population during World War II. Women adopted mannish tailoring for suits and dresses, and the wearing of pants was more universal than in the thirties. Slack suits and jumper suits were a favorite garb for women working in factories and on farms, driving buses, and operating elevators. Rationing of materials became necessary, and woolens in particular were needed for the army; in 1942 the War Production Board issued ruling L-58, which limited the dimensions and design of garments manufactured for civilian use. A man's double-breasted suit could not include a vest. Jackets were shortened, and vents, patch pockets, and belts were eliminated. Civilian as well as uniform trousers were made without cuffs. Women's dresses were reduced in yardage by some fifteen percent and were made without such "extravagant" items as turnover cuffs, patch pockets, balloon sleeves, matching sashes, double yokes, attached hoods, and shawls. Skirt widths were restricted to 72–80 inches, and hem and belt widths were limited to two inches. Some categories were exempt from these restrictions — infants' clothing, bridal gowns, maternity dresses, religious vestments, burial gowns. Throughout the war, skirts were skimpy in appearance and worn just below the knee. In London, where clothing was more tightly rationed and the hazards of war were more imminent, girls achieved some variety in their meager wardrobes by changing hair arrangements and makeup two or three times daily. The tantalizing luxury of nylon hose, which had been proffered in 1939, was speedily withdrawn as nylon was channeled to parachute construction and to wardrobes of military personnel. Nylon stockings became a prized black market item and as negotiable as cigarettes in return for scarce commodities and favors. White cotton shirts and underwear for men became virtually unobtainable during these years. In 1945 nylon garments for civilian use again appeared on the market; shirts made of nylon soon became very popular because they did not wrinkle, were easily washed, and required little or no pressing.

The Parisian high fashion center went into comparative eclipse when France fell to the Nazis in 1940. Many couturier houses were closed — among them Vionnet and Chanel. Mainbocher closed his Paris shop and moved to New York to establish himself in new quarters on 57th Street. Among his new clients was Mary Martin, for whom he designed the costumes in *One Touch of Venus* in 1942. New American designers were coming to the fore in the fashion field — Claire McCardell, Norman Norell, and Charles James. Norell won the first American Fashion Critics' Award for outstanding design in 1943; McCardell received the second award in 1944. In California, Adrian was achieving distinction as a costume designer for motion pictures.

The broad-shouldered, utilitarian wartime silhouette, complete with "wedgie" shoes, platform soles, or sensible oxfords, tended to make a dainty female look a little like a football player. The men fared better, however; well-padded shoulders did help to make a Tarzan out of a skinny Casper Milquetoast. *Vogue* valiantly continued to mirror what was left in the way of "fashion" during these years. A mid-century review in its editorial pages comments:

> The war brings Centura [the twentieth-century female] back to earth with a jolt, and by 1942 she has worked out for herself a satisfactory way to look — a frugal, spare-silhouetted American primitive look that Martha Graham helps her to visualize, and Claire McCardell and Capezio help her to achieve: her dress a jersey tube with a décolleté daytime neckline (or a skimpy jersey jumper over a skimpy leotard) [Figure 37]; her Phelps belt and bag bold, with brass emblems; her feet flat on the ground.[1]

Capezio's contribution to this look was flat slippers similar to ballet shoes, typically worn with leotards. The leather belt was three inches wide, and the bag was suspended nonchalantly on a shoulder strap, leaving the hands free to carry parcels when the whole world was in transit and often walking instead of riding.

MEN'S FASHIONS

Men's styles continued in the silhouette of the thirties. In civilian clothing, shoulders were broad and padded, waists were nipped in to a semifitted line, lapels were wide and usually peaked, and double-breasted models were still in the majority. The jacket front was loosely draped to give a full effect, and the air was casual, with perhaps only a single button buttoned at the waistline. Pinstripes and Glenurquart plaids were popular. Since many men were in uniform, social gatherings were likely to present a mixture of military and civilian attire. Comfort and informality were stressed, and there was less formal dress for the duration of the war.

Hair Styles and Grooming

Men's haircuts were short and clean-cut during this period. Hair might be parted on the left or right side, or be combed straight back in a pompadour. A style much used in the Army was the "butch" haircut, or crew cut, a very short allover cut that left the hair standing in a brush less than one inch long. It had the practical value of being easy to shampoo and care for, and discouraging to vermin in combat circumstances. Occasionally one saw a neat, small mustache, but men were generally clean-shaven and there were almost no beards.

Hat Styles

The black silk top hat was still correct for wear with formal evening attire or with a cutaway coat for formal daytime occasions. A homburg or derby might also be worn for formal or semiformal affairs. Probably the most universally worn style during this period was the soft felt fedora with a fairly wide snap-brim pulled down over the eyes (Figures 6, 8). The porkpie hat with crown creased down to a squared-off level was still in favor for sporty outfits and campus wear. A tweed cap with a bill was also popular for sports wear. In summer the straw boater and the Panama hat were still worn, and even more popular was the dark coconut straw hat with a wide pleated puggree silk band. (Military hats and caps are discussed under the heading of "Uniforms.")

Underwear, Loungewear, and Sleepwear

Standard underwear for men was a combination of boxer shorts of white or patterned cotton and a sleeveless knitted lisle undershirt (Figure 1). Shorts might also be of cotton jersey, very brief, with an elastic waistband. The war created shortages in rubber and metal; from 1942 to 1945 shorts were designed with side ties to replace waistband elastic and buttons instead of snap fasteners. As in the thirties, the undershirt was frequently omitted under an opaque shirt. Pajamas in various styles were the most-popular garment for sleeping. They were made of cotton, rayon, or silk, plain or patterned. The top was either a slipover style, usually with a V-neck, or a jacket buttoned down the front, which for a while had no collar (Figure 1). Lounging robes came in the traditional style, mid-calf in length with a shawl collar, lapover front, and tie sash (Figure 2), or in a shorter version called the lounge suit. The suit shown in Figure 3 consisted of blue-gray flannel slacks and a flannel jacket of tan with a blue and brown check. A page in *Men's Wear Review* devoted to men's robes reported:

The practical rayon-and-worsted gabardine robe made its debut a couple of years ago. . . . Gabardines are found both lined and unlined and with yoke and sleeve lining, in solids, in color tone combinations, in stripes, in plaids and novelty checks.[2]

Models were shown in light blue with a darker blue stripe; one in maroon with a blue stripe; one in dark green trimmed with lighter green plaid on the collar, pockets, sash, and cuffs; and another in maroon with a light blue piping around the collar, down the front, and on the pockets and cuffs, and with a tasseled sash. Brooks Brothers advertised a natural pongee dressing gown piped in maroon or navy blue. Also shown were smoking jackets styled like dinner jackets with satin-faced shawl collars in a polka-dot pattern or a fancy stripe, and sometimes with frog closings rather than buttons.

Neckwear

Shirts for formal dress continued to be of fine white cotton or linen, with pleated front and turnover collar, or with stiff white piqué bosom and detachable wing collar. During the war, white cotton dress shirts became very scarce; nylon shirts appeared on the market as the war ended. Shirt collars were rather wide, with a broad slope or deep points at the front closing; collar tips were usually unfastened, but sometimes they were held down with a bar tie pin or buttoned down. Pinstriped shirts were popular. The all-purpose shirt appeared, with a loop fastening at the top button, which permitted it to be worn open as a sport shirt without a tie, or closed to a high neckline and combined with a tie. Bright-colored Hawaiian prints for sport shirts were popular. Pullover polo shirts, of soft cotton jersey, with round crew neck or pointed turnover collar, might be worn with a sports jacket. For formal evening dress, a white piqué bow tie with pointed tips or butterfly shape was worn. The four-in-hand or ascot was worn for formal daytime affairs; a black bow tie or four-in-hand was worn for informal evening occasions. Four-in-hands were still wide, as they had been in the thirties; diagonal stripes were probably the most-popular pattern. Bow ties frequently had pointed tips. The Prince scarf, with divided ends that wrapped around the neck and tied in front resembling an ascot, was worn informally for lounging or to fill in the open neck of a sport shirt.

Day Wear

Formal day wear continued to consist of the cutaway coat, gray waistcoat, white dress shirt with detachable wing collar, ascot, striped trousers, and black dress shoes (Figure 4). For business or informal town wear, the double-breasted suit was still the most-popular style (Figures 5, 6). Shoulders were broad and well padded, and lapels were wide. A rather loose fit was the fashion, with a drape across the chest.

Single-breasted models were also prevalent, in two- or three-button styles, usually worn with only one or two buttons fastened (Figure 7). Trousers were full, nineteen or twenty inches wide at the cuff, and pleated at the waistband. For a while during the war years they were made without cuffs, and pleats at the waist were omitted. Trousers were long enough to break over the instep, and the hemlines slanted from front to back. Glen plaids and pinstripes were popular. Summer suits of washable cotton fabrics were in favor (Figure 8). Coats were a little longer in 1945 than in 1940. The outlandish "zoot suit" affected by teen-agers in the late 1930s and the early days of the war featured a coat almost to the knees and highly exaggerated accessories (Figure 9). As previously mentioned, vests were omitted from men's double-breasted suits during the war years by order of the War Production Board.

Evening Wear   The war curtailed formal dress to a considerable extent. When white tie and tails were worn for the most-formal evening occasions, midnight blue was preferred to black. For semiformal dress, a favored style was a white tuxedo jacket, single- or double-breasted with shawl collar (or a white mess jacket), worn with black dress trousers, braid-trimmed, and a black bow tie. The midnight blue double-breasted evening jacket continued to be as popular as it was in the thirties. A homburg in dark blue or black was a preferred hat for semiformal evening attire. For summer or resort wear, a dark straw hat with white silk band or a light straw with black band might be worn with evening dress.

Sportswear   For active sports the usual outfit was a sport shirt of cotton, flannel, or lightweight wool worn with slacks (Figures 10, 11). A slipover polo shirt of cotton or wool jersey with short sleeves and round neck or turnover collar was also popular. Long-sleeved sport shirts in military style were in evidence and came in colors such as maroon, gold, dark green, or navy blue. Novelty sports jackets abounded, in varying styles (Figure 12). There was a slack suit with a two-tone jacket — the back, collar, and sleeves were in a contrasting color or plaid (Figure 13). The unlined flannel blazer was a perennial, in plain colors or stripes. The bush jacket of the thirties was still worn. For warm weather and beach wear, Bermuda shorts, just above the knee, were popular (Figure 14). "Cabana sets" of matching sport shirts and shorts in exotic South Sea prints were the last word in style for the beach (Figure 15). With suit vests eliminated, sweaters were worn more than ever. Slipover sleeve-less sweaters with V-necks took the place of vests in casual outfits combining slacks and odd sports jackets (often plaid or checked). This combination of jacket, sweater, and slacks was very popular on college campuses. Long-sleeved sweaters with round or V-necks or turtlenecks were also worn. The cardigan sweater was a perennial style.

Coats and Wraps

The Chesterfield coat in black or midnight blue continued to be correct with formal and semiformal dress in daytime or evening. For general wear, there were broad-shouldered overcoats in single- and double-breasted styles (Figure 16). The balmacaan and raglan topcoat were still popular (Figure 17). All these models were wide in the shoulder and loose in fit. The military trench coat was omnipresent and considered very dashing for all-purpose wear as well as for rain protection (Figure 18). New short jackets were appearing on the scene. A fur-collared model is shown in Figure 19. The hip-length heavy plaid wool lumber jacket, which was belted and had patch pockets, was good for cold weather outdoor activities. The short Eisenhower jacket, with a built-in belt at the waistline, which had been designed for General Eisenhower to wear in the European battlefield, proved to be a very practical and comfortable style and was taken over for civilian use when the war ended (Figure 22). A Lord and Taylor advertisement in *The New Yorker* shows it as a uniform as well as in a tweed version worn by a golfer:

> You may not know it, Lieutenant — but you've started something! That battle jacket, that you're making history in, is ready to lend a hand with your post-war plans, too. How do you like it in tweed?[3]

The style continued to be popular for sports wear. It even appeared in London in black with a satin-faced shawl collar for semiformal evening wear, but this model did not gain general acceptance.

Uniforms

The look of uniforms had changed considerably since World War I. The high-necked tunic with standing collar had been converted to the World War II single-breasted, four-button jacket with turnover collar and lapels. The full knickers (resembling jodhpurs) of the doughboy had been replaced by long trousers that tucked into combat boots (Figure 20). The wide-brimmed, high-crowned campaign hat (with the "Montana peak") was seen early in World War II but disappeared before the war ended. The soft, folding overseas cap was still in use, now called the "garrison cap." The shape of the steel helmet worn in active combat had changed from the rather shallow, wide-brimmed contour of World War I to a broader crown and a very narrow brim that dipped to cover the back of the neck. The Sam Browne belt was discarded about 1944. Throughout the war, research experts were busy, testing and improving specific uniforms for special assignments. Parachute jumping, tank and submarine operation, arctic maneuvers on skis, tropical jungle fighting, all required garments designed for special conditions — high altitudes or underwater pressures, extreme heat or cold, storm and moisture. Out of these experiments came a great array of specialized clothing — nylon jump suits, thermal suits, wet suits, fiber helmets, parkas — far too varied to be included here. Each branch of the armed services had three basic uniforms: a service uniform, a field uniform, and a dress uniform.

> By the beginning of the 20th century uniforms were divided into two types: dress uniforms for peacetime wear; and field uniforms to provide comfort, concealment, and protection in combat. The post-World War II service and field uniforms of all countries are simple, practical, and relatively economical, while dress uniforms, which are still ornate and still a source of *esprit de corps*, are worn less often and are seldom required except for career soldiers [Figure 21].
>   . . . World War II saw the abandonment of breeches and boots, the Sam Browne belt, and the campaign hat. The garrison cap returned to favor, and trousers were tucked into leggings or combat boots. Late in the war the olive-drab Eisenhower jacket [Figure 22] became service dress for enlisted men and supplemented the officers' blouse and pink trousers. The wearing of dress and mess uniforms was suspended.[4]

In the Air Force, in winter officers and men wore forest-green trousers, coats, and visor caps. Officers' service uniforms were forest-green coats and lighter drab ("pink") trousers. They wore drab shirts, black or drab ties, and russet shoes (Figure 23). In the Army, in winter men wore drab shirts with olive-drab coats and trousers, black or drab ties, and russet shoes. Officers' service uniforms were olive-drab coats, lighter drab ("pink") trousers, and olive-drab visor caps. Enlisted men wore overseas caps. The Marine Corps winter uniforms were of forest-green wool, worn with drab shirts, black ties, and black shoes. For dress occasions, the Marines wore dark blue jackets with gold buttons (single-breasted with standing collar), light blue trousers with scarlet stripes, and white caps and belts. In the Navy, in winter, officers and chief petty officers wore navy blue double-breasted suits with six gold buttons, white shirts, black ties, and black shoes. In summer, they might wear single-breasted white or khaki suits. An officer's summer dress white uniform had a standing collar; this style remained the same as in World War I (see chapter 1, Figure 28). The naval officer's uniform in the tropics had a shirt with turndown collar and short sleeves (Figure 24). Visor or overseas caps might be worn with the khaki uniform, but only the visor cap was worn with the white uniform. Officers wore gold sleeve braid. In winter, enlisted men wore navy blue jumpers that had three white stripes on their large collars

(Figure 25). They wore all-white cotton summer uniforms. Enlisted men wore washable round white cotton hats.[5]

All branches of the service wore cotton khaki uniforms in the summer. All branches might wear "fatigues" (blue denim shirts and dungarees) for dirty work that was hard on uniforms. Colors for service and field uniforms were generally subdued, soft, and grayed to blend with the terrain during combat. The basic color for Army uniforms throughout World War II was olive-drab (a grayed greenish-tan); for the Marines and Air Force it was forest-green (a dark olive green). Army uniforms changed to "army green" (a little brighter than forest-green) in 1954; Air Force uniforms changed to slate blue in 1950. Coast Guard uniforms were the same as the Navy's, navy blue and white, with different insignia. An officer's rank was indicated by insignia worn on the shoulder straps and, in the Navy, by gold stripes on the sleeve cuff. The following table gives the insignia for the various ranks in the American armed forces.[6]

Army, Air Force, and Marines		**Navy and Coast Guard**	
Insignia	*Rank*	*Rank*	*Stripes**
Five silver stars	General of Army, AF	Fleet Admiral	1 — 4 — 0
Four silver stars	General	Admiral	1 — 3 — 0
Three silver stars	Lieutenant General	Vice Admiral	1 — 2 — 0
Two silver stars	Major General	Rear Admiral	1 — 1 — 0
One silver star	Brigadier General	Commodore	1 — 0 — 0
Silver eagle	Colonel	Captain	0 — 4 — 0
Silver oak leaf	Lieutenant Colonel	Commander	0 — 3 — 0
Gold oak leaf	Major	Lieutenant Commander	0 — 2 — 1
Two silver bars	Captain	Lieutenant	0 — 2 — 0
One silver bar	First Lieutenant	Lieutenant (jg.)	0 — 1 — 1
One gold bar	Second Lieutenant	Ensign	0 — 1 — 0
Silver bar with 3 enamel bands	Chief Warrant Officer (W-4)	Chief Warrant Officer (W-4)	0 — 1 — 0 (1 break)
Silver bar with 2 enamel bands	Chief Warrant Officer (W-3)	Chief Warrant Officer (W-3)	0 — 1 — 0 (2 breaks)
Gold bar with 3 enamel bands	Chief Warrant Officer (W-2)	Chief Warrant Officer (W-2)	0 — 1 — 0 (3 breaks)
Gold bar with 2 enamel bands	Chief Warrant Officer (W-1)	Chief Warrant Officer (W-1)	0 — 0 — 1 (3 breaks)

*Navy and Coast Guard stripes are of gold embroidery; first figure is number of 2-inch stripes, second is number of ½-inch stripes, third is number of ¼-inch stripes.

In addition to insignia of rank, emblems of metal or cloth were worn on caps, upper sleeves, or lapels. The following commentary gives some further regulations for wearing these markings:

These emblems identify the wearer's rank or grade, branch of service, duty assignment, or honors. Insignia may also take the form of a wound stripe, a length-of-service stripe called a "hash mark," or a *fourragère*, a braided cord looped over the [left] shoulder.

Officers in the United States Army and United States Air Force wear insignia of rank on each shoulder, in the form of small gold or silver bars, oak leaves, eagles, or stars. Army officers wear branch-of-service insignia on blouse lapels, and, on some uniforms, insignia of rank and branch of service on their shirt collars. Enlisted men of both services wear cloth chevrons on both arms as insignia of rank. In the army, they wear metal branch-of-service insignia on their blouse lapels.

Naval officers wear gold stripes on their cuffs or shoulder boards. On some uniforms, they wear miniature metal insignia, similar to those of army officers, on their shirt collars. White stripes on the cuff are the seamen's insignia of rating. The petty officers' insignia of rating, an eagle and chevrons, appear on the upper sleeve.[7]

Cap devices are worn on the left side of the garrison cap. For officers, the cap device is the United States coat of arms, a spread eagle; for enlisted men, a smaller coat of arms on a disk. Medals and citations are usually worn on the upper left-hand side of the blouse, above the pocket. The regulations for Army insignia also apply to the Marine Corps; those for the Navy apply to the Coast Guard. To lighten this rather involved discussion, one might ask, "Would you rather be a colonel with an eagle on your shoulder, or a private with a chicken on your knee?" (*Ziegfeld Follies* tune, 1918).

Footwear

Men's shoes for civilian wear were much the same as they had been in the thirties. For formal evening dress, black patent leather pumps were correct. For formal day wear and informal evening dress, plain black calf shoes with straight tips — oxfords or a new slip-on style — were appropriate. For business and town, plain brown or black oxfords were worn. The Blucher shoe, or half-boot with a strap buckled high on the instep, was still in evidence. The new Norwegian slip-on moccasin, or "loafer," was gaining in popularity for both casual and town wear. Two-toned oxfords of brown and white in various styles were still popular for sports wear. The chukka, or "flight boot," of soft suede, ankle-high, was also popular. Heavy crepe soles were still favored for sports. At the beach, one might see a variety of styles — sandals, canvas shoes with cork or rope soles, Japanese thongs. Ration stamps were required to buy shoes during the war years, since leather was being conserved for the army. Synthetic materials were being utilized for soles as well as uppers; inexpensive shoes might have cardboard insoles. Growing children were likely to be the first members of the family to get new shoes, while their fathers wore old ones.

During the war years, accessories for men remained about the same as in the thirties. For formal or informal dress, a fine white linen handkerchief was worn folded in the breast pocket. For informal wear, the handkerchief might be colored or have a colored border. White mufflers were worn with formal evening attire; black mufflers with informal evening dress. In cold weather, men wore wool, rayon, or silk mufflers, in plain colors, plaids, or patterns, and sometimes fringed. For evening dress, a boutonnière was often worn in the lapel — a white carnation for formal occasions, a red one for informal affairs. In place of evening waistcoats, silk cummerbunds (wide pleated waistbands) were still popular, usually in plain blue or red, or in checks, plaids, or stripes. Gloves for formal evening dress were of white kid; for formal day dress they might be of gray mocha or chamois, for general wear of pigskin in tan, brown, or black. Pocket accessories included leather billfolds or wallets, credential cases, key cases, cigarette cases, and folding pocket knives. The "Zippo" windproof cigarette lighter of plain stainless steel was a great favorite with soldiers. Vest pockets might accommodate a fountain pen and automatic pencil and perhaps a small packet containing a pocket comb, stainless steel mirror, and nail file. Wristwatches were available in shockproof and waterproof models. Pipes and cigars were seen more frequently than in the twenties and thirties (perhaps Winston Churchill's ever-present cigar helped to promote this trend). All men in uniform wore "dog tags," two metal identification tags, circular or oblong in shape, on a chain around the neck. They also carried an identification card in their wallets. Canes and spats for dress were seen very infrequently, perhaps more often in England than America. The plain black umbrella with a crooked handle had become the symbol of conservatism or appeasement, since it was identified with Chamberlain and his capitulation to Hitler at Munich in 1938. Men's jewelry continued to be the same as in the thirties. Pearl studs and cuff links were worn for formal evening dress; gold, enamel, or colored stone studs and links for other occasions. Rings and fraternity or lodge pins were worn. A gold or silver bar tie clip held the four-in-hand to the shirt front. Trousers were held up by suspenders or belts. Hand-tooled leather belts were popular, but belts also appeared in bright woven fabrics, such as a red, gold, and blue ribbon.

WOMEN'S FASHIONS

In World War II, more women than ever before were wearing service uniforms. Thousands more were working in factories, helping with war production, and wearing slacks or coveralls. In civilian clothing, probably the most-striking aspect of the wartime silhouette was the wide, square shoulder line. Almost every garment had generous shoulder pads, not only tailored suits and coats, but even negligees, shirtwaists and blouses, cocktail dresses, and evening gowns.

Hair Styles and Makeup

During the war, women presented a rather curious combination of masculine and tailored efficiency topped by very feminine coiffures, as though hair styles were the one area in which they could maintain their femininity. Some women still wore the short or medium-length bob of the mid-thirties. Most women had fairly long hair, and the flowing shoulder-length bob, which had appeared in the late thirties, was the prevailing mode throughout the war years. It was worn in a variety of styles, usually softly waved and loosely curled. The pageboy bob curled under neatly in a loose roll. The hair was more often than not parted — on either side or in the middle — and combed back in a semi-pompadour to fall to the shoulders in loose curls. It might be held in place by a ribbon or band running under the hair, behind the ears, and tied on top of the head. The hair in front was frequently worn in bangs — curled, waved, or straight — or in a cluster on the forehead. A full, high pompadour effect was sometimes achieved by pushing the hair forward in a puff secured by a bow or a hair clip, or by swirling the front and side hair upward and pinning it in three or four full, spiral curls. Pinned-on bows or flower clusters were popular hair ornaments, quite often worn for daytime dress as well as evening. When war duties required less-fanciful hair treatments, the hair was pinned up on top of the head in rolls, or braided into pigtails, and the entire mop was pushed into a service or working cap. The sight was quite common, however, of a WAC or a WAVE with a neat service cap perched on top of a curling shoulder-length bob.

Styles in makeup called for a frankly and brightly made-up mouth, little or no rouge, and eye makeup for dress occasions. Fingernails were painted in brilliant colors, and quite often toenails were also painted. Nail polish came in such shades as Black Red, Gingerbread, Lollipop, Butterscotch, Sugar Plum, Blackberry, and Red Flannel. The advertisements said: "The lacquer-luster and color-brilliance of precious Chen Yu will turn your nails into gorgeous jewels! Choose from twenty lacquer shades — each breath-taking!"[8] Nails and lips, of course, were supposed to match or harmonize with the costume. Another novelty of wartime cosmetics was leg makeup (complete with painted-on seams) to take the place of the nylon hose, which had become unavailable.

Hat Styles

Women were going hatless more than they did in the thirties. Those in service wore their own particular brand of service cap, and women in war work often caught up their hair in kerchiefs wrapped turban style or tied under the chin as a babushka. All the hat styles of the thirties were still in fashion — the slouch felt hat, the snug cloche, the turban, the broad-brimmed straw hat, and the smaller straw sailor. Berets were still popular — large and small, draped, pancake flat, or round and bulbous, and sometimes trimmed with a jeweled clip or a fur pompom. The most frequently seen style was a small, frivolous confection of ribbon and flowers attached to a minimum base, sometimes just a disc of felt or straw. Even the smallest hat had a tiny veil. Small hats were often tilted forward over one eye. Off-the-face hats were still worn — with a folded-back brim, or simply a platter pushed to the back of the head. Several styles of bonnets were in vogue, with curving brims over the forehead. Hats with matching accessories were in style — a striped taffeta bonnet with matching ascot, a striped jersey turban with matching scarf (Figure 29), a big red-and-white polka-dot picture hat with matching polka-dot gloves, or a checked straw hat with matching straw handbag. Snoods were more popular than ever, much used to contain the long bobs and keep them neat (Figure 52). Sometimes snoods were trimmed with small bows or sequins.

Underwear, Loungewear, and Sleepwear

The customary undergarments for women were panties and a brassiere. The elasticized two-way stretch girdle was very popular as a control for the hip and waistline. The pantie girdle had appeared, with built-in legs, which eliminated panties as a separate garment. A full bosom was appreciated, and brassieres were designed to mold and lift. New on the market was a wired brassiere that could be worn without straps. The advertisements were glowing: "A revolutionary new bra wired for witchery. At last . . . a bra that speaks glamour's own language . . . with flexible padded-in-plush wire to define your breasts in their most flattering terms. . . . The wire is removable for easy laundering."[9] The most-popular style for slips was still the fitted model with brassiere top in silk or rayon satin. Half-slips, or petticoats, were also worn. Housecoats were usually long and full-skirted, as in the tricolor wraparound model shown in Figure 26. A page from *McCall's* devoted to lounging attire in 1946 showed a negligee in primrose pink crepe with fitted bodice, floor-length flared skirt, lapped front, tie sash, wide shoulders, three-quarter-length gathered sleeves, and a loose hood. A short bed jacket in turquoise satin also had a hood; the accompanying comment was, "These loosely fitting hoods are ever so becoming." A pale yellow nightgown, floor-length, had a bare midriff — "You just tie the fronts together casually."[10] The article also showed a suit of lounging pajamas in black brocade. It had a long, tunic jacket with long, straight sleeves and wide, square shoulders. The trousers were rather straight and slim, in contrast to the skirtlike fullness of pajamas in the thirties. Man-tailored pajamas were also popular for sleeping attire.

Day Wear   The silhouette of the forties preserved the natural figure, except for the exaggerated broad shoulders. Bodices were fitted, and a small, natural waistline, combined with a full bosom and trim hips, was admired. Skirts came just below the knees and were full or slightly flared more often than straight (Figure 27). Even the uniform skirts had a little flare to them. Tailored suits were popular (Figures 28, 29, 30, 31) and might have matching topcoats—boxy and straight, or fitted reefers. Pleated skirts, swing skirts (circular), and dirndl skirts were worn with shirtwaists or with full, gathered peasant blouses (Figure 53). The shirtwaist dress, buttoned down the front (Figure 64), was a popular style. Rayon prints were favored for dress occasions (Figure 33). Two-color combinations—such as black and fuchsia, black and beige, or cocoa and turquoise—were frequently used.

For afternoon wear and cocktail parties, the "little black dress" continued to be a staple of the wardrobe (Figure 34). Accessories were much emphasized for giving variety to a severely plain basic black dress. *Vogue* presented suggestions for making "One Dress into Ten," as shown in Figure 32:

> You begin with one short black dinner sheath—neck low, sleeves short—and you ring ten changes on it this way:
> 1. Bank large pink roses at the neck, gird waist with a sash of pink and violet chiffon.
> 2. Tie on an apron of flower print, add scarf [draped over head as snood] and gloves to match, fill in neck with beads.
> 3. Hook on a full overskirt of black net and veil your head and face with more of the net.
> 4. Add a snood and long gloves of gay print.
> 5. Tie on a chiffon sash with floating panels.
> 6. Pull on a sweater-blouse of black satin, tuck in the neck a sequin-dotted tulle scarf.
> 7. Add a brief lace peplum and lace gloves.
> 8. Cover with loose jacket of jet-dotted net.
> 9. By day, wear a grey-and-black tweed jacket, by afternoon—a brilliantly striped satin one.
> 10. Or just wear the sheath as is—with your best jewels and cut-steel buckles on your pumps.[11]

No afternoon outfit was considered complete without a hat and gloves (Figures 35, 36).

Figure 37 shows the dramatic changes in silhouette from the late thirties to the end of the forties.

During the war, an evening dress was more likely to be a dressy *Evening Wear* cocktail style than a floor-length formal. Even for such affairs as weddings, arrangements were often made on the spur of the moment — perhaps to take advantage of a weekend leave — and there was no time to plan an elaborate formal ceremony. Often a bride might wear a pastel suit or a light crepe afternoon dress. When formal dress was worn, the styles were less décolleté than in the thirties. Shoulders and backs tended to be covered up. Evening formals frequently had little jackets. The majority had sleeves — puffed or cap, or long and fitted (Figures 38, 39, 40, 41). Shoulders were square and padded in evening gowns, just as in other garments. One much-photographed model was Adrian's "Roan Stallion," designed in 1945 (now in the Metropolitan Museum collection), with a boat neck, wide padded shoulder line, and slim skirt. It was made of black crepe with a wild print of a single rearing horse in red and white splashed diagonally across the front (Figure 37). The dinner suit, which had been introduced by Schiaparelli in the late thirties, was still a favorite model for evening wear (Figure 42). A suit designed by Adele Simpson in off-white wool had a double-breasted jacket, with large sequined revers, and a pencil-slim slit skirt. The "little-girl look," which was current in the thirties, was still in vogue. There were sheer formals in dotted swiss or organdy, with fitted bodices, full ruffled skirts, and puffed sleeves. There was a Gibson Girl style that combined a full striped or checked taffeta skirt and a sheer white blouse with long, full sleeves. In 1940 and again in 1946 there was a trend toward paddling hips, sometimes with the addition of panniers under the full skirt (Figure 43). In 1946 some strapless and off-the-shoulder styles were seen.

Slacks or some variety of trousers were worn for many different activ- *Sportswear* ities during the early forties. They were seen in the war production plants and at the supermarket, as well as on the beach (Figures 44, 45, 46). Their versatility and practicality were lauded in the *Ladies' Home Journal*:

> If you are a trouser type — slim enough, straight enough and, above all, not bulgy at the hipline — you can have a whole trouser wardrobe: the basic gray flannel slacks, jacket and a skirt to match for marketing, driving and general outdoor wear; denim overalls for housework, corduroy slacks and shirts for outdoor or indoor work (or picnics or camping); smart flannel slacks or soft crepe pajamas for afternoon or dinner wear.[12]

Of course, across the years many women who were not really trousers types wore them anyway and gave Ogden Nash the inspiration for his immortal rhyme:

> Sure, deck your lower limbs in pants
> Yours are the limbs, my sweeting
> You look divine as you advance
> Have you seen yourself retreating?[13]

(He wrote this gem without having been exposed to the stretch pants of the fifties and sixties, which were to reveal every curve and bulge!) A variation in the jacket-and-slacks suit was a combination of slacks, a full-sleeved shirtwaist, and a fitted sleeveless jerkin or weskit. The many kinds of playsuits that had appeared in the thirties were still in evidence — one-piece suits (Figure 47), shorts and shirts with button-on skirts, culottes, sarongs, midriff tops, and halters. Sweaters were popular for sports, worn with pleated, circular, or flared skirts. Sweater sets of matching pullover sweater and cardigan were campus favorites. Embroidered or sequined sweaters might be worn for dress occasions. An oversized Sloppy Joe sweater worn with blue jeans was the prevailing outfit for teen-age girls. A Sloppy Joe sweater worn with a swing skirt and bobby-socks was the favorite uniform for jitterbugging. Bathing suits were brief one-piece maillots (Figures 48, 49), or two-piece styles with bra or halter tops, often in exotic prints (Figures 50, 51).

Coats and Wraps

Coats were fitted with flaring or full skirts, or they might be straight and boxy, or swagger (flared from the shoulder). All of them had broad, square shoulders. Dressy coats might have full fur collars, usually rather wide on the shoulders. Fur coats usually had swagger lines and also had square shoulders. The tailored and fitted double-breasted reefer in tweed was very popular (Figure 54). Some fitted models appeared without collars. A redingote style was in fashion, single-breasted with a flaring skirt, and sometimes worn as an ensemble over a silk or rayon print dress. Fitted coats frequently had tie closings at the waistline (Figure 55). Straight coats might be three-quarter-, seven-eighths-, or full-length (Figure 56). Often they completed a three-piece suit ensemble. Short box jackets were popular. Fabric coats came in brilliant colors — such as bright red, blue, or green, with red particularly favored. A swagger coat had raglan sleeves and a zip-out fleece lining. Some capes were worn. A short shoulder cape might be part of a suit ensemble. A floor-length cape with a hood might be worn as an evening wrap. Short fitted jackets were also in evidence, with or without collars. The most-popular style in evening wraps was the floor-length fitted coat in black velvet, with a flaring skirt, and usually with a white satin lining.

Every branch of the armed services had female volunteers in World War II. They did not fight at the front but performed innumerable necessary tasks behind the lines. Women's service uniforms were generally of the same basic color as those of the men in the same division. Air Force and Marine uniforms were of forest green, Army uniforms were of olive drab with lighter drab skirts, and Navy uniforms were navy blue and white. The standard style for most uniforms was a single-breasted jacket, trimly fitted, and a slightly flared skirt just below the knee in length.

In the Air Force, in winter women wore two-piece forest-green wool uniforms, drab shirts and ties, russet shoes, and forest-green visor caps or overseas caps. In summer they wore cotton khaki dresses. The Women's Auxiliary Ferrying Squadron (WAFS) wore brown goatskin suits and hoods lined and edged with alpaca pile (with goggles on the hoods), mouton collars, zippered jackets, trousers with zippered legs, brown gauntlets, and brown boots. The Women Flyers of America wore overalls of olive-drab cloth or cotton, hoods tied under the chin, and Army russet shoes. In winter the Women's Army Corps (WACs) wore two-piece uniforms of lightweight wool, olive-drab jackets and lighter drab skirts; beige shirts and ties; and russet shoes, bags, and gloves (Figure 57). The overcoats worn with this uniform were of 15-ounce serge. In summer, the WACs wore service dresses of light tan cotton oxford cloth, and their dress uniforms were white. They wore overseas caps or visor hats tilted downward to the right. Their field uniform consisted of olive-drab coveralls with "cargo pockets" on the upper legs, khaki gaiters, Army russet shoes, and steel helmets (Figure 58). In winter the Marine Corps Women's Reserve (MCWR) wore forest-green wool suits, beige shirts and ties, and russet bags and shoes. Their visor hats were forest green with red cord trim and silver insignia. In summer they wore green-striped cotton suits. In the Navy, the Women Appointed for Volunteer Emergency Service (WAVES) wore navy-blue skirts and jackets of wool gabardine in winter, with white shirts, navy blue scarves, black shoes, and white gloves (Figure 59). They might wear either overseas caps or soft-brim hats with high crowns. In summer they wore gray-and-white striped seersucker dresses. All-white uniforms were worn for dress.

Army Corps nurses wore olive-drab uniforms, tan shirts and scarves, brown leather bags and shoes, and olive-drab visor caps. The regulation officers' overcoats were of olive-drab cloth, double-breasted, worn over white uniforms, with olive-drab garrison caps, white shoes and stockings, and brown wool gloves. The Army nurses' field uniform was similar to that of the WACs (Figure 58). The Navy Corps nurses wore navy blue double-breasted uniforms, gilt buttons and sleeve stripes, white or navy pie caps with black ribbon headbands, white shirts, black scarves, and white skirts with white shoes or navy skirts with black shoes (Figure 61). The Medical Corps nurses and Red Cross nurses wore white washable uniforms and nurses' caps; dark blue wool hem-length capes with dark red linings, fastened at the neck by hooks and eyes and at the chest by black frogs; and white shoes and stockings (Figure 62). The Red Cross nurses' aides wore French blue denim caps and jumpers, and white cotton short-sleeved shirtwaists. Red Cross field workers in the Naval and Military Welfare Service wore brown cloth uniforms and garrison caps, tan shirts and ties, and brown shoes and bags. The American Women's Voluntary Services (AWVS) wore dark blue uniforms with gilt buttons; blue hats (similar to Civil War style); white shirts; blue scarves; brown shoes, purses, belts, and straps; white cotton gloves; brown moccasin-styled shoes; and tan stockings.[14]

Footwear

Shoe styles during the war were similar to those of the thirties. Heels were generally rather low and sturdy, with a Cuban heel the most popular. Toes were blunt, round, or squared-off; and open toes were very prevalent. A cartoon of that era showed a young lady asking for ski boots with open toes! Shoes had a snub-nosed, foreshortened look; they came high on the instep and were designed to make the foot look shorter. Since leather was scarce, shoes began to appear in a variety of stretch fabrics, often in combination with leather—gabardine, maracain, covert cloth, and linen. Many models were seen in patent leather and suede. Flat, comfortable shoes were worn for war work. Canvas sneakers and ballet-type slippers with very low heels were frequently worn. Service uniform shoes were generally laced oxfords with Cuban heels. Saddle oxfords were worn for sports and for war work. Norwegian loafers were worn by women as well as men. Sandals with wedge heels were very popular. Shoes for formal dress were often sandals with ankle straps and three-inch heels. However, Cuban heels were also worn for dress occasions. Platform soles, which gave added height to the wearer, were still popular. Sling-back styles (with a strap holding the shoe on the back of the heel) were seen more and more as the war ended. A new style in oxfords was the monk's shoe, with a plain toe and a strap that buckled across the instep.

Accessories

Costume jewelry during the war continued to feature rhinestones or colored imitation stones. Settings might also be of mother-of-pearl or of opalescent milk glass. In addition to the usual necklaces, bracelets, and earrings, one saw jeweled clips and hair ornaments. Pearl necklaces remained a perennial favorite, particularly with sweaters or plain black dresses. Jewelry was also made of novelty materials—new synthetic plastics, wood and raffia, leather, or shells. Handcrafted metal jewelry appeared in abstract shapes influenced by the nonobjective trend in the fine arts. Dog-collar necklaces fitting the base of the neck were popular. A single heavy bracelet or multiple narrow bangles might be worn. Wristwatches were an ever-present necessity. Scarves and kerchiefs were very prevalent and appeared in festive colors and bright prints. They were worn as ascot ties around the neck, as snoods around the hair, or as babushkas tied under the chin. Purses were large and capacious, and the shoulder-strap model, which could be slung over one shoulder to leave the hands free, was one of the most-popular styles. It was a standard item in a military uniform. Smaller handbags were often made up in fabric to match a scarf or hat, perhaps in striped taffeta, colored straw, or a flowered print. This era was a great one for matching accessories, and gloves followed the trend. They were seen in many fanciful styles, in satin or lace, in polka dots, stripes, or floral prints. The contents of a purse might include a wallet or billfold; a key case; a compact containing face powder, and sometimes rouge and lipstick; or a makeup kit in a smaller purse style to hold a comb, lipstick, powder, and eye makeup. Cigarette cases and lighters were also carried, and perhaps a fountain pen and pencil set. The wide Phelps belt of metal-studded leather was very popular and was frequently worn with a matching shoulder-strap bag. Bright cummerbunds were also in style, and there was a fashion for varying plain dresses by tying on a decorative silk or rayon print apron or peplum. Women's umbrellas were short-handled. Occasionally muffs were carried, small and round or flat and pillow-shaped.

CHILDREN'S FASHIONS

Styles for children during World War II reflected those of their parents. The silhouette for both boys and girls tended to have square shoulders and a natural waistline.

Boys' fashions had changed little since the thirties. Knickerbocker pants were no longer on the scene. Small boys wore short pants until they were about eight years old. They might go into long trousers as soon as they started school. For dress occasions, a small boy might wear an Eton jacket and long trousers or short pants (Figure 63). For play he might wear coveralls or overalls of denim or corduroy. An older boy wore a replica of his father's tailored suit, or he might wear a mix-and-match outfit of slacks and a sports jacket. For school and play, boys wore slacks with sport shirts or with cotton knit polo shirts. Brightly striped polo shirts were a perennial favorite. A plaid flannel shirt was popular for cold weather. A combination of slacks, shirt, and pullover sweater, with or without sleeves, was a popular school outfit. Blue jeans were standard wear for active work or play. A variety of sports jackets were worn by boys — windbreakers, plaid wool lumber jackets, leather jackets, two-tone coat-sweaters (Figure 63). Boys' shoes were generally oxfords in tan, brown, black, or saddle styles. Socks were short, a little above the ankle. For the most part boys went hatless, but an older boy might wear a soft felt fedora for dress.

During the war there was a fad for mother-and-daughter outfits (Figure 64). Girls' dresses had fitted bodices; full skirts, which were gathered, pleated, or flared; and wide shoulders with gathered sleeves. Pinafores were popular, worn over dresses with puffed sleeves and full gathered skirts. Jumpers worn over long-sleeved blouses were also in fashion. Box-pleated skirts, frequently seen in plaid wool, were worn with shirtwaists or sweaters. Suits might have bolero jackets or fitted jackets with or without collars. Girls also wore dirndl skirts with peasant blouses. Shoes for dress were low-heeled black patent leather pumps or strap styles. Schoolgirls wore plain dark oxfords, saddle oxfords, or loafers. They wore knee-high socks or anklets. A small girl's hair style might be a Dutch bob with bangs, braids tied with ribbon bows, or a simply styled shoulder-length bob. In hats, girls wore calottes (skull caps, or "beanies"), small berets, or Breton sailors in straw or felt with turned-up brim.

Typical Materials, Colors, Motifs, and Trimmings

The war period was one of contrasts. Service uniforms were subdued in color but were made of fine wools and the best materials. Civilian clothing was likely to be made of ersatz or synthetic materials, but often came in high colors and strong values. Nylon had appeared on the market in 1940 but was channeled into war production. Rayon came to the fore and was rapidly replacing silk; it was now available in various blends with cotton or wool, which were proving very serviceable, and these new fabrics were being utilized for both men's and women's clothing.

Materials for men's suits were worsted, flannel, and tweed. Glen plaids, pinstripes, and herringbone weaves were in fashion. Popular shades for Glen plaids were medium gray, tan, gray-green, or gray-blue. Pinstripes might be white on navy blue or gray, or tan on dark brown. A rayon-and-cotton blend was used for washable summer suits. Seersucker was also still favored for summer. Shirts were more likely to be in pastel stripes or colors than white. Popular colors for sport shirts were tan, gold, navy blue, French blue, maroon, or deep green. Plaids, stripes, or checks were perennially popular for sport shirts or separate jackets. Hawaiian prints in splashy floral, leaf, or aquatic designs and brilliant colors were made into summer sport shirts. The South Sea batik prints favored for beach wear were usually in shades of brown and tan.

For women's clothing, rayon fabrics were more prevalent than ever, and many new blends had appeared. Rayon crepe and rayon jersey were popular fabrics for afternoon dresses. Printed rayons were particularly fashionable for dressy occasions. For cool weather, plaid wool was a favorite. Wool jerseys, corduroy, and velveteen were much used. Cotton and rayon fabrics were available in splashy border prints, which made up well in bordered dirndl skirts. Taffeta patterned in stripes, checks, or plaids was on the market and was very popular for hats and scarves as well as for formal dresses. Stripes and plaids were also much used for housedresses in seersucker, gingham, madras, and chambray. Sheer cottons, such as dotted swiss and organdy, were popular for summer dresses, in formal or informal styles. It was probably no accident that, with the Star-Spangled Banner waving on all sides, a favorite color scheme was red, white, and blue. An outfit often seen was a navy blue suit with a white piqué blouse and hat and perhaps a red bag and shoes, or red gloves and flower. The mother-and-daughter outfits shown in Figure 64 are of red-white-and-blue striped seersucker. Other popular colors were fuchsia, purple, plum, gold, bright or dark green, and turquoise or a deeper blue-green.

In trimmings, sequins were among the most-used decorations. They appeared on snoods, scarves, collars and cuffs, belts, bodice fronts, and peplums. Another trim that appeared frequently were metal studs clipped into belts or fabrics. Appliquéd leather was also seen, for example, gold kid on a black velvet evening wrap. For dressy outfits, jeweled belt buckles, buttons, or clips might be used. Rhinestones also might be cleated into the fabric as a permanent trim, perhaps at the neckline or on a wide cummerbund. For casual dresses, rickrack braid was a popular decoration, and so were eyelet embroidery ruffles. Matching accessories were all the rage — hats matching bags or gloves or scarves, belts matching handbags and possibly shoes.

SUGGESTIONS FOR COSTUMING PLAYS IN THE PERIOD

In re-creating the era of World War II, the costumer will need to find old models of suits and dresses with a broad-shouldered look. Men's jackets should have wide lapels, peaked or notched, and preferably should be double-breasted. Trousers should be generous in width, pleated at the waistband, and may or may not have cuffs. Four-in-hands should be wide — two or three inchess — and bow ties might have pointed ends. For evening wear, a white dinner jacket with shawl collar or a white mess jacket would be appropriate, or a midnight blue double-breasted dinner jacket. A Glen plaid or pinstripe double-breasted suit would be typical for the period.

It is an obvious suggestion to look for uniform and military accessories at an Army and Navy surplus store, but remember that Air

Force blue and the current Army green uniforms were adopted some time after World War II. Air Force uniforms should be forest green and Army uniforms olive drab. The color of a visor cap may be changed by slipping a fitted cover over the crown. In all branches of the service, an overseas cap may usually be worn if a visor cap is not available.

The look of the war period in women's wear required that almost any garment have generous shoulder pads inserted to shape and extend the shoulder seams — blouses, shirtwaists, negligees, evening gowns, and housedresses as well as tailored coats and suits. Slack suits would be appropriate for casual wear. A jerkin or fitted vest worn over a long-sleeved shirtwaist with slacks makes an interesting variation. Box-pleated plaid skirts worn with sweaters or dirndl skirts with peasant blouses are typical combinations for informal outfits. Printed rayon suits or dresses are appropriate for afternoon or town wear. A plain black, navy, or dark crepe dress may be enhanced with rather flashy accessories — scarf, costume jewelry, tie-on apron or peplum, cummerbund, frivolous hat or fanciful gloves — and accessories are frequently matched to a point that seems overdone. Shoulder-strap purses are appropriate. Hair styles are most often shoulder-length and frequently adorned with flowers, velvet bows, or jeweled ornaments. Hair may be covered by a kerchief, turban, snood, or babushka. Shoes are round or square-toed, or open-toed, and heels are most often Cuban height and rather sturdy. Platform soles, wedge heels, and ankle straps are evocative of the period. A treasure hunt through thrift shops and secondhand clothing stores may still turn up many of these items.

TITLE	AUTHOR	PERIOD
Anna Lucasta	Philip Yordan	1944
Arsenic and Old Lace	Joseph Kesselring	1941
Best Foot Forward (M)	C. Holm, H. Martin, R. Blane	1940
Blithe Spirit	Noel Coward	1941
Born Yesterday	Garson Kanin	1945
Caine Mutiny Court Martial	Herman Wouk	WWII
Carmen Jones (M)	Oscar Hammerstein	1943
Command Decision	William Haines	WWII
Dark of the Moon	H. Richardson, W. Berney, W. Hendl	1945
Deep Are the Roots	Arnaud D'Usseau, James Gow	1945
The Deputy	Rolf Hochhuth	1942–43
The Diary of Anne Frank	F. Goodrich, A. Hackett	WWII
Dream Girl	Elmer Rice	1945
George Washington Slept Here	Moss Hart, George Kaufman	1940
Harvey	Mary Chase	1944
The Hasty Heart	John Patrick	WWII
Home of the Brave	Arthur Laurents	WWII
Incident at Vichy	Arthur Miller	1942
Lady in the Dark (M)	Kurt Weill, Ira Gershwin	1941
The Male Animal	James Thurber, Elliott Nugent	1940
Member of the Wedding	Carson McCullers	1945
Mister Roberts	Thomas Heggen, Joshua Logan	WWII
My Sister Eileen	Joseph Fields, Jerome Chedorov	1940
Night of the Iguana	Tennessee Williams	1940
No Time for Sergeants	Ira Levin	WWII
On the Town (M)	B. Comden, A. Green, L. Bernstein	1944
One Touch of Venus (M)	Odgen Nash, Kurt Weill	1943
Over Twenty-One	Ruth Gordon	1944
Pal Joey (M)	R. Rodgers, L. Hart, J. O'Hara	1940
Skin of Our Teeth	Thornton Wilder	1942
South Pacific (M)	R. Rodgers, O. Hammerstein	WWII
Stalag 17	Donald Bevan, Edmund Trzcinski	WWII
State of the Union	Howard Lindsay, Russel Crouse	1946
The Subject Was Roses	Frank D. Gilroy	1946
Talley's Folly	Lanford Wilson	1944
The Teahouse of the August Moon	John Patrick, Vern Sneider	WWII
There Shall Be No Night	Robert E. Sherwood	WWII
The Voice of the Turtle	John Van Druten	1943
The Wall	Millard Lampell	1940–43
Watch on the Rhine	Lillian Hellman	WWII
Wonderful Town (M)	B. Comden, A. Green, L. Bernstein	1940
Zoot Suit	Luis Valdez	1942–44

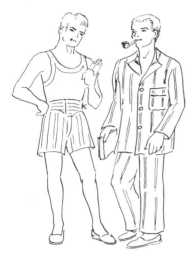

1. Left, boxer shorts and tank top. Right, wartime pajamas without collar or cuffs. 1943.

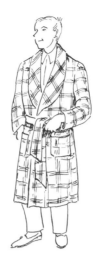

2. Wool robe: blue plaid on tan ground. 1944.

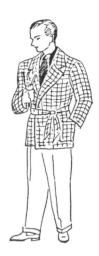

3. Lounge suit: lightweight flannel in tan, brown, and blue check. 1944.

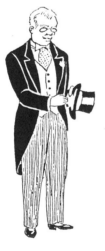

4. Formal day wear: Oxford gray cutaway; gray waistcoat; silk ascot. 1942.

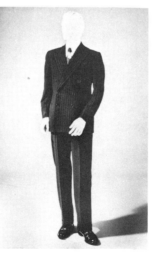

5. Two-piece suit in navy blue wool with white pinstripe; double-breasted, three-button jacket; cuffed trousers. By Silverwoods of Southern California, 1945. (Division of Costume, Smithsonian Institution.)

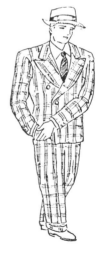

6. Double-breasted lounge suit with broad shoulders and snug hips. 1940.

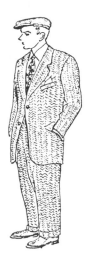

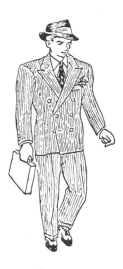

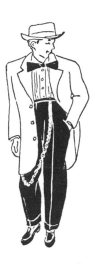

7. Summer suit of lightweight tweed; tan shirt; figured foulard tie. 1941.

8. Double-breasted summer suit of washable cotton. 1946.

9. Teen-age "zoot suit" with long jacket; huge bow tie; long key chain. 1942.

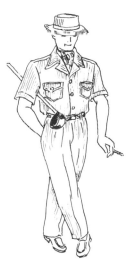

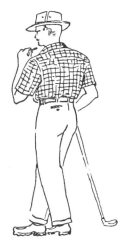

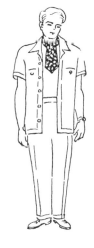

10. Two-piece suit of lightweight corduroy for sports wear. 1942.

11. Golfing outfit: checked sport shirt; slacks; Panama hat. 1946.

12. Sports outfit: short-sleeved jacket; slacks; polo shirt; ascot. 1945.

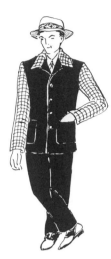

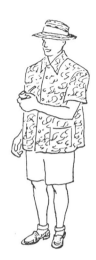

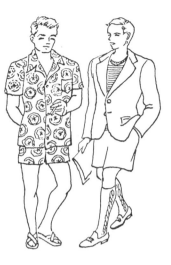

13. Gabardine slack suit: jacket has plaid back, collar, and sleeves. 1942.

14. Sports outfit: cotton print shirt; Bermuda shorts. 1946.

15. Beach wear. Left, batik shirt and shorts. Right, jacket and Bermuda shorts. 1940.

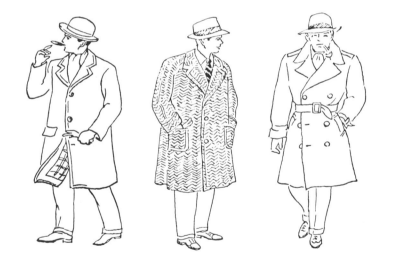

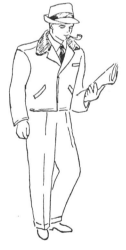

16, 17, 18. Single-breasted tweed overcoat with plaid lining. 1946. Raglan topcoat in herringbone tweed. 1940. Tan raincoat adapted from Army trench coat in water-repellent twill. 1941.

19. Wool sports jacket with sheepskin lining and dark brown mouton collar. 1944.

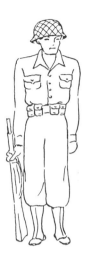

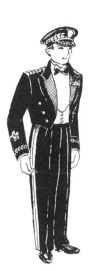

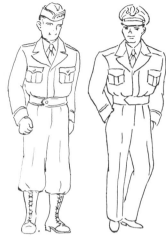

20. Army combat uniform: khaki blouse and trousers; cartridge belt; gaiters.

21. Army general's mess dress uniform: dark blue with gold trim.

22. Army field dress: olive drab "Eisenhower jacket" and trousers; field boots.

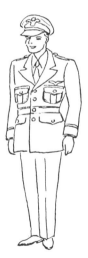

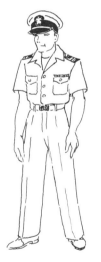

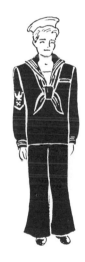

23. Air Force officer's uniform: olive drab coat; taupe trousers.

24. Naval officer's tropical white long uniform; white shoes.

25. Sailor's uniform: navy blue or white with braid trim; black tie; black shoes.

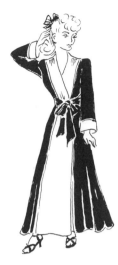

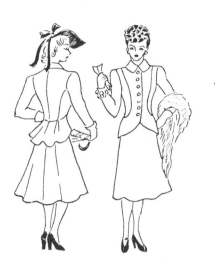

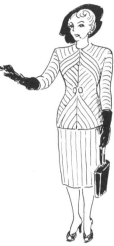

26. Tricolor wraparound housecoat of rayon crepe: black, white, and red. 1942.

27. Velveteen suit, front and back view: flared back, jacket and skirt. 1939.

28. Tailored wool suit in bold stripe; black hat, gloves, and bag. 1942.

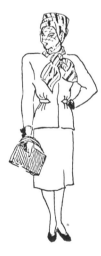

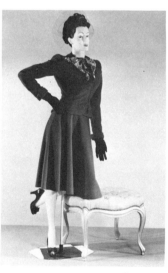

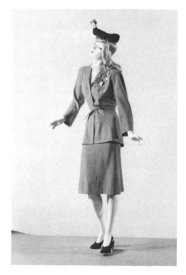

29. Blue-gray wool suit; striped velvet hat and scarf. 1945.

30. Two-piece suit of green wool. By Sophie Gimbel, 1943. (The Costume Institute of The Metropolitan Museum of Art. Gift of Saks Fifth Avenue.)

31. Two-piece suit of red wool. By Omar Kiam, 1943. (The Costume Institute of The Metropolitan Museum of Art. Gift of Omar Kiam.)

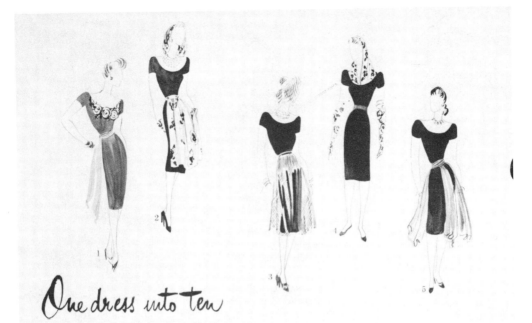

One dress into ten

Here's a 10-to-1 shot that will pay off all spring and summer. You begin with one short black dinner sheath—neck low, sleeves short—and you ring ten changes on it this way:

1. Bank large pink roses at the neck, gird waist with a sash of pink and violet chiffon.
2. Tie on an apron of flower print, add scarf and gloves to match, fill in neck with beads.
3. Hook on a full overskirt of black net and veil your head and face with more of the net.

4. Add a snood and long gloves of gay print.
5. Tie on a chiffon sash with floating panels.
6. Pull on a sweater-blouse of black satin, tuck in the neck a sequin-dotted tulle scarf.
7. Add a brief lace peplum and lace gloves.
8. Cover with loose jacket of jet-dotted net.
9. By day, wear a grey-and-black tweed jacket, by afternoon—a brilliantly striped satin one.
10. Or just wear the sheath as is— with your best jewels and cut-steel buckles on your pumps

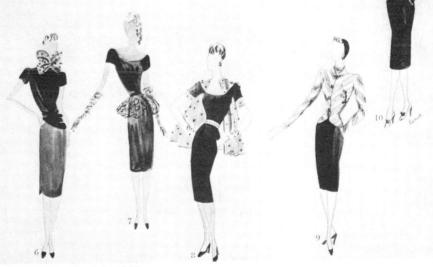

32. Page from *Vogue*, April 1, 1943.

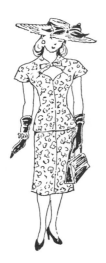

33. Two-piece afternoon dress in printed rayon crepe; large straw hat. 1945.

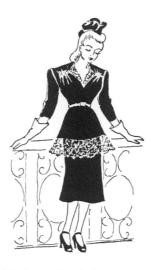

34. Street-length formal frock in rayon crepe with venise lace trim. 1941.

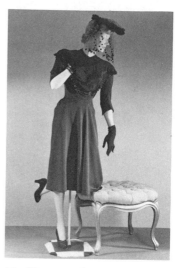

35. Afternoon dress of blue crepe. By Juana de Garzon, 1942. Hat of blue felt. By Titania du Plessix. (The Costume Institute of The Metropolitan Museum of Art. Gift of Henri Bendel, Inc.)

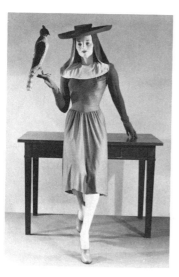

36. Afternoon dress of red wool jersey. By Nettie Rosenstein, 1942. Hat of red wool jersey. By Madame Pauline. Gloves of red wool jersey. Shoes of red leather. By Palter De Liso. (The Costume Institute of The Metropolitan Museum of Art. Gift of Nettie Rosenstein.)

37. Women's fashions, prewar to postwar.
   Left to right: Fitted suit by Schiaparelli; doll hat with veil. 1937.   Evening gown by Schiaparelli: bias-cut black crepe with shocking pink bolero. 1938.   Evening gown by Adrian of black crepe with bold printed pattern in red and white, called "Roan Stallion." 1945.   Fitted suit in chartreuse wool; shoulder bag; fedora hat. Mid-1940s.   Seated, hooded jumper in gray jersey, by Claire McCardell; worn with red leotards, red ballet shoes, red leather belt and bag. 1942.   "New Look" suit by Christian Dior: jacket of beige tussore silk; full, calf-length, black wool skirt. 1947. (The Costume Institute of The Metropolitan Museum of Art, and The Brooklyn Museum. Photograph by Milton H. Greene.)

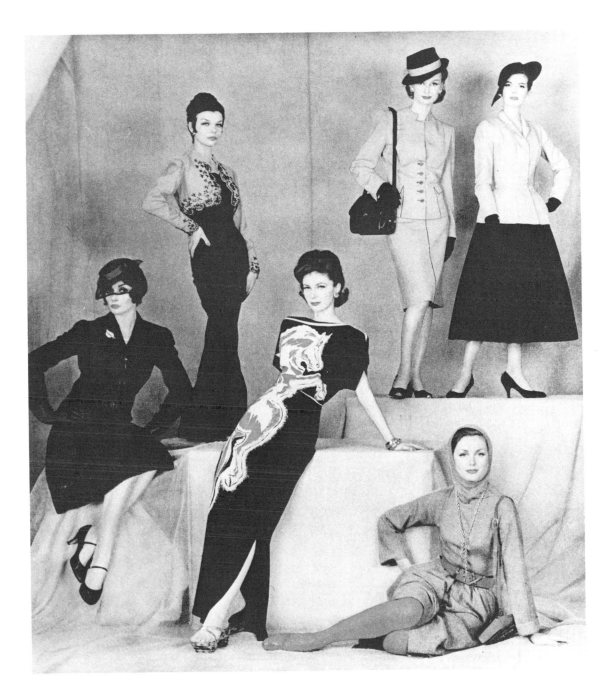

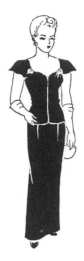

38. Two-piece black rayon jersey evening gown; satin gloves and bag. 1944.

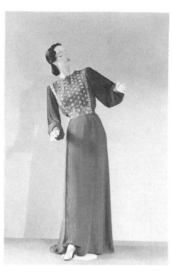

39. Dinner dress of geranium-red pleated Tuscanna. By Jessie Franklin Turner, 1942. Red-and-gold sandal. (The Costume Institute of The Metropolitan Museum of Art. Gift of Jessie Franklin Turner.)

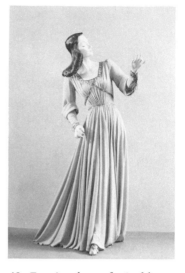

40. Evening dress of mist-blue Tuscanna, called "Primavera" after Botticelli. By Jessie Franklin Turner, 1942. Gold and mist-blue satin sandal. (The Costume Institute of The Metropolitan Museum of Art. Gift of Jessie Franklin Turner.)

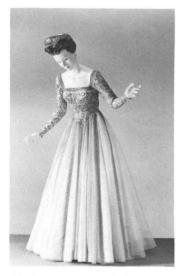

41. Evening dress of white marganza embroidered in two tones of gold; white taffeta underskirt. By Nettie Rosenstein, 1942. Turban of gold tissue. By Madame Pauline. White satin sandals. By Ansonia, N. Y. (The Costume Institute of The Metropolitan Museum of Art. Gift of Nettie Rosenstein.)

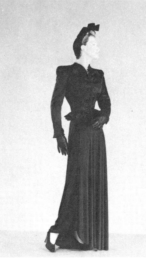

42. Dinner dress: navy satin jacket, navy jersey skirt. By Mark Mooring, 1942. Navy silk crocheted hat and gloves. Navy crepe shoes. By Delman. (The Costume Institute of The Metropolitan Museum of Art. Gift of Bergdorf Goodman.)

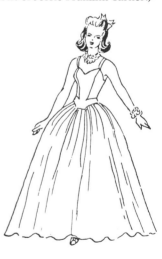

43. Taffeta evening gown; pannier hip pads extend the full skirt. 1940.

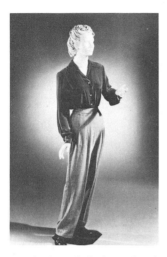

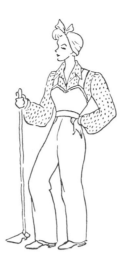

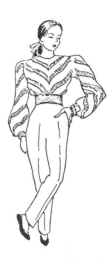

44. Plaid wool slacks with side zipper and side-seam pocket. By Dennison, 1942 – 43. Purple crepe blouse with turnback cuffs 1948 – 49. (Division of Costume, Smithsonian Institution.)

45. Denim overalls and shirtwaist, for kitchen, garden, or factory. 1942.

46. Cabana slacks of lime linen; sky-blue awning-striped shirt. 1946.

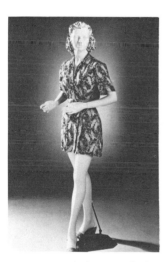

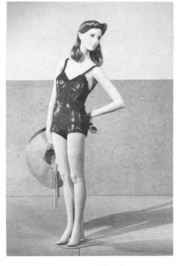

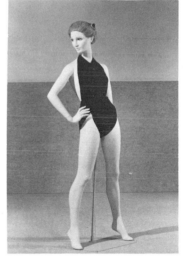

47. One-piece playsuit of white and coral print: shirt top with short sleeves, button front; full shorts with tucks released at thighs. Playsuits of this type were often worn with an overskirt. 1940s. (Division of Costume, Smithsonian Institution.)

48. Sequined wool bathing suit. American, Bonwit Teller, 1940. (The Costume Institute of The Metropolitan Museum of Art. Gift of Mr. and Mrs. Burton Tremaine.)

49. Bathing suit of wool and rayon in diaper design. By Claire McCardell, 1944. (The Costume Institute of The Metropolitan Museum of Art. Gift of Mrs. A. Moore Montgomery.)

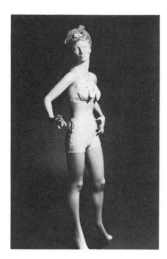

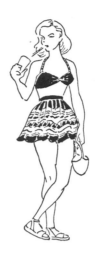

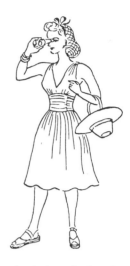

50. Two-piece white bathing suit: pants lace up both sides; halter top ties in back and adjusts by a decorative tie in front. Early 1940s. (Division of Costume, Smithsonian Institution.)

51. Two-piece cotton swim suit, Guatemalan design; rubber cap. 1942.

52. Sunback dress for beach or sports wear; wedge sandals. 1940.

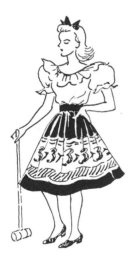

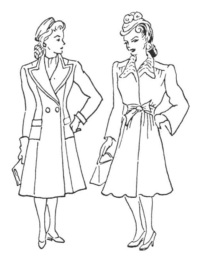

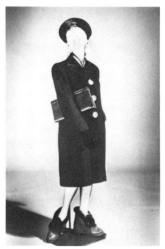

53. Dirndl skirt in bright cotton print; white peasant blouse. 1943.

54, 55. Double-breasted, reefer-style spring coat in soft beige tweed. 1942. Wool town coat with mink collar. 1941.

56. "Chesterfield" coat: brown wool, with velvet trim on collar and pocket, braid trim on pocket. Central Michigan, early 1040s. (Division of Costume, Smithsonian Institution.)

WOMEN'S UNIFORMS, WORLD WAR II

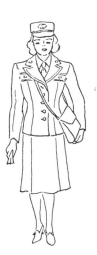

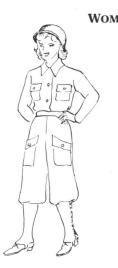

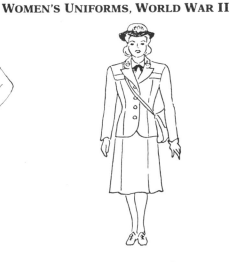

57. WAC (Army) uniform: khaki suit and "Hobby hat"; brown shoes.

58. WAC field uniform: khaki shirt, trousers, and gaiters; steel helmet.

59. WAVE (Navy) uniform: navy blue suit; navy tie; white shirt; black shoes.

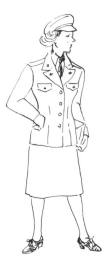

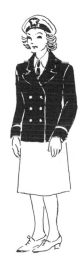

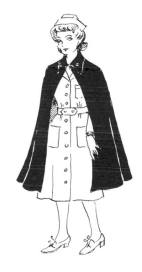

60. Army nurse's tropical service uniform: beige jacket, skirt, and cap.

61. Navy nurse's service dress: blue coat, white skirt, white cap, white shoes.

62. Army nurse's white hospital duty uniform; navy cape with red lining.

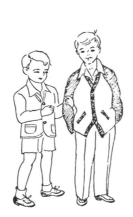

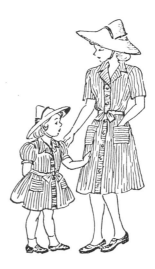

63. Left, boy's jacket suit. Right, school outfit of two-tone sweater and twill slacks. 1945.

64. Mother-and-daughter matching dresses of striped seersucker. 1946.

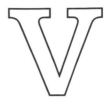

The Postwar Era
and the "New Look"
(1947 — 1952)

THE SECOND WORLD WAR was finally over, and Americans could relax a little and think about clothes once more, after several years of austerity. Wartime rationing and scarcities faded into memory as the Office of Price Administration rulings on most items were lifted by the end of 1946. Factories converted from wartime production and began to produce items for the home and for individual consumption. It was again possible to purchase nylon hose, to get a pair of shoes without counting out ration stamps, to find men's white shirts on the counters, and to buy a man's suit with trouser cuffs and a vest if that is what one wanted. With a sigh of relief, women reverted to their more-feminine roles and welcomed the new silhouette launched by Christian Dior in the spring of 1947. They must have grown very tired of being so sturdy and efficient for the preceding few years. With Paris designers again leading the way, the football shoulders shrank to a natural size and sloped in appealing helplessness. Waistlines were almost as tiny as in grandmother's day, back in 1900, and the frills and flounces just as charming and fluttery. Bosoms and hips were as round and buxom as Lillian Russell's (or Jane Russell's), and the ballet-dancer skirts swished over wonderfully full petticoats. The heels on shoes went to spiky heights, really quite impractical, and once again it was ostensibly the man's job to keep his feet flat on the ground, do the heavy work, and take care of the female sex. However, women would never truly go back to being the clinging vines of the Gay Nineties. Some of the old customs had disappeared forever during the fighting of two World Wars. Men no longer leaped forward to open a door or carry a package, and gone were the days when a woman might hope that a man would give her his seat on a bus or subway train. The absurd notion that a "woman's place was in the home" could not be recaptured. It had been dealt a death blow when women began receiving sizable weekly paychecks. Sky-rocketing costs of living made it more or less imperative for the woman of the house to retain her place as wage earner in addition to her role of homemaker.

CONCERNING THE PERIOD

The primary task of this era was to make an adjustment to the landmark events of 1945 — the launching of the United Nations, the defeat of the Axis powers, and the explosion of the first atomic bombs. It was necessary to convert from a wartime psychology and a wartime economy as swiftly and painlessly as possible.

At home, Americans were busily replenishing their furnishings. Streamlined household appliances were once more on the market. Laundry was easier than ever before with automatic washing machines and electric clothes dryers. In the kitchen, time and energy could be saved with electric garbage disposal units, improved stoves and refrigerators, freezers, electric dishwashers, mixers and blenders, pop-up toasters and grills. Shortcuts to cooking were provided by frozen foods, packaged mixes, and instant coffee.

Houses were designed with more open spaces, often with no wall between the kitchen and the living room. Entire exterior walls were made of glass, in effect bringing the outdoors into the house. Public taste turned toward the sprawling single-story ranch-style home or the split-level house, which combined half-stories in interesting arrangements: for example, the living room might be a few steps lower than the kitchen-dining area, with the bedrooms or recreation rooms a half-level up or down. Exposure to Japanese architecture and interior decoration during the war in the Pacific doubtless influenced many Americans to seek the more-spacious and uncluttered lines of modern architecture and decor. After the war, the trend toward modern interior decoration increased markedly. The free-form plastic chairs of Charles Eames, Loewy's furniture designed in simple geometric shapes, canvas sling chairs, and slender steel legs on tables and chairs (what one decorator called "mosquito modern") appeared everywhere.

Mass production, which made items of everyday living readily available at reasonable prices, also had the drawback of making every home look very much like its neighbor; and a man's suit was a replica of those worn by thousands of others across the country. Suburban developments of tract houses — little boxes that all looked alike — helped complete the picture. The resulting loss of identity sent many people (if they could afford it) to a psychiatrist's couch in search of their lost selves.

In the arts, the movement toward abstract expressionism was at its height. Some leading painters in this nonobjective styles were Jackson Pollock, who dripped paint in intricate patterns on his canvases; Hans Hofmann, who influenced many younger painters through his school in Greenwich Village; Arshile Gorky; Willem de Kooning; and Mark Rothko. Since the method of working was accidental and subconscious, this style of painting often seemed to depend on luck or intuition. Capturing public attention were Raoul Dufy's free-and-easy Impressionistic paintings, with crisp line drawings superimposed on hazy splashes of background color. His technique was found to be theatrically effective and was adopted by many stage designers. Picasso was producing caricatures in sculpture, such as his grotesque *Baboon and Young* in 1951 and his series of ceramic owls.

Popular music and dancing held to much the same rhythms as had prevailed in the war years. Long-playing records with a speed of 33 1/3 revolutions per minute appeared on the market in 1946, and their production soon became a major industry. The big swing bands that had held sway since the mid-thirties were on their way out. Television was shifting the spotlight to popular singers. The first regularly scheduled television programs were launched in 1948. In that initial period, many shows were transferred from radio to the television screen — musical programs such as "Your Hit Parade," "Voice of Firestone," and "The Kate Smith Hour" and comedians Jack Benny, Eddie Cantor, Burns and Allen, and "Amos 'n' Andy." Singers Perry Como and Dinah Shore had their own shows dating from that era. New comedians were Milton Berle, Jackie Gleason, and Sid Caesar. Durable variety programs were inaugurated by Arthur Godfrey (another veteran from radio), Garry Moore, and Ed Sullivan. Lucille Ball first appeared in "I Love Lucy" in 1951, and Dave Garroway's "Today" show started in 1952.

The motion picture industry was threatened by the advent of television and the fact that the public could now stay home and watch a free show. Innovations to combat this trend included drive-in movie theatres in the open air, where entire families could stay in their cars and watch a film, and wide-screen and three-dimensional motion pictures. The year 1952 saw the first Cinerama, using a 146° curved screen and stereophonic sound, and the first 3-D films, for which the audience wore Polaroid glasses. The latter was a novelty that lasted only a year or so and was replaced by other wide-screen processes such as CinemaScope and VistaVision, which got rid of the inconvenient glasses. Male screen idols of this era included the old reliables of the war years — Clark Gable, Gary Cooper, Spencer Tracy, James Stewart, Humphrey Bogart, Gregory Peck — and newcomers Marlon Brando and Burt Lancaster. Pinup girls Betty Grable, Rita Hayworth, and Lana Turner were still very popular. Joan Crawford, Marlene Dietrich, Katharine Hepburn, and Bette Davis held their well-earned positions as top stars. New faces, young but destined for box-office success, were Elizabeth Taylor and Marilyn Monroe. A new appreciation for ladylike elegance (which went well with the "New Look" in fashion) put a seal of approval on such well-bred stars as Grace Kelly, Loretta Young, and Greer Garson.

GENERAL CHARACTERISTICS OF COSTUME

Against a background of rapid change and feverish activity, the silhouette in clothing was also changing. The "New Look" (for both men and women) had an Edwardian flavor. An usual, the men were slower to shift their tastes in wearing apparel. The female revolution in fashion arrived in 1947; it was not until 1952 that male styles began to change to a slimmer look. One guess as to why people wanted to revert to the fashions worn by their grandparents in simpler, slower times is that they needed some old-fashioned assurances and patterns to cling to in the new atomic age.

In the spring of 1947, Christian Dior's Paris opening created a sensation by its radical departure from the square-shouldered, short-skirted look of the war years. Dior's models caught the public fancy, and this "New Look" was hailed with delight and excitement by such arbiters of fashion as *Vogue*:

> The opening of Christian Dior's new Paris couture house on February 12 not only presented an extraordinarily beautiful collection; it gave the French couture a new assurance in its own abilities; and because the luxury trades are economic necessity in France, Dior's flashing success was in Paris, more than fashion. It was on a par with current political and economic news. Here — once again — things were done on a grand scale; the clothes were elegant, built for a woman's figure; the pretty new mannequins were *soignées*, certain, had been taught to wear the costumery (every one over its own waist-indenting guêpière). There was on opening day such an air of contagious confidence in the atelier and salons of the new house that shortages of heat, light, and transportation were forgotten in the pure pleasure of the grand luxe première. There were no "easy little dresses," no flashing theatrical designs. Rather, each model was constructed with a deep knowledge of dressmaking, to give you an exaggeratedly feminine figure, even if nature has not. Dior . . . draws from the era of Madame Bovary for hats picture pretty or with motoring scarf drapery — wasp-waisted Gibson Girl shirtwaists, pleated or tucked — the caped Inverness coat — the dress rounded with scarf drapery across the back — slow-sloped, easy shoulders — variations of the belt-back jacket — wrapped and bound middles — barrel (almost hobble) skirts — longer, deeply draped shadow-box décolletage — padded hips.[1]

The new styles depended on firm undergirding. Of primary importance was the guêpière or "waist-cincher," a tiny girdle that took inches off the waistline. Hips were frequently padded, and for the full-skirted models a bouffant petticoat was also essential. Skirts went down almost to the ankles; some were very slim, others extravagantly wide. Dior was an expert craftsman, with a shrewd flair for publicity and a well thought-out philosophy of design. In his memoirs he comments:

> We were emerging from a period of war, of uniforms, of women-soldiers built like boxers. I drew women-flowers, soft shoulders, flowering busts, fine waists like liana and wide skirts like corolla. But it is well known that such fragile appearances are obtained only at the price of a rigorous construction. . . . I wanted my dresses to be constructed, molded upon the curves of the feminine body whose sweep they would stylize.[2]

Other leading French designers of this era were Jacques Fath, Nina Ricci, Balmain, and Cardin. Molyneux closed shop after the war, and Schiaparelli left the fashion field in 1950. Balenciaga, from Spain, was gaining prominence and was destined to be perhaps the most-outstanding designer of the fifties and sixties. Givenchy opened his couture house in 1951. New designers were appearing in Italy in the late forties — Pucci in Florence and Simonetta in Rome. The Italian designers have been most noted for casual fashions and sportswear. In Ireland, after her opening in 1950, Sibyl Connolly was producing elegant designs in native linen. In America leading fashion designers were Mainbocher, Philip Mangone, Charles James, Tina Leser, Norman Norell, and Claire McCardell. James Galanos started a design establishment in Los Angeles in 1951.

Men's styles retained the broad silhouette of the war era until the mid-fifties, beginning to break away to natural shoulders, longer lapels, longer coats, and tapered trousers about 1952. This "Ivy League" look had for some time been admired and maintained by college men on the eastern seaboard, at such conservative strongholds as Harvard, Princeton, and Yale. The new fashions for men actually paralleled the trend of the women's "New Look" in recapitulating the first decade of the century, with a quiet, slim elegance that was typical of Bond Street in London and of Madison Avenue in New York. In the years immediately following World War II, most men contented themselves with the "New Bold Look," which still had wide shoulders, wide lapels, and pleated trousers.

MEN'S FASHIONS

The period between World War II and the mid-fifties, when the atomic and space age began to take shape, was a time of transition from the image of the broad-shouldered he-man who fought the war to a new silhouette, slender and with a faintly Edwardian flavor. During this interlude jackets still had fairly broad, padded shoulders and wide lapels, but they were single-breasted more often than double-breasted.

Colors for casual dress were brighter than they had been at any time in the twentieth century. For example, sport slacks might be bright yellow or orange, and might be combined with an African print shirt. There was a vogue for dinner jackets in bright red or tartan worsted. Four-in-hands during the late forties, for those who had any sartorial dash, were in bold, vivid prints.

Hair Styles and Grooming

As during the war years, a man's hair was worn rather short, clipped over the ears, parted on the right or left side, or combed back in a pompadour. The brush cut, or crew cut, was popular, wherein the hair stood up in short bristles, and so was the feather cut, which was just a little longer. Most men were clean-shaven; a very few wore small mustaches. Good grooming was considered important, and after the war a number of new grooming aids appeared on the market. Men became good customers for after-shave lotions, deodorants, and cologne, in addition to their shaving creams, hair oils and creams, and shampoos. For some, electric razors helped to make the task of shaving easier.

Hat Styles

The high silk hat was now worn only for the most formal "white-tie" occasions. The homburg or derby in black, midnight blue, or dark gray was preferred for daytime formal or evening semiformal affairs. The most-popular hat for town or business wear was the snap-brim fedora. There was one felt model with a flat-topped crown. The Tremont hat, with tapered crown and narrow brim, appeared in 1950. The porkpie hat, with square-creased crown, was still around for country and campus wear. The flat tweed cap with visor was back in fashion for sports or casual wear. In the summer the old perennials were worn — the straw boater (now with a narrow brim), the Panama hat, and the dark coconut straw with puggree silk pleated band. For sports wear, a new variety of visored cap had appeared, similar to a jockey or baseball cap with a somewhat higher crown; a winter version in heavy wool might be worn on the ski slope, a summer model in cotton or straw on the beach.

Underwear, Loungewear, and Sleepwear

Standard male undergarments were cotton boxer shorts or knitted briefs worn alone or with a sleeveless lisle undershirt. Striped shorts were popular. Long knitted underwear for winter was still available, but was now made in separate pull-on tops and bottoms with elastic waistbands. Thermal underwear had been developed during the war and was found to be very suitable for cold-weather sports such as hunting and skiing. Pajamas were worn for sleeping; they were made of cotton, rayon, or silk, plain or printed (Figure 1). Lounging attire included the standard robe of mid-calf length as well as one of hip-length. Leisure jackets were available in tartans. The short beach robe of cotton with terry cloth lining and matching trunks illustrated in Figure 14 was of red-white-and-blue checks. The set included a longer matching robe with shawl collar, "if you prefer more cover-up." New on the market were "T.V. jackets," loosely fitting coats of cotton blends or lightweight wool resembling extra-long sport shirts with long sleeves and patch pockets.

White cotton shirts were available once more, after the wartime short-ages. Shirts made of nylon or cotton-Dacron blends had gained great popularity; they were easy to launder and required little if any press-ing. The stiff-bosomed piqué shirt with detachable wing collar and white piqué bow tie were still worn with a tailcoat for formal dress. For black-tie dress occasions a turnover collar was usually worn. The semiformal dress shirt often had a pleated front and long pointed col-lar tips, and might be of fine white cotton, linen, silk, or nylon. Collars came in several styles — wide, and flaring away from the tie; with long, slender points; button-down; or narrow, with curved tips to be pinned under the tie knot. Dress shirts might be pastel colored, or have a pinstripe or small check. Sport shirts were frequently made in bright colors, bold stripes, checks or plaids, and Hawaiian or African prints (Figure 12). In the late forties four-in-hands were often wild and bright, still fairly wide, and might have a hand-painted single motif in a prominent position below the knot. Diagonal stripes were as popular as ever. By 1952 a very narrow bow tie, with pointed or straight ends, had come into fashion. Four-in-hands also appeared in narrower styles, with pointed or straight ends. White silk mufflers were worn with for-mal evening attire. Colored mufflers, plain or patterned, might be worn with topcoats in cold weather. Ascots or scarves were often used to fill in the neck of an open-collared sport shirt or leisure jacket.

Neckwear

For formal daytime occasions, men rarely wore the traditional outfit: cutaway coat in oxford gray or black, white dress shirt with wing or starched turnover collar, ascot or four-in-hand, black-and-gray striped trousers, light gray waistcoat, spats, black dress shoes, and high silk hat. More often the cutaway was replaced by the British lounge coat in black (a two-button single-breasted jacket with peaked lapels), which was worn with a matching black vest, striped trousers, white dress shirt with turnover collar, black dress shoes, and homburg or derby. The war had changed the public taste regarding formality in dress; the general approach was more casual. A dark business suit might be worn for almost any dress-up daytime affair. By 1952 the well-tailored gray flannel suit had become the uniform of the rising young executive on

Day Wear

Madison Avenue, that stronghold of the entertainment and advertising world; the favorite shade was charcoal. On Wall Street the preferred shade was a dark blue, or "banker's blue." In the late forties, shoulders were still wide and padded, and trousers were pleated at the waistband and full at the cuff (nineteen inches). By 1952 a natural shoulder, unpadded, was being worn by a few men, and some trousers were tapered to a narrower cuff (about sixteen inches). This slender silhouette became the prevailing mode for the late fifties and sixties. Double-breasted models with peaked lapels were still worn (Figure 2), but single-breasted styles were more popular (Figure 3). For informal and casual wear, Glenurquart plaids and herringbone tweeds were favored, in fairly lively colors such as gray and blue, gray and green, and tan and brown. For the most part, vests that matched the suits had disappeared. In 1952 there was a fad for brilliant vests, often gaily patterned, for informal daytime and evening wear (Figure 4). New on the market were lightweight permanent-press blends of wool and Dacron for summer or year-round wear (Figure 5).

Evening Wear   White tie and tails were still worn for the most-formal evening occasions (Figure 6). A desire for comfort prevailed, and most evening affairs called for semiformal dress. The midnight blue tuxedo jacket was still popular, as was the white dinner jacket, now available in lightweight synthetic fabrics (Figures 7, 8). They were worn with white dress shirts, often pleated, with turnover collars, black bow ties, black or midnight blue trousers with braid stripes, and black patent leather dress shoes. More color had appeared on the evening scene, and by 1950 dinner jackets might be dark red flannel or tartan (Figure 9). The dress trousers worn with the plaid jacket had a stripe of matching tartan braid. Bright cummerbunds and matching bow ties might be worn with a plain black or white jacket. Evening waistcoats added a festive note in 1952 with their bright colors and patterns — for example, a red-gold-and-black striped waistcoat was worn with a midnight blue tuxedo jacket; a dark red-and-green paisley print waistcoat with a black jacket.

Sportswear   For country wear and spectator sports, men favored combinations of separate jackets and slacks. In the late forties, they were often light in color. The tan camel's-hair jacket was a favorite, worn with gray or brown slacks. Pullover sweaters were frequently worn in place of vests (Figure 10). A crew-necked knitted polo shirt or a turtleneck sweater might also be worn with the sports jacket and slacks ensemble. Separate jackets in lively checks, madras, or tartans were in favor. There was a vogue for two-toned shirts or jackets — for example, the body might be plain and the sleeves plaid, or the front might be dark and the back and sleeves light. Sweaters were very popular, and cardigans were often worn in place of jackets. Bulky knit pullover sweaters were new and popular, some of them in bright pattern weaves. The Cowichan, or Siwash, style in a bold black or red pattern on white, made by the Indians of British Columbia, was favored for winter sports. For country wear, active sports, and work, "Levi's" were gaining in popularity — Western-style trousers with narrow tapered legs (made by Levi Strauss). In the summer, Bermuda shorts were frequently worn instead of slacks (Figure 13). For the beach there were cabana sets (Figure 14), terry cloth robes, boxer trunks in vivid prints (Figure 15), and briefs in nylon, Hawaiian prints, or knitted wool. There were various styles of leisure jackets — the bush jacket of the thirties, a new collarless single-breasted model, and a loose smocklike jacket with a tie-belt and patch pockets.

Coats and Wraps

The traditional Chesterfield topcoat for evening or daytime formal wear came in black, midnight blue, and oxford gray models, with a black velvet collar and usually with a fly front. A dress overcoat with a fur collar was available for evening wear (Figure 16). Topcoats appeared in both single- and double-breasted styles (Figure 17) and might be plain tan or gray, herringbone tweed, or various checked or plaid patterns — for example, gray with a blue check overlay, or tan with a red check overlay. The Chester was a new style of topcoat with a half-belt in back. The raglan-sleeved topcoat was a perennial favorite. The polo coat of tan camel's hair, double-breasted with wide lapels, was still worn for sports and travel. A water-repellent winter coat, double-breasted and belted, with a sheepskin lining and a mouton collar, was a popular model. There were all-purpose topcoats and raincoats with zip-in pile linings for conversion to winter wear. Several short jackets were available — the Eisenhower jacket was still popular for sports wear, as were the windbreaker and the lumber jacket. A sturdy blue denim jacket might be worn for work (Figure 18). The suburban coat (also called the car coat, tow coat, or duffle coat) was new on the market in 1950; it was a warm jacket of deep-piled wool, hip-length, with loop-and-toggle closings, and with a hood that could be worn over the head or folded down to form a collar.

Uniforms

The United States armed forces fighting in the Korean War were equipped for operation in very cold weather. In addition to the standard uniforms described for World War II, the soldiers in Korea wore sheepskin-lined hooded parkas and heavy gloves (Figure 19). Steel helmets were worn on top of wool caps with ear flaps. The fighting forces were drawn from the Army and the Marines; hence uniforms might be olive-drab or forest-green. The color of the Air Force uniforms was changed to gray-blue in 1950.

Footwear

The shoe styles of the early forties continued to be worn in this era. For formal dress, black patent leather pumps, oxfords, or slip-ons were appropriate. For semiformal occasions, black patent or calf dress shoes were worn. For town or business, plain dark oxfords or Norwegian loafers in black, brown, or dark blue were favored. New shades were cordovan (a deep red-brown) and olive (a greenish-brown). The monk's shoe, with plain toe and strap across the instep, was in fashion. The high-rise Blucher half-boot and the ankle-high chukka boot were still being worn. Two-toned shoes were still popular for casual and sports wear — saddie shoes in brown and white, black and white, or tan and brown. Loafers were also available in two-toned models. For sports wear there were woven leather moccasins and crepe-soled shoes, and beach shoes of raffia, blue denim, and linen. The shape of men's shoes changed in 1952 to conform to the general trend toward slimmer lines — toes, which had been rather square and bulky, became tapered and more pointed; plain toes and high-rise vamps were preferred fashions.

Accessories

Men's jewelry included rings, wristwatches, collar pins, tie clips, and cuff links and studs for dress shirts (white or gray pearl for formal wear, gold or set with colored stones for semiformal). Handkerchiefs were white for formal wear, and might be of plain color or have a colored border for informal wear; they were worn in the breast pocket with a two-point fold showing. Contents of pockets might include a leather wallet or billfold, credential case, cigarette case, key case or key chain, pocket comb, fountain pen and automatic pencil, and folding penknife. White or light gray gloves were worn for evening; gloves for general wear might be black, brown, or gray. Light tan gloves were popular. A man might carry the traditional black umbrella with crooked handle, but walking canes were almost never seen. Trousers were held up with belts or suspenders. Suspenders were available in sets with matching garters, or sometimes with matching socks. Boutonnières, usually white or red carnations, were worn in the lapel for evening.

WOMEN'S FASHIONS

The "New Look" featured a pinched-in waist, rounded shoulders and bosom, and ample hips — frequently padded. Skirts descended dramatically in 1947 from their wartime length just below the knees to a hemline at mid-calf or just above the ankles. Bouffant petticoats helped to extend the wide skirts. Heels were high and slender. The typical stance for the period was that of a ballet dancer—chin up, shoulders and back erect, figure poised gracefully with one toe forward and pointed. It is somewhat difficult to fix a cut-off date for the transition from this style to the next, the "shapeless shape," in which the female figure was once more ignored. Some commentators state that the New Look lasted five years; others say it continued until 1957. The straight sack or chemise dress made its first appearance in 1953. For women who preferred a neatly fitted style rather than the loose lines of a shift or chemise, the 1947 silhouette was carried over into the sixties, with a less-corseted waistline and shorter skirts.

Hair Styles and Makeup

The shoulder-length bob of the war years gave way to a shorter cut in 1947. The preferred look in the postwar period was a neatly curled cap of hair, styled close to the head. The "poodle cut" was an allover cap of short ringlets. The Italian, or feather, cut was longer, about four inches in length, and styled in loose curls often brought forward around the face. A pompadour style with wide marcel waves was popular. Soft bangs or curls on the forehead were frequently worn. Some women kept their longer hair but wore it styled in neat rolls on the neck, or in a chignon or French roll on the back of the head. Teen-agers were fond of the "pony tail," in which the longer hair was swept back into a single lock or flowing mane. It was held rather high on the back of the head with a rubber band or tied with a scarf and left to cascade down the back. This hair style was particularly effective for dancing and is still popular with ballet dancers. The extravagant hair ornaments of the war years, the velvet bows and artificial flowers, had disappeared. An evening coiffure might be enhanced with a tiny hat with veil.

Makeup was concentrated on the eyes and lips during this era. Little rouge was worn, but eye shadow and eye liner were much used. There was a vogue for "doe eyes," a bold line drawn above the upper lashes, extended outward and curved upward to give the eyes an exotic, slightly startled look. Colors in lipstick and nail polish were a little softer, after the hard brilliance of the wartime shades. A new range of pinks was available, in shades such as "Spice Pink" and "Pink Tang."

Hat Styles

The hat styles of the thirties and forties carried over into this era; small, frivolous hats with veils seemed to be the most-prevalent variety. Among the popular fashions were draped and crushed berets; pillboxes; fitted cloches—some with shallow crown and down-curved brim, others with deeper crown and upturned brim; tiny bonnets in various shapes with curving brims framing the face; wide-brimmed hats in felt or straw; the perennial slouch felt (also in suede); the straight-brimmed straw sailor hat and the Breton sailor with upturned brim. There was a matador hat, similar to the style worn by bullfighters, and several versions of a cone-shaped or coolie hat (in straw, felt, or velvet). For winter, there was a calotte that tied under the chin. A close-fitting hat made of feathers was a popular fashion for dress occasions. There were diminutive half-hats, curving over the top of the head (sometimes accommodating a chignon or French roll at the back of the neck) or cupped over the back of the head to frame a pompadour wave or cluster of curls on the forehead. Theatre or cocktail hats might be the merest disc or halo or "bicycle clip" of velvet or satin embroidered with sequins or beads. Dressy hats might be trimmed with bird wings or ostrich tips. Veils were omnipresent, sometimes a filmy adornment of the hat frame, and again swathed completely about the head and face. A wide-mesh "see-through" fashion of veiling the entire face was very smart in the early days of the New Look. The peekaboo effect was sometimes heightened with a sprinkling of chenille dots.

Underwear, Loungewear, and Sleepwear

Corsets were once more essential items for achieving the fashionable silhouette. Several new models appeared on the market, the most-popular being the small "waist-liner" to diminish the middle (Figure 20), about which *Vogue* commented:

> This year, with your new clothes, a waistline becomes a necessity. . . . One small "waist-liner" gives simply a thin strip of indentation about your waist, could be sewn into each of your dresses. Others define the waist, and the area above and below, give a gentle rounding of the hips. And others, with brassière attached, will minimize the diaphragm as well as the waist.[3]

These waist-cinching bands could be worn alone or combined with a short girdle. Longer girdles extended three or four inches above the waistline to achieve the center pinch, or there were all-in-one combinations that included a brassiere. Silk or rayon panties or briefs were worn over the girdle, unless it was a panty style. Brassieres were made with uplift lines and were now available with foam rubber padding for figures that needed such enhancement. The "Merry Widow" long-line and strapless brassiere, with feather boning, appeared in 1952; it was designed by Warner Foundations for Lana Turner to wear in the motion picture of that name. Lingerie was very feminine, usually lace-trimmed, and was now available in nylon as well as silk and rayon. Full-length slips were made with fitted brassiere-like tops. Waist-length bouffant petticoats were made of stiff nylon or taffeta, crinoline or horsehair net, with fitted hip yokes and flaring hem ruffles; an inner ruffle of eyelet embroidery or softer fabric kept the stiff hemline from snagging nylon hose (Figure 21). Housecoats and hostess gowns for lounging or informal entertaining at home were quite elegant, usually well fitted at the waistline, and might have a lapped front (Figure 22) or a long zipper closing up the front. Of a practical nature was the calf-length loose duster with flaring lines, for wear about the house. The short robe of quilted satin was also popular for cool weather (Figure 23). Toreador pants were a sophisticated choice for lounging or entertaining (Figure 24). Another leisure outfit was a fitted tunic with a flaring skirt ending at mid-thigh worn over tapered trousers. For sleeping, the traditional pajamas and long nightgowns were still being worn. Gowns might be quite elaborate and highly trimmed (Figure 25). Innovations were elasticized midriffs and frills or skirts made of permanent-pleated nylon. College girls often wore knee-length nightshirts.

Day Wear

For daytime wear, skirts were from eleven to fourteen inches from the floor. Bodices were well fitted and usually tightly belted. Early in the period, shoulder pads were still used to some extent, but they were smaller than those of the wartime days. Some styles utilized the basque (or long-torso) bodice, with a full skirt set on at hip level, but the lines followed an exaggerated hour-glass figure. Skirts were pleated, gathered, gored, or cut with a circular flare. New synthetic stiffening materials such as Pellon (a felted nylon) might be used as a lining to hold the full skirts out. Such linings were also sometimes used to give a rounded hipline to the peplum of a tailored jacket (Figures 26, 27). Suits had a sculptured look reminiscent of the late nineteenth century (Figures 28, 29). Shirtwaist dresses were in great favor, with bodices buttoned to the waistline, wide revers or fly-away collars, and pleated, gathered, or widely flaring skirts (Figures 30, 31). Redingote outfits with coat-dresses worn over harmonizing dresses were popular (Figure 33). Old-fashioned Gibson Girl shirtwaists — usually of fine white fabric, tucked, pleated, ruffled, and lace-trimmed — were worn with skirts that might be full and wide or straight and slim. Dirndl skirts and low-necked, gathered peasant blouses were also still in fashion. Woven Guatemalan fabrics in striking Indian patterns were frequently utilized for the skirts. Middy blouses with well-fitted waistlines were being worn by college girls. Jumpers were also popular on campus. Some slender styles in dresses or separate skirts had added fullness at the hip, which gave a peg-top line to the skirt. A preview of the late fifties is seen in an early version of the chemise by Norman Norell (Figure 32). Sleeve styles varied considerably; in addition to the set-in sleeve, the raglan and dolman (or bat-wing) sleeves were much used. Jacket dresses were popular; the jacket might be a short, buttoned spencer style, or a bolero, or fitted with a flaring peplum. Large patch pockets were frequently used for decoration. Sunback dresses were still very much favored for summer, strapless or with shoulder straps or halter tops, and sometimes with matching cover-up stoles or jackets.

Evening Wear   After the austerity of the wartime years, when formal dress was worn infrequently (and generally disapproved of), women welcomed the chance to dress up once more for evening occasions. The most-radical departure from the foregoing styles in formals, which had been floor-length since the early thirties, was the new ballet-length formal, seven to twelve inches from the floor (Figure 34). Another change was a return to baring the back and shoulders, after several years of keeping them covered with jackets, sleeves, or higher necklines (Figures 35, 38). The strapless ballerina-length ball gown was the most-prevalent style during this postwar era (Figure 36). It was frequently black, even on the young teen-age set. Some models had halter tops; some had little jackets to cover up the bare backs when desired. Stoles were very popular throughout the period, and might be of fabric matching the gown, of velvet, lace, or jersey, and might be trimmed with fringe or sequins. Floor-length evening gowns were also in evidence, full-skirted or slim. Dior's dramatic black velvet strapless sheath was much photographed when it first appeared (Figure 37). Ankle-strap evening sandals with high, spike heels were very popular. Some platform soles were still being worn. A flirtatious note was added to the evening scene with the reappearance of small folding fans, often made of such frivolous materials as satin or lace. Costume jewelry was important with the bare-necked styles. Earrings might be quite extravagant in size and styling — for example, flaring clusters of rhinestones on fine wires, or entire bouquets of small flowers, or several translucent plastic bubbles suspended from each ear. There was a brief vogue for paste-on jewels, affixed to the bare neck, bosom, or back with an adhesive.

Sportswear   For spectator sports, a tailored suit might be worn, or a blouse and skirt or sweater and skirt, or a jumper and blouse. A shirtwaist dress, a coat dress, or a dress with matching jacket might also be appropriate. One sporty outfit that was frequently seen was a slim tweed skirt worn with a rather short, boxy, or flaring sport coat with wide revers and huge patch pockets, cinched in with a wide leather belt. A beret, small pillbox, fitted cloche, or slouch felt hat might be worn, although many women frequently went hatless for informal occasions.

For active sports, the range of play clothes was ever increasing. The sets of matching shorts, shirts, and wraparound or button-on skirts, which had been worn since the mid-thirties, were still popular.

There were also romper-style cotton playsuits with elastic midriffs. For tennis there was a neat one-piece suit with a short pleated skirt (Figure 39). There were halter tops and sarongs. New styles in pants included the closely fitted toreador pants (Figure 24), cabin-boy breeches that laced below the knee, pedal-pushers of mid-calf length with a slit leg, clam-diggers (resembling rolled-up blue jeans — Figure 40), and ankle-length tapered slacks. For beach or resort wear, triangular ponchos were a new fashion. The one-piece bathing suit, or maillot, was still a favorite for swimming, and was now available in various fabrics made stretchable with Lastex (Figure 41). Two-piece suits were briefer than ever, and frequently the trunks had a short skirt attached. Both styles could be seen in strapless models, with a built-in boned brassiere. For evenings in the snow country, *Vogue* was showing ankle-length and floor-length tweed skirts, knitted camisole tops, sleeveless sweaters with gathered necklines or long-sleeved turtlenecks, slacks of bold plaid wool and of fake pony fur, poncho-like tops made of fringed steamer rugs, and short cardigan-style leather jackets.

Coats and Wraps

Coats came in a wide variety of styles during the postwar era. There were coats cut on princesse lines, with closely fitted waistlines and full flaring skirts, such as Dior's Cossack coat (Figure 42). The fitted models might have wide lapels, cape collars, or shoulder capes. The double-breasted reefer was still in style, with more flare to the skirt and fuller, shorter sleeves with large cuffs. There was a Chesterfield coat for women, boxy with a slight flare and full sleeves, made of light fabric with black velvet turnover collar and wide black cuffs. The pyramid, or tent, coat flared from narrow shoulders to a very wide hemline. There was a voluminous wraparound greatcoat with bloused fullness in the raglan sleeves. A novel style appeared with a dropped yoke and balloon sleeves. A bloused, rather short sleeve with a push-up cuff was popular. New in this era was the three-quarter-length sleeve, usually with a full turnback cuff, which was worn with elbow-length gloves. Shorter boxy or flared coats, hip-length or three-quarter-length, might be worn loose or tightly belted over a slim skirt. There were light-weight summer coats with short sleeves, more for decoration than warmth, some of them in silk or sheer cottons. Raincoats had become glamorous in waterproofed silk and taffeta, and might be patterned in polka dots or checks. There were many styles in short jackets — boxy, flared, or fitted. Capes were also popular; they might be hem-length with armhole slits, hip-length, waist-length, or shoulder-length. Fur coats were luxurious and styled on the same extravagantly flowing, flaring lines as the cloth coats — mutation mink in blue or white, Alaskan sealskin, ocelot or leopard, Persian lamb, or gray squirrel (Figure 43). Fur jackets and stoles were also very popular.

Footwear   During the postwar era, sandals were particularly popular, high-heeled for formal dress and flat-soled for leisure wear. Shoes were made in a great range of styles from flat ballet slippers to high spike heels. Flat heels were generally worn for sports and play, Cuban heels for street wear, and high heels for late afternoon and evening dress. Toes were still rounded, but the effect of footwear was lighter and slenderer than the sturdy, solid shoes of the war years. The craze for open toes had subsided, although many styles still left the toes showing; the heels were just as likely to be open now. Rather simply styled pumps with medium heels were popular for general wear. Ankle-strap sandals were favored for cocktails and evening, sometimes with platform soles. Shoes were now available in vivid colors — red, blue, pink, and yellow — and in open-work lace or fabrics such as velvet. Flat-heeled shoes resembling ballet slippers for leisure wear sometimes had a jeweled trim. Wedge heels were still worn for sports and play. Mexican huaraches of woven leather were another play-shoe style. Saddle oxfords and canvas sneakers were worn for active sports. Nylon hose were once more available for everyone. They came in proportioned lengths, in misty pastels as well as a range of beiges and grays, and for dress occasions might have fancy clocks on the heels or ankles. There were also knee-high ribbed hose and anklets for sports wear.

Accessories With necklines, shoulders, and arms left bare by the strapless styles, costume jewelry became a very important part of the New Look. Rhinestones were especially popular, and sparkling colored stones were set in dangling chandelier earrings, dog-collar necklaces, bib necklaces of intricate design, wide link bracelets, ornamental scatter pins, jeweled hair clips, chignon ornaments or tiaras, and jeweled buttons. Pearls were also in fashion, frequently worn in multiple-strand necklaces or bracelets. Plastics were being used for jewelry, in plain bold designs for button earrings and long strands of beads (white was particularly effective with a dark costume) or molded into flower forms. Bracelets were worn in sets of multiple bangles or in single wide bands, links, or chains; charm bracelets with dangling ornaments were in fashion. Artificial flowers were used to enhance a plain dress, a large single rose often placed at the neckline or waistline. Gloves were worn again for dress occasions. They came in many lengths — wrist, bracelet, gauntlet, elbow, or opera — and might be brightly colored or patterned. Wrist-length gloves, as well as the traditional elbow- or opera-length, were popular for cocktail and evening wear. Long, rectangular stoles, in a variety of soft and gracefully draped fabrics, were worn throughout the period to cover bare shoulders and arms. Folding fans had been rediscovered as an attractive and flirtatious addition to an evening costume. A new accessory was the small decorative cocktail or hostess apron, a frilly wisp of organza, lace, and ribbon, which could be tied over a cocktail dress — guarding against spots, perhaps, but also enlivening the party scene. Belts were wide and dashing, sometimes contoured in corselet style or curved to follow the waist or hipline. They might be ornamented with metal trim or stone settings. Shoulder-strap bags were still being carried. New fashions in purses included the box-shaped bag made of leather, straw, or fabric, and the duffel bag, a pouch closed with a drawstring, in fabric or leather. Smaller, flat clutch bags without handles, carried in the hand, were gaining in popularity. Muffs were sometimes carried, usually matching a fur-trimmed jacket or coat. Umbrellas were available again in a long-handled, slender style, although the short, stubby umbrella was also still in fashion. The passion for matching sets of accessories that was typical of the early forties had subsided. An article about Celeste Holm reports:

> In accessories Celeste believes very strongly in just two of a kind. She likes to have a hat matching her gloves, or shoes matching a bag, but no more than two matching accessories for an ensemble.[4]

CHILDREN'S FASHIONS

Children's wear kept pace with the general trend in fashions during the postwar years. Girls' dresses and coats took on the princesse lines of their mothers' garments — with fitted waistlines and wide, flaring skirts. The vogue for mother and-daughter dresses in the same style, which started during the war, continued. Identical dresses for big and little sisters were also popular. There was an upsurge of "Alice in Wonderland" dresses with full skirts, puffed sleeves, and ruffled pinafores when the Disney motion picture of *Alice* came out in 1951. School girls might wear Gibson Girl blouses with full skirts, or middy blouses with pleated skirts, or jumpers (Figure 44). Little girls might wear slacks or leggings with their coats in cold weather. Girls' shoes were oxfords, loafers, or Mary Jane strap styles. There was also an ankle-strap sandal (low-heeled) for little ones. Older girls were wearing ballet-style flat shoes. Girls wore knee socks or anklets.

Boys of any age (from one or two years) now wore long trousers, although they were likely to be in short pants until the age of six. Dress-up suits might have Eton jackets without collars or regular suit jackets with collars and lapels. A boy's dress coat might be double-breasted tweed with a matching tweed cap, beanie style with very small visor. Little boys wore coveralls or overalls for play. Schoolboys might wear sport shirts and slacks with pullover sweaters, cardigan sweaters, sports jackets, or windbreaker jackets with zipper closings. Boys' shoes were oxfords, saddle shoes, loafers, or tennis shoes. Cowboy suits with fringed jackets were popular for play.

TYPICAL MATERIALS, COLORS, MOTIFS, AND TRIMMINGS

New synthetic materials were appearing on the market constantly. In addition to nylon, the Du Pont Company was now producing two new fibers — Orlon (acrylic) and Dacron (polyester). A random list of synthetic blends and new fabrics in 1952 included: insulated lining material for coats or jackets made of acetate satin; Millium, a lining fabric of rayon combined with metal insulation; washable flannel of blended wool and nylon; washable corduroy of rayon and combed cotton; hand-washable taffeta made of 100 percent acetate; and crush-resistant, water-repellent velvet made of rayon and cotton. Cottons were "Sanforized" (pre-shrunk) and "disciplined" (processed to make them wrinkle-resistant); some were "glazed" to give a surface sheen resembling sateen. Jersey worsted was processed to give added body and firmness and became "sag-proof." Orlon added to wool, cotton, or rayon had the effect of making these fibers wrinkle-resistant and washable. Many of these blends were superior to the natural fibers in that they were longer wearing, lighter in weight, cooler or warmer, resistant to wrinkles, easier to clean and wash, and wearable with less pressing. Colors were a little softer than in the war years — avocado green, jade green, champagne, maize, turquoise, slate blue, suntan beige, rust, and many pinks, such as spice pink, shrimp, apricot, mauve, and lilac. Two-color combinations were popular — navy and white, black and beige, coral and brown, red and white. Permanent-pleated fabrics were available in nylon chiffon, jersey, and a linen blend. Printed silks and nylon jerseys, checked and plaid taffeta, shantung and surah were popular for dressy outfits. Quilted cottons were made into skirts, and quilted satins into lounging robes. Crepes were still very popular. For ball gowns filmy sheers such as nylon tulle, organza, and laces were much used, as well as rich velvets, brocades, and satins. Stripes, checks, plaids, and polka dots were popular patterns. Floral prints were not as large or as flamboyant as those of the thirties and early forties; they had become smaller and daintier. Eyelet embroidery and floral-embroidered sheers were favored for summer dresses. Trimmings included fringe, ball fringe, braid, passementerie, sequins, beads, rhinestones, and ornamental or jeweled buttons.

SUGGESTIONS FOR COSTUMING PLAYS IN THE PERIOD

Men's wear in this period began to approach the slender fashions of the sixties. Conservative characters would still be wearing the broad-shouldered suits of the war years, with trousers wide at the cuff. Younger or forward-looking men might adopt the Ivy League silhouette, with narrower, natural shoulders and tapered trousers. The gray flannel suit — particularly charcoal gray — is typical of these years. A tan camel's-hair sports jacket or a madras jacket with separate slacks would be appropriate for informal wear. For evening, a white or red dinner jacket, or a plaid one would be in order. A bright striped or figured vest might be worn for informal daytime or evening occasions.

The most-important concern in achieving the New Look silhouette for women is to provide the proper foundation garments to create an hour-glass figure—a waist-cincher girdle, long-line strapless bra, and one or more bouffant petticoats. Many of the New Look styles are still available in thrift shops or tucked away in closets or attics. Ankle-strap sandals help to give the flavor of the period. Stoles are very typical, and so are wrist-length gloves and folding fans for evening dress. Veils covering the entire face suggest the coquettish attitude of the era. The stance should always be ladylike and graceful, as though one were poised to start dancing—none of the wide-legged slouch of the sixties. Makeup giving the startled upswept "doe eye" line to the upper lid and arching the eyebrows will also help to recreate the New Look. Hair styles should be small neat caps, close to the head.

TITLE	AUTHOR	PERIOD
All My Sons	Arthur Miller	1947
The Autumn Garden	Lillian Hellman	1949
Bell, Book and Candle	John Van Druten	1950
Brigadoon (M) (modern scenes)	Alan Lerner, Frederick Loewe, Arthur Schwartz, Dorothy Fields	1947
Call Me Madam (M)	Irving Berlin, Howard Lindsay, Russel Crouse	1950
Chips with Everything	Arnold Wesker	Postwar
The Cocktail Party	T. S. Eliot	1950
Come Back, Little Sheba	William Inge	1950
The Consul (M)	Gian-Carlo Menotti	1950
The Country Girl	Clifford Odets	1950
Darkness at Noon	Sidney Kingsley	1951
Death of a Salesman	Arthur Miller	1949
Detective Story	Sidney Kingsley	1949
Dial "M" for Murder	Frederick Knott	1952
Dylan	Sidney Michaels	1949–53
Goodbye, My Fancy	Fay Kanin	Postwar
Guys and Dolls (M)	Frank Loesser, Jo Swerling, Abe Burrows	1950
The Hidden River	Ruth and Augustus Goetz	Postwar
Kiss Me, Kate (M) (modern scenes)	Samuel and Bella Spewack, Cole Porter	1948
Light Up the Sky	Moss Hart	1948
Lost in the Stars (M)	Maxwell Anderson, Kurt Weill	1949
The Medium (M)	Gian-Carlo Menotti	1947
A Raisin in the Sun	Lorraine Hansberry	Postwar
Raisin (M)	Robert Nemeroff, Charlotte Zaltberg, Judd Woldin, Robert Brittan	early 1950s
The Rehearsal	Jean Anouilh	1950; 18th cen.
The Rose Tattoo	Tennessee Williams	1951
The Seven Year Itch	George Axelrod	1952
Street Scene (M)	Elmer Rice, Kurt Weill, Langston Hughes	1947
A Streetcar Named Desire	Tennessee Williams	1947
The Telephone (M)	Gian-Carlo Menotti	1947
Venus Observed	Christopher Fry	1949

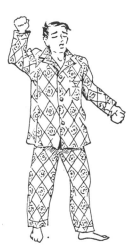

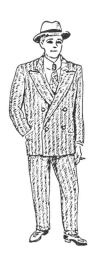

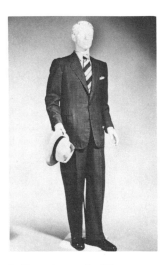

1. Printed rayon pajamas. 1947.

2. Double-breasted suit of navy blue; peaked lapels. 1947.

3. Two-piece suit of brown, beige, and blue plaid: single-breasted, three-button jacket; cuffed trousers. Worn in Connecticut and Massachusetts. By Witty Brothers, 1949. (Division of Costume, Smithsonian Institution.)

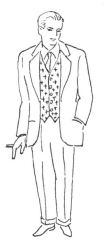

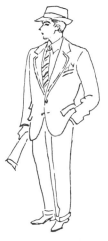

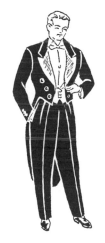

4. Tan tweed jacket; yellow vest with red-and-black figure. 1952.

5. Single-breasted summer suit of lightweight cheviot. 1951.

6. Evening tailcoat with satin-faced lapels; white tie; white waistcoat. 1950.

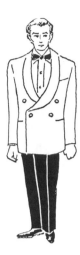

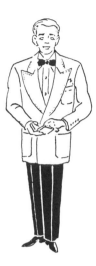

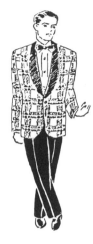

7. Double-breasted white dinner jacket of Celanese. 1952.

8. Double-breasted white flannel leisure jacket with peaked lapels. 1948.

9. Dinner jacket of tartan worsted with black shawl collar. 1950.

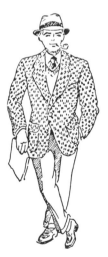

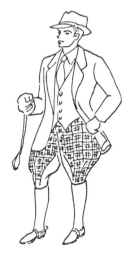

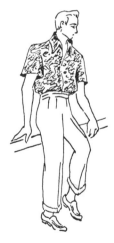

10. Rough tweed jacket; sleeveless sweater; flannel slacks. 1947.

11. Riding habit: brown jacket; tan vest; plaid jodhpurs; brown boots. 1950.

12. Dark African print cotton shirt; yellow linen slacks. 1950.

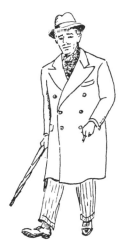
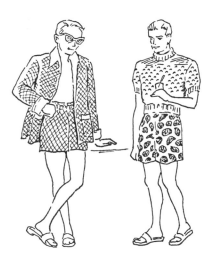
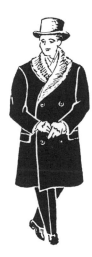

13. Dark flannel sports jacket; white Bermuda shorts. 1949.

14, 15. Checked cabana set: terry-lined jacket; cotton swim trunks. 1952. Boxer swim trunks; popcorn weave pullover sweater. 1948.

16. Black dress overcoat with fur collar. 1950.

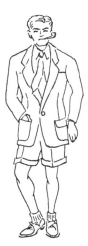
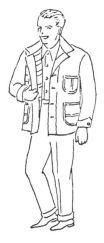
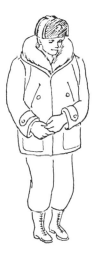

17. Double-breasted worsted overcoat with peaked lapels. 1947.

18. Work jacket of blue denim with striped blanket-cloth lining. 1952.

19. Korean War outfit: hooded battle jacket lined with sheepskin. 1952.

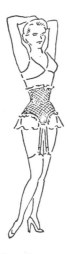

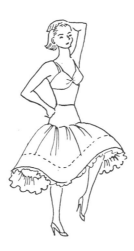

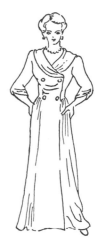

20. "Waistliner" corset of nylon satin. 1947.

21. Bouffant petticoat of taffeta and crinoline with eyelet-ruffled hemline. 1951.

22. Housecoat of blue-gray rayon satin. 1948.

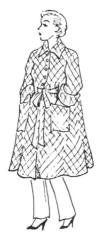

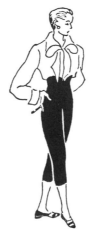

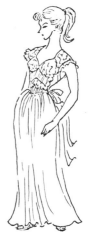

23. Lounging robe of blue quilted satin, swing-back; crepe trousers. 1951.

24. Lounge wear: white linen blouse; black velveteen toreador pants. 1950.

25. Nightgown of silk crepe, trimmed with Alençon-type lace. 1950.

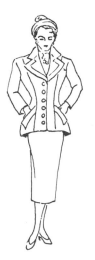

26. Tailored suit of lightweight wool. 1950.

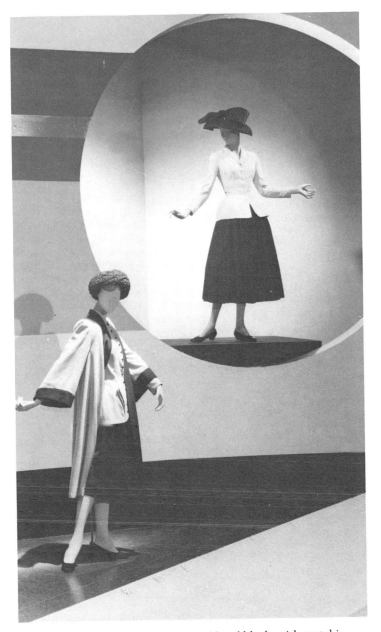

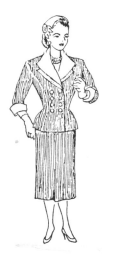

27. Tailored suit of nylon-Orlon pinstripe with white collar and cuffs. 1952.

28. Left, coat and suit ensemble in gold and black, with matching accessories: melton cloth coat and gabardine suit jacket have heavily padded shoulder line; skirt is short and straight. American, Philip Mangone, 1947. Right, "New Look" suit: jacket of beige tussore silk, closely fitted with padded hips, accenting bosom and waistline; full, calf-length, pleated wool skirt. French, by Christian Dior, 1947. (The Costume Institute of The Metropolitan Museum of Art. Gifts of Bloomingdale Brothers, Inc., and Mrs. John Chambers Hughes.)

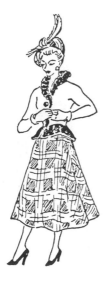
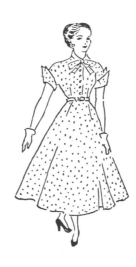
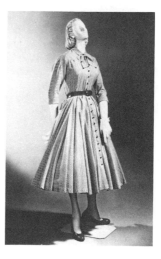

29. Fath suit: green wool jacket with astrakhan trim; plaid skirt; plaid hat. 1947.

30. Afternoon dress of dotted swiss with six-gore skirt. 1948.

31. Dress of red-and-white checked cotton: full circular gathered skirt; three-quarter-length sleeves with turnback cuffs; button-front closure; red plastic belt. Worn in California and Nevada. By Gray, 1950. (Division of Costume, Smithsonian Institution.)

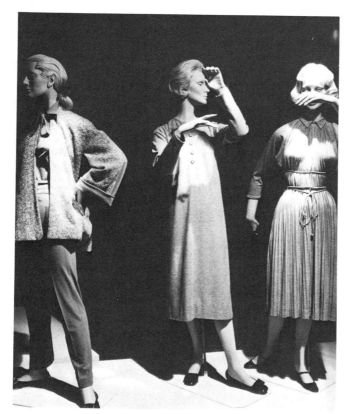

32. Left, three-piece travel costume: jacket, slacks, and blouse of cocoa jersey and brown-and-white Donegal tweed. By Vera Maxwell, 1948. Center, chemise dress of gray heather wool jersey. By Norman Norell, 1952. Right, day dress of sand and dark gray, heather-textured wool jersey: shallow knife pleating anchored at high neckline; narrow, turndown collar; bat-wing sleeves with raglan mounting; narrow bias-tube belt confining front pleats at raised waist. By Claire McCardell, 1949. (The Costume Institute of The Metropolitan Museum of Art. Gifts of Vera Maxwell, Mrs. Lester Hano, and Miss Kay Hafner.)

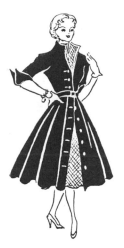

33. Redingote worn over navy-and-white checked rayon taffeta dress. 1952.

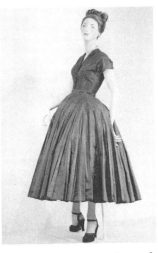

34. Two-piece dinner dress of purplish navy blue silk taffeta. By Christian Dior, 1947. (The Costume Institute of The Metropolitan Museum of Art. Gift of Christian Dior.)

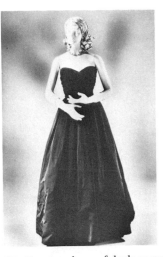

35. Evening dress of dark green silk: long skirt; strapless bodice; fabric wrapped around with random pleats. 1950s. (Division of Costume, Smithsonian Institution.)

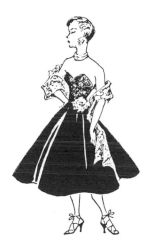

36. Ballet-length black satin evening skirt; lace bodice and stole. 1951.

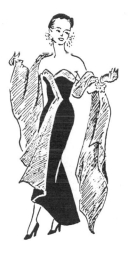

37. Dior evening sheath of black velvet, with peau de soie trim and stole. 1950.

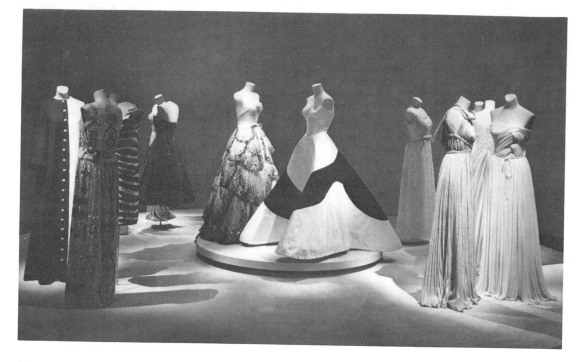

38. Evening fashions from the late forties to the mid-sixties.
   Left to right: Evening dress of heavy silk crepe in black and white; rhinestone-studded ball buttons from neck to hem. By Hannah Troy, 1966.   Overblouse and slim skirt of printed chiffon overlaid with matching opalescent sequins in shades of pink, yellow, and black in a modernistic geometric design. Italian, by Emilio Pucci, 1964.   Fur evening dress: ivory Indian lamb and black Russian broadtail, appliquéd in a zebra pattern. American, by Emeric Partos, 1965.   Short, strapless evening dress of ruby-red velvet. By Dior, 1955.   Strapless ball gown, called "Junon," with enormous petaled skirt of irridescent sequins in peacock shades of blue and green on pale blue net. By Dior, 1949.   Ball gown of white satin and faille with black velvet appliqué; strapless bodice; very wide, stiffly contoured "cloverleaf" skirt. By Charles James, 1953.   Reception dress of rose-pink net and matching stole, embroidered and ornamented in silver. Worn at the White House by Mrs. Joseph Kennedy. By Marc Bohan for Dior, 1962.   "Directoire-style" ball gown of pleated cloth of gold, banded with a classic girdle; worn with voluminous wrap of wine-purple velvet. French, by Chaumont, 1948.   Classic ball gown of peach-colored silk jersey; strapless bodice molded by intricate pleating and draping. French, by Grès, 1963. (The Costume Institute of The Metropolitan Museum of Art.)

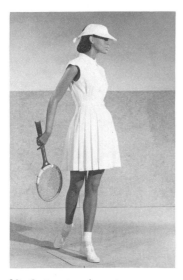

39. Cotton tennis costume. American, by Fred Picard and Bobbie Yeoman, 1947. (The Costume Institute of The Metropolitan Museum of Art. Gift of Bloomingdale Brothers, Inc.)

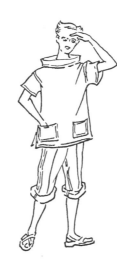

40. Beach wear: boat shirt, clam-digger pants of sailcloth. 1950.

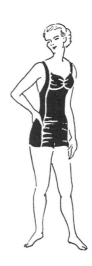

41. Maillot swimsuit of black nylon woven with Lastex. 1947.

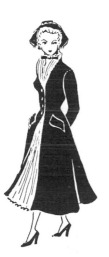

42. Dior Cossack coat of black wool over pleated green silk taffeta dress. 1947.

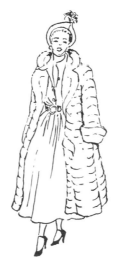

43. Gray squirrel coat over gray silk taffeta Shantung shirt dress. 1950.

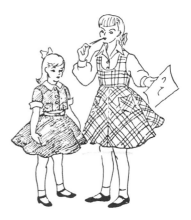

44. Girls' outfits. Left, jacket dress. Right, white blouse and plaid jumper. 1952.

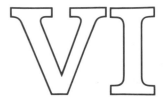

The Late Fifties:
Dawn of the Space Age
(1953 — 1960)

ON OCTOBER 4, 1957, the first satellite, Sputnik I, was launched by the USSR and went into orbit around the Earth. That historic moment signaled a giant shift in human orientation to the universe, similar to the change in perspective caused by the ideas that the Earth was round, that it turned on an axis, and that it revolved around the sun. From that day forward people were no longer chained to this planet but were suddenly liberated to go wandering into the outer reaches of space. What people were wearing on Earth seemed negligible in this new frame of reference — and, oddly enough, what was being worn in the new Space Age often appeared to be just that — negligible. After 1957 hemlines started creeping inexorably upward and within a few years stood at an all-time high in the history of costume. Street dress rivaled the state of undress that had formerly been restricted to the beaches, boudoirs, and burlesque houses.

CONCERNING THE PERIOD

Americans had been so certain that the United States held first place in scientific research as well as in technical invention and superior mechanical ability, that the entire populace experienced a rude shock when Russia "won the race into space." For those who saw the significance of that first satellite launching, it mattered little whether Sputnik had started from a pad in Russia, America, China, or France — it represented one more unbelievably thrilling leap on the part of the human race.

Throughout the fifties, the United States enjoyed prosperity under the administration of the Republican President, Dwight Eisenhower, the very popular General and Commander of the American forces in

Europe during World War II. It was a relatively peaceful interlude, although the Cold War was an ever-present reality, and actual fighting existed in Korea until 1953 and then in Vietnam. In 1959 Alaska and Hawaii were admitted to the Union as the 49th and 50th states. The United Nations grew tremendously (in size if not in power), doubling its membership to include 101 nations by the end of 1960. Sixteen newly independent nations from Africa were admitted during the 1960 session. The rising influence of the dark races in the world arena was reflected on the domestic front in America during the late fifties. Dr. Martin Luther King, Jr., came forward as a champion of the Black cause, and his strong leadership inspired many nonviolent demonstrations across the country — such as freedom marches, restaurant sit-ins, and freedom rides on buses. By the end of the decade Congress had passed civil rights legislation guaranteeing voters' rights and promoting school integration.

The swift economic expansion that began after World War II continued throughout the fifties. A network of freeways was built to crisscross the country, bridging over or bypassing the large cities. During the 1950s there was a mass exodus from the cities to the suburbs, and one-third of the nation's population became commuters. Large outlying shopping centers grew up to serve the suburban communities, and many cities found their downtown business districts deserted. Compact cars, foreign and then domestic, appeared on the scene, and jet airplane flights were inaugurated in 1958. Electronic computers were adopted for industrial use in mid-decade, and soon these miraculous inventions were keeping mass records and sorting out data with incredible swiftness in every sizable institution. As the machines took over, one more area of life was streamlined and dehumanized, frequently leaving the citizen powerless to reach or blame anyone in case of error. The only recourse seemed to be to bend, spindle, or mutilate a punched card.

In science, research continued into the nature of the atom, and atomic bombs were tested by the United States, the USSR, and Great Britain. Mounting public alarm over the danger of radioactive fallout and the contamination of the atmosphere led to the formation in 1957 of the International Atomic Energy Agency. If the world's health was being endangered on one side, it was being improved on another. During this decade the list of antibiotic "wonder drugs" was expanded, tranquilizer pills appeared, a polio vaccine was developed, and open-heart surgery and organ transplants became commonplace. The discovery in 1958 of the laser beam had far-reaching implications. This intensely hot and powerful beam could not only cut through the hardest steel but also relay messages to the moon. During the 1950s the first atomic-powered electric generating plant was opened, and the first atomic-powered submarines, cruisers, and aircraft carriers were launched.

In the home, the fireplace as the living center had been replaced by the television set, that fascinating new toy before which the whole family sat enthralled for hours at a time. Other popular electronic playthings were stereophonic high-fidelity record players and tape recorders. Pocket-sized transistor radios were carried everywhere. The newest item in the kitchen was the wall oven, now divorced from the surface cooking units of the stove, and equipped with automatic controls. Air conditioners became standard equipment for homes as well as for public buildings. Interior decoration continued in the modern mode of functionalism, with increasing use of glass, plastics, and tubular steel. In extreme treatments, these interiors were rather stark and perhaps too clinical for comfort. By the late fifties reaction against the austerity of this cold functional style took several pathways: one was through the use in home decoration of Pop art, which caricatured the garish realities of the neon world outside; another was a recapitulation of the rococo scrolls and curlicues of Art Nouveau from the turn of the century.

The arts of painting and sculpture also underwent rather marked shifts during the fifties. Among the schools of painting that broke with the abstract tradition were Pop (popular) art and Op (optical) art. Pop art matched the banality of commonplace subjects with the banality of commercial art methods. Young artists turned to a macabre kind of realism with such vulgarities as Jasper Johns's bronze beer cans and Robert Rauschenberg's stuffed goat framed in a rubber tire. The Op artists worked in precise geometric patterns and arranged violently contrasting colors so that the eye of the observer tended to jump back and forth restlessly from one area to another.

Popular music in the mid-fifties turned from sweet and hot jazz and the rhythms of swing to the monotonous four-four beat of "rock 'n' roll." Rock singer Elvis Presley was the new teen-age idol. The young people in revolt against the established culture patterns — the "beatniks" of the fifties and the "hippies" of the sixties — adopted folk singing with guitar accompaniment and used this medium for their songs of social protest. Through the performances of Harry Belafonte, calypso numbers from the West Indies gained great popularity. Latin American dances were still in fashion, and new varieties in the late fifties included the cha-cha, the mambo, and the bossa nova. As the decade ended, the favorite dance by all odds was the Twist, which concentrated on swiveling hip motion.

The decade of the fifties was the "Golden Age" of television. The medium was new and experimental, and large budgets were devoted to live shows employing the best available talents in directing, playwriting, and acting. "Playhouse 90," "Studio One," and "Omnibus" presented excellent dramas week after week for several seasons. In the movies, leading stars included two outstanding beauties whose private lives were just as sensational as their professional careers — the blonde, curvaceous Marilyn Monroe and the dark-haired, violet-eyed Elizabeth Taylor. Leslie Caron and Audrey Hepburn popularized a slim, gamin style of appealing half-boyish prettiness. New male idols were Rock Hudson, Tab Hunter, Paul Newman, and William Holden. Marlon Brando and Elvis Presley portrayed brooding, pouting young men who wore leather jackets or turtleneck sweaters, or went bare to the waist.

The theatre of the fifties evidenced some new trends. European playwrights contributed plays about lonely and lost souls, such as Shelagh Delaney's *A Taste of Honey*. The school of "angry young men" was represented on Broadway by John Osborne's *Look Back in Anger*. A lively group of theatres sprang up off Broadway, in Greenwich Village, and on the lower east side in Manhattan. The Phoenix repertory theatre, one of the most successful, opened in December 1953. Many of these small theatres were devoted to experimental and original scripts, some representing the "Theatre of the Absurd." They were enigmatic, sometimes allegorical plays, often with a surrealist flavor. Among the playwrights contributing to this genre were Edward Albee, Jean Genet, and Samuel Beckett. The off-Broadway theatres served as showcases for budding young talents, many of whom went on to become Broadway stars. In the mid-fifties ambitious permanent repertory theatres were established at Stratford, Connecticut, and Stratford, Ontario, for the production of Shakespeare's plays.

As the arts and the theatre veered toward the absurd — and sometimes the vulgar and unaesthetic — fashion evidenced some of the same tendencies, with styles that went in many different directions, often ignoring the human figure and distorting it in an unappealing way.

GENERAL CHARACTERISTICS OF COSTUME

Men's fashions during the fifties shifted gradually from the square, broad-shouldered look of the forties to the slender Ivy League silhouette, which began to emerge in 1952. By 1960 unpadded natural shoulders, narrow lapels, tapered trousers, and narrow-brimmed hats were being worn by most men. The charcoal gray flannel suit was the uniform of the young executive on the rise. The last word in style for the well-dressed man was a hand-tailored suit of Italian raw nubby silk. Evening clothes took on more and more color, and dinner jackets became available in wine, gold, Bermuda blue, silver gray, and Moroccan beige.

The silhouette of women's clothing through the fifties was divided between the hour-glass figure of the New Look and the newer unfitted line, or "shapeless shape." In 1953 the pinched-in waistline began to disappear with the advent of semifitted suits with short, boxy jackets (Figure 32). Looser lines also appeared in bloused-back styles and dresses with dolman sleeves. Cocoon-shaped jackets and coats and waistlines dropped to the hips or raised to an Empire line just under the bust were also showing up in the Paris collections, although they did not gain general acceptance until the late fifties. It was not until 1957 and 1958 that three rather radically new models appeared in full force — the straight chemise, or sack; the free-swinging trapeze, or tent dress; and the puffed-out bubble, or harem skirt (Figure 35).

MEN'S FASHIONS

London tailors continued to be the arbiters of men's fashions, but Italian designers such as Pucci were contributing designs for sportswear and casual fashions, and California designers were also styling beachwear and sports clothes for men. The jet set were having their suits tailored to order in Rome and Hong Kong.

Hair Styles and Grooming

Men's hair was still worn short and clipped over the ears, parted on the left or right side or combed back in a pompadour. Crew cuts or brush cuts were still popular. Most men were clean-shaven, but a few wore small, neat mustaches. Teen-age rock 'n' roll fans imitated the longer haircut and sideburns worn by Elvis Presley, and this hair style was a part of the look of the leather-jacketed motorcycling crowd. There was a fad for a shingled style combed into a flipped-up point on the back of the head, called a "ducktail." The Bohemian element known as "beatniks" were beginning to sport even shaggier haircuts and to let their beards grow, in some instances to a luxurious bushiness. Impeccable grooming was an attribute of the "man in the gray flannel suit," whereas the "beat generation" was affecting a deliberate sloppiness, unkempt and unwashed, as part of its revolt against the "Establishment."

Hat Styles

For evening wear, a black, dark gray, or midnight blue homburg hat was appropriate. With formal evening attire of white tie and tails, a black silk top hat was worn. For daytime, a derby or homburg might be worn. A fedora with a low crown and narrow brim was the most generally worn, all-purpose hat. The Tremont, with its sloping crown, or a Tyrolean model, with a brush, might be worn for casual or sports occasions. The flat tweed cap with a rather small visor was increasingly popular for sports wear. In the summer the dark coconut straw hat with silk puggree band was worn for dress as well as informal occasions. The straw boater, now made with a narrow brim, was still worn for summer. For beach wear, a variety of novelty straw hats was available, from visored jockey caps to broad-brimmed floppy models (Figure 18).

Underwear, Loungewear, and Sleepwear

Men's underwear continued to consist of boxer shorts or briefs, worn with or without a sleeveless or short-sleeved lisle undershirt. For lounging, there were smoking jackets in velvet or brocade, and a new short kimono-style robe (Figure 1), in addition to the traditional lapped-front bathrobe. Pajamas were the standard garment for sleeping and were now available with short trousers for summer; for cool weather there was also a knitted balbriggan style (Figure 2).

Neckwear

The stiff-bosomed white dress shirt with detachable wing collar was worn only for the most-formal occasions, with white tie and tails. For informal evening wear, the soft-bosomed white dress shirt of cotton, nylon, or Dacron, with pleated front and turnover collar was customary. By the late fifties it was possible to get evening shirts with ruffled as well as pleated bosoms. For town or business wear, shirts were plain white or pastel, or might have a small check or pinstripe. They were now available in wash-and-wear fabrics. Turnover collars were narrow, with pointed or rounded ends; the button-down collar was popular. Sport shirts came in a variety of fabrics and styles. Short-sleeved shirts for summer might be pullover knits, or they might be made of block-printed imported cottons, Indian madras, seersucker, or a drip-dry blend. Sport shirts were frequently worn open at the throat, without a tie. Four-in-hands varied in width but were generally narrower and more conservative (more subdued in color and smaller in pattern) than in the forties. A slender tie (about one and a half inches wide) was worn with the narrow-lapeled Ivy League suit. Some men wore bow ties, which became long and narrow in shape by the mid-fifties. Evening bow ties were usually black, but might also be bright and patterned to match a cummerbund (Figure 9). Ascots were worn for formal day attire or to fill in the neck of an open-collared sport shirt or lounging robe.

Day Wear

Formal day wear consisted of the traditional cutaway coat in black or oxford gray, worn with striped trousers and ascot tie or four-in-hand. A British lounge coat in black or oxford gray might be substituted for the cutaway. For town or business wear, a flannel suit in charcoal gray, black, or dark blue was preferred. Especially elegant (and expensive) was the fashionable lightweight suit of Italian Dupioni silk (Figure 3). For casual wear men wore lighter colors — shades of blue, gray, and brown — or mixed combinations of separate sports jackets and slacks. In 1953 jacket lapels were of medium width, but were notched rather than peaked, as they had been in the forties. By the mid-fifties the slimmer, Ivy League silhouette was becoming more prevalent. Lapels became longer and narrower in the late fifties. Trousers were growing slimmer, with or without pleats at the waistband, and were tapered to cuffs that varied in width from fourteen to sixteen inches (Figures 4, 5, 6). New fabrics made summer or year-round suits more comfortable than ever before.

> The biggest change in modern men's clothes has been the introduction of man-made fibers. Used alone or in blends they have made possible a new degree of comfort and ease of care. Outstanding examples are the new, lightweight clothes containing Du Pont "Orlon." They're as cool and comfortable as you'll ever want. . . . The sport jacket and slacks will hold their press even in damp weather. Hung up overnight, they'll shed wrinkles. The shorts, sport shirt, and dress shirt will wash, dry quickly, and can be worn again with little — if any — ironing.[1]

Dacron and worsted blends were popular for tropical weight summer suits (Figure 7). Wash-and-wear shirts and pajamas were a godsend for travelers. In 1953 and 1954 the more-daring members of the business community wore Bermuda shorts to their offices during the summer heat, but this innovation was short-lived. In 1958 London introduced a new flared silhouette, with pinched-in waist, flared jacket tail, and bell-bottomed trousers, forecasting styles of the sixties. Bright vests added color to the scene in the mid-fifties.

> After World War II, the vest seemed nearly as extinct as the whooping crane or the dodo — or the two-pants suit — but it has come back with, according to experts, a vengeance. The vests that well-dressed men, especially young college sports, are wearing today make a fellow wonder if Solomon hasn't finally caught up with the lily, or maybe is even a little ahead of it.[2]

Evening Wear   For formal evening dress, the traditional black tailcoat was worn with black trousers, white piqué stiff-bosomed shirt with wing collar, white bow tie, white waistcoat, black silk top hat, and black patent leather pumps. The black or midnight blue tuxedo was still appropriate for informal evening dress, but more and more color was creeping into the evening scene. Dinner jackets might be of white rayon gabardine; or of red, green, or gold flannel (Figures 8, 9); or tartan. The newest styles for evening featured colorful jackets of Italian raw silk in shades such as claret, gold, Bermuda blue, silver gray, cognac, or Moroccan beige (Figure 10), worn with black silk trousers. Bright cummerbunds and matching bow ties continued to be worn. In 1954 *Esquire* showed cummerbund and tie sets in bright red, teal blue, and gold shantung; in red-and-green Indian madras; in gold-and-rust or red-and-white striped silk repp; and in red-and-gray, blue-and-wine, or red-and-white diagonal checks.[3] Colorful waistcoats in stripes, patterned prints, or brocades were worn with plain, dark dinner jackets. A backless waistcoat was now available with an adjustable strap across the back waistline.

Sportswear

Men's outfits for spectator sports and casual wear usually consisted of separate sports jackets and slacks (Figures 5, 11). For campus wear, the striped blazer was still popular (Figure 12). Also good for campus was a wash-and-wear blouse-and-jacket combination (Figure 13) with Velcro fastenings (the new synthetic snap-closing that resembled a cocklebur). For active sports there were many styles in sport shirts — knits, pullovers, and models with tails to be worn loose or tucked into slacks or shorts (Figures 14, 15, 16, 17). Beach wear was colorful and varied.

> There's a real international look about this summer's beach clothes. In addition to typically American summertime classics, West Indies influence is seen in bright, bold, calypso styles [Figure 18]; Tyrolean lederhosen make an unexpected appearance as cotton play shorts; India madras is used for just about everything; and the brief swim trunk, long a favorite on the Riviera, is now in style for active swimming here. Bright-banded hats top off a list of beach fashions that make 1957 the most colorful season yet.[4]

Well-tailored Bermuda or walking shorts, with knee-length hose, were frequently worn for informal dress in the heat of summer (Figures 17, 19). For winter, a ski costume now might be made of nylon as well as of wool (Figure 20). In Western style, there were fringed suede shirts and suede pants (Figure 21). Bulky knit sweaters were increasing in popularity during this era, with men as well as women.

Coats and Wraps

The Chesterfield in black, oxford gray, or midnight blue was worn with formal and informal evening dress. The reversible black-and-tan raincoat shown in Figure 22 might be worn on inclement evenings. Topcoats for general wear included the traditional models — single-breasted tweed with raglan sleeves, balmacaan, and dressy tailored styles. One of the most-luxurious fabrics for overcoats was vicuna, a soft South American wool, which came to national attention (or notoriety) in 1957, when Sherman Adams, President Eisenhower's White House aide, received a vicuna coat as a political gift — an episode that ended his Washington career. The military-style trench coat was still a popular model for rain or all-purpose wear (Figure 23). Multipurpose coats included a reversible rain-or-shine coat that was tweed on one side and waterproof poplin on the other, and a summer-or-winter coat with a zip-in alpaca or Orlon fleece lining. Very smart in 1958 was an ensemble of suit and matching topcoat in Glenurquart plaid. Shorter jackets in several lengths were gaining in popularity. The waist-length models included the Eisenhower jacket and the windbreaker with elastic cuffs and waistband (sometimes reversible with waterproof lining). Suede or smooth leather jackets in this length were popular, in red, blue, green, and tan, as well as black. Short jackets were also made in the new plastics and in vinyl, which gave much the same effect as leather. There was also an intermediate-length jacket, about 32 inches long, slightly longer than a suit jacket. For suburban living, one of the most-popular garments was the car coat, suburban coat, or duffle coat, about 36 inches long and warmly lined with alpaca, nylon, or Orlon fleece (Figures 24, 25). All these jackets might have zipper closings. Various models had fly fronts, four-buttoned closures, or toggle-and-loop closings; some also had detachable fleece-lined hoods.

Footwear

Men's shoes changed from rounded toes and low-cut vamps during the early fifties to slender, rather pointed toes, and high-rise insteps near the end of the decade. Shoes for evening wear followed this trend. Black patent leather pumps were still worn for formal evening attire, but informal dress shoes might be patent leather or calf oxfords, or high-rise slip-ons, sometimes with a monk's shoe instep strap. For daytime wear, there were slender-toed oxfords and Norwegian loafers. The Blucher half-boot came just below the ankle, and the chukka boot came above the ankle. Ankle-high desert boots in soft suede for leisure wear were looser at the top than the chukka boot and very comfortable. Suede shoes were popular in the mid-fifties, particularly in a deep blue shade. Harlem's natty dressers sported blue suede shoes, and there was a popular song about them. Shoes for sports wear included two-toned saddle oxfords, loafers, crepe-soled shoes of suede or fabric, and canvas tennis shoes. For lounging, in addition to the traditional mules and low-cut leather slippers, there were ankle-high slip-on boots of soft leather with long pointed toes, reminiscent of the Middle Ages.

Accessories

Accessories for men during the fifties were about the same as in the preceding decade. Jewelry included studs and cuff links for evening dress, made of pearl or smoked pearl for formal dress, and of gold, enamel, or colored stones for informal dress occasions. Men might wear rings and fraternity or lodge pins. They still fastened their shirt collars (when they had rounded tabs) with bar tie pins, and fastened four-in-hands to the shirt front with tie clasps. A new means of securing the four-in-hand was the tie tack, similar to a dress shirt stud. Wristwatches now came in waterproof, dustproof, shockproof models. Handkerchiefs were white for dress occasions, but might be pastel or bordered for informal wear. The customary fold for the early fifties was straight across and parallel to the breast pocket; in the late fifties a diagonal fold allowed two points to show in the pocket. A man's coat pockets might contain a fountain pen (or ball-point pen) and automatic pencil set, pocket comb and nail file, address book, folding penknife, wallet, and key case. Leather wallets or billfolds were equipped with multiple plastic folders that housed snapshots of the family, Social Security card, driver's license and automobile insurance forms, membership cards in professional organizations, medical insurance cards, charge account plates, and a battery of credit cards. Men still carried cigarette cases and lighters; despite the publicity that smoking was a principal cause of lung cancer, the majority continued to smoke cigarettes. In addition to the traditional leather belts, there were several styles of novelty belts, such as striped elastic, paisley-print fabric, and hemp, perhaps with flip-top buckles or hook-and-ring closures. Gloves for general use were worn only for warmth; they might be made of pigskin or goatskin in black, brown, gray, or tan. White gloves were worn for formal evening occasions, and white or gray gloves for daytime formal events. Scarves or mufflers were worn with topcoats in cold weather and were plain or patterned, of light wool, rayon, or silk. The styling of the man's black umbrella with a crooked handle did not change from one decade to the next; it might have a Malacca handle in the fifties. An omnipresent object carried by office workers or professional men was the attaché case, a rectangular leather case in which business papers were carried. Serving the same function was a flat leather briefcase zippered on three sides. Goggles were worn by the motorcycling younger set, and might be pushed back on the forehead when the rider was off the Honda. Dark sunglasses were worn on the beach and for driving in the bright sunshine, or around town in the daytime to hide the red eyes of a hangover. For a traveler, a very usual accessory was a 35mm camera in a leather case with shoulder strap.

WOMEN'S FASHIONS

The major change in women's styles in the fifties was the relaxing of the pinched-in waistline and the closely fitted bodice of the New Look. Finally, in 1957, came the straight chemise, or sack dress, with no waistline at all.

> In the spring of 1958 when women took off their winter coats, eager-eyed males were confronted by young women who looked like toothpaste tubes.

The view was infuriating. Fashion experts explained that the new mode was the "loose look" or the "relaxed silhouette," but men would not be mollified. To them it was the "sad sack," the "sag bag," the "waistless waste" and a host of other epithets. So widespread was the uproar that Adlai Stevenson, addressing a meeting of 2,000 members of the Democratic party's women's organization, found time to comment: "The source of the chemise is Moscow. Its purpose is to spread discontent. . . ."[5]

Two other radical departures from the New Look that appeared in 1958 were Yves St. Laurent's "trapeze" model, which had a free-swinging tent-shaped back and a high-belted front; and several versions of the "bubble," or "harem skirt," with a full hemline gathered and tucked up to form a puffball or bloused effect from the waist to the knees. In 1954 Dior introduced the "H-line," a sheath dress with a straight long-torso jacket; and in 1955 an "A-line," a semifitted look with a slight flare to the hemline, which became a popular silhouette (Figure 32). Among the leading Parisian designers were Cardin, Givenchy, and Ricci. Chanel reopened her salon in 1954, after fifteen years of retirement from the fashion world. She reintroduced her trademark — a straight knitted suit with a long overblouse and a simple cardigan jacket. Probably the most-outstanding couturier of this era was Balenciaga, who was particularly noted for his classic-looking coats. His designs were bold and elegant, his workmanship impeccable. Not all the innovations in silhouette during these years were attractive or flattering to the wearers. Frequently the new styles ignored the basic shape of the human figure, giving the effect of a meal sack or a cocoon. An Empire waistline combined with gathers in front often made a woman look pregnant, no matter how slim and svelte her figure. One absurdly wide-necked, wide-collared fashion in coats appeared to be falling off the wearer. As skirts went higher and higher, it became more important for a woman to have attractive legs and knees. Some hats even conspired to make the wearer look ridiculous.

One wonders if fashion has not, along with all artistic activity, suffered from a general phenomenon referred to as alienation and also as the "dehumanization of art". . . . Fashion . . . has come full circle and created a new essentialism: that of the cold, architectural, unapproachable goddess. . . .

In a sense this dehumanization of women via fashion is quite in order, is almost fitting. It is . . . in the vein of the logic of the modern world and takes part in a general trend toward a universal style, called by some critics a non-style, namely functionalism. Thus women conceived by the Parisian couturiers do quite well in front of Swedish or Danish backgrounds, in the midst of modern furniture, squares, lines, and geometric color shapes as well as utensils which look like surgical instruments.[6]

Exaggerated treatment, almost a caricature, extended to all elements of the costume, including hair styles and footwear. By the late fifties coiffures were being teased and puffed out to elaborate bubbles, while shoes often had four-inch heels of needle-slender steel and toes were elongated to sharp points.

Hair Styles and Makeup

The small, neatly curled and waved caps of hair that were characteristic of the New Look continued through the mid-fifties. The medium short bob was worn in loose waves with curled ends, parted or swept back in a pompadour, sometimes curled under in a short pageboy effect, with or without bangs. The short "poodle cut" was still popular, worn in ringlets all over the head. The Italian cut gave a feathery effect of short wisps on the forehead and around the face — an elfin or "little-boy" style. Another short, feathered hair style featured the "ducktail" in back, for girls as well as boys. About 1956 a trend toward built-up and built-out hair styles started. Heads began to look larger, as new bouffant and bubble coiffures appeared. This effect was achieved by back-combing or teasing the under hair and arranging the outer layer in bold waves and curls, then lacquering the surface with hair spray to hold the structure in place. The "beehive" was a conical variation of the bouffant style. Evening coiffures became more and more elaborate and reached exaggerated heights. Wigs and wiglets were coming into fashion by the late fifties. It was simple and easy (although expensive, since a good wig might cost $150) to change the color or style of one's hair, or to acquire an elaborate coiffure for the evening, by slipping on a dressed wig. Smaller hairpieces, chignons, or braids might also be pinned on to give fullness or height. The "pony tail" continued to be popular with the younger set throughout the fifties. Their long straight hair was usually pulled back and secured by an elastic band or a ribbon on the crown of the head, then fell down the back in a single lock.

Makeup in the early fifties continued in the style of the New Look — gentle pinks and soft reds for lipstick; little or no rouge; and accented eyes with the startled "doe-eyed" look, upper lids lined in an upswept curve at the outer ends. Late in the decade, makeup began to change to subtler colors, grayed and softened. Lips were toned down and eyes were played up even more than in the New Look, and rouge was omitted entirely. Some suggestions for off-beat makeup were given by *McCall's* beauty editor in 1959:

These tricks we show you how to do are frankly daring, purely for glamour. All of them take note of this year's beauty look: pale skin, pale lips, eyes newly emphasized, color used unexpectedly. . . .

Pale lips — both maidenly and provocative when they're outlined by a deeper shade. Use one of the new "whited" sticks or a white lipstick under your ordinary shade.

Nails — new opaque polishes in shades either pale or vibrant to match your prettiest dress (suntan, pale pink, aqua, French blue, violet, olive green).

Movie-star eyes — they're yours! New false lashes, attached to a plastic strip tinted in eye-shadow color, go on in a moment with a special adhesive.

Who doesn't crave wider, brighter eyes? They'll seem to be if you extend your eye liner out beyond the corners, then brush stark white eye liner between the lines.

Be daring with color — Picasso is. A brilliant blue eye liner, plus a minty green shadow, can do miraculously flattering things to your eyes.

Wonder if a blonde feels specially glamorous? You can find out in a jiffy. Look extra special on special evenings with a temporary spray.

Special tricks for special evenings: Sprinkle metallic glitter on your hair. It brushes out easily, does wonders for a brunette. Tip the ends of your hair with silver spray. Try a glitter-sprinkled beauty patch at the corner of your eye. Or paste a colored sequin at the outer corner of your brow. As a change from conventional mascara, use an offbeat, flattering green. For eyes with a new kind of sparkle: gold or silver shadow that is carried up to the brows.[7]

Hat Styles

Womens' hats in the early fifties continued to be small, compact, and frivolous to fit the neat, small-headed coiffures of the New Look. Styles included a variety of berets, half-hats, doll hats, tiny halos or discs trimmed and veiled as cocktail hats, turbans, small straight-brimmed sailors, and Breton sailors with turned-up brims. As the styles veered toward the look of the twenties in the latter part of the decade, cloches became increasingly popular and appeared in various materials, such as felt, suede, or velvet. Part of the outfit made popular by Jacqueline Kennedy when she became the First Lady in 1961 was a pillbox hat sitting on top of a bouffant coiffure (Figure 33). When the hair styles became teased and puffed out in bubbles and beehives, hats were worn less frequently — they might crush and ruin an elaborate, lacquered coiffure. In the late fifties, several exaggerated shapes appeared — bowlers with high, bulbous crowns, stovepipe hats with small brims, wiglike turbans made of tulle roses or curled ostrich plumes. There was a vogue for fur hats in 1958, which carried over into the sixties (Figure 54).

Underwear, Loungewear, and Sleepwear

As long as the New Look persisted, waist-cinching girdles continued to be worn. When the waistline relaxed and all but disappeared with the chemise and tent styles of the late fifties, waist-liners became unnecessary. Strapless evening gowns and some sunback daytime styles required the strapless, boned style of brassiere, such as the Merry Widow. Full-skirted dresses still needed stiff, bouffant, ruffled petticoats to extend the skirts. As skirts went to the knee and above, petticoats or slips grew shorter. Straight half-slips with elastic waistbands became more popular. For sleeping, a shorter nightgown came into fashion — the waltz-length gown, slightly above mid-calf in length. Short lounging robes and peignoirs in waltz-length were worn with the shorter gowns (Figure 26). Pajamas were also being made with "shortie" trousers, just below or above the knee. A very popular new style was the "baby doll pajama," which had a sleeveless, loose, flaring top worn over very short bloomer panties — the entire outfit just below the hip in length. Short, flaring dusters were in fashion as housecoats, made of lightweight fabrics for summer and of quilted satin or cotton for winter wear. Lounging pajamas were still popular for leisure wear, but the trousers were slim and tapered rather than having the skirtlike fullness of the thirties. Even more popular than pajamas were toreador pants or tapered slacks worn with blouses or tunic tops (Figure 27). Tights and leotards of stretch jersey, long the standard garb of ballet dancers, had been discovered by the general public and were worn increasingly for leisure dress, combined with a short tunic or jumper, or a tie-on skirt or apron. Stretch pants made of the new elasticized fabrics were also a favorite garment for wear around the house, as well as on the street. The suburban scene was often enlivened by the rather bizarre spectacle of a housewife who had tied a kerchief over a head full of two-inch curlers, thrown a duffle coat over shirtwaist and stretch pants, and dashed to the supermarket for a jar of instant coffee and several frozen TV dinners.

Day Wear

During the early fifties, dress styles continued in the New Look silhouette, with fitted bodices and flared skirts. Dirndl skirts and blouses were still popular. The "broomstick dress" in ruffled tiers was favored for square dancing (Figure 28). The perennially popular shirtwaist dress appeared in several versions, in dressy sheer fabrics for summer, in wash-and-wear synthetics with permanent accordion-pleated skirts, and even in brocade for evening wear. Sunback dresses were still in fashion, and might be worn with a cover-up jacket or a matching stole (Figure 29). Fitted sheaths and suits were worn throughout the fifties by those who preferred a defined waistline (Figures 30, 55). Some of them were based on Oriental styles (Figure 31). Suits were the first garments to break away from the tightly fitted waistline (Figure 32). Loosely fitted boxy jackets appeared in 1953 (Figure 34), and the box jacket suit became one of the most-popular styles in the country when it was worn as a favorite costume by Jacqueline Kennedy (Figure 33). The straight-line Chanel suit with a long overblouse and a cardigan jacket was a perennial favorite, appearing most often in jersey (Figure 35). The imported Italian knit suits in two- and three-piece styles proved to be most-practical garments for general wear — handsome, dressy, durable, and requiring no pressing (another "natural" for travelers). The "walking suit," with a loose, three-quarter-length jacket, was an elegant style appearing in the late fifties (Figure 54). A bloused back was a feature of some suits and dresses (Figure 36, 37). In 1958 several new styles in dresses appeared — the controversial chemise, the trapeze, and the bubble (Figures 35, 38, 39, 40). The chemise created a furore when it first appeared, lasted a year or so during which time the mass market was flooded with many poorly designed models, then disappeared. It returned, however, in the sixties in several durable styles of better design. Sweaters were very popular in the fifties and have continued to be so. The cowl collar was a new touch introduced by Givenchy (Figure 41). Bulky knits were favored.

Evening Wear   Throughout the fifties the strapless evening gown with tightly fitted bodice and very full skirt, either floor-length or ballerina-length (Figures 42, 43), continued to be a very popular style. (See also chapter 5, Figure 38.) The gown worn by Queen Elizabeth II of England at her coronation in 1953 was in this style and much photographed — a simple, beautiful gown of tulle with a pearl-and-jewel embroidered lace overskirt, designed by the queen's dressmaker, Norman Hartnell (Figure 44). The eyes of the fashion world were upon the elegant gowns worn for the coronation; they were much publicized and were designed by London's leading couturiers — Norman Hartnell, John Cavanagh, and Hardie Amies. For the most part they were white, strapless gowns with bouffant skirts, in fabrics such as tulle, organdy or organza, crepe, satin, lace, or brocade, trimmed with gold embroidery, sequins, pearls, beads, or jewels. There were some slimmer styles with trains reminiscent of the bustle era, in brocade or embroidered satin. The coronation itself was a glittering spectacle, and there were many accompanying balls. One reporter commented:

> Shown here in full panoply are some of London's leading beauties. While a French or Italian aristocrat can achieve a studied and sophisticated magnificence, nobody looks as born to a ball gown as does the British lady, with her assured carriage and family jewels. Since her dress is regarded primarily as a background for jewels, not many gowns are needed for even a crowded calendar. As one lady explained, a basic ball gown can be varied one night with diamonds, a second with rubies and a third with emeralds. A newly popular fashion for the coming season is colored gloves

to match stones. Even with all the glitter coming out for the season, there is no chance of anyone outshining her majesty, whose family owns the world's largest collection of historic jewels.

Tiaras may be worn to any function the queen attends if the invitation calls for white ties for men; if it specifies black tie, the tiara is left home since the queen may come bareheaded. At the coronation a peeress (anyone with the rank of baroness or above) should wear a coronet, whose design is prescribed by court etiquette. Ordinary ladies may wear a tiara.[8]

In America, a similar formal elegance might be seen at such occasions as a debutante coming-out ball. For the most part, however, American women preferred short formals for evening dress, styles that could be worn to a cocktail party in the early evening and then on to dinner and the theatre (Figure 46). Semiformal attire, halfway between cocktail or dinner dresses and floor-length formals, included ballerina styles and separate ankle-length evening skirts, pencil-slim and with slit hemlines, worn with a variety of tops: loose straight camisoles or flaring smocks, blousons, sleeveless jewel-necked shells, and jeweled or sequined cashmere evening sweaters. The chemise, bubble, and sheath models were all appropriate as short formal dresses. A strapless sheath, short or ankle-length, in satin or brocade with a matching jacket was popular as a theatre suit. In 1958 waistlines began to rise to the Empire level, just below the bust (Figures 35, 47).

> The high-waisted trend that marks this season's clothes sweeps around the clock to after-five fashions. Evening gowns and cocktail dresses hew to the Empire line, with only a handspan of fabric between the neckline and the lifted waist. From these abbreviated bodices flow skirts that are shaped like bells, formed like cones or fluted like classic Greek columns.[9]

Sportswear

For spectator sports, women in the fifties might wear box-jacket suits, two- or three-piece jersey outfits, dress-and-jacket ensembles, or shirtwaist dresses. Skirts and sweaters, shirtwaists, or blouses might be worn. In the early fifties skirts might be full and gathered, flared, or circle-cut; later in the decade they were usually straight, peg-top, or pleated. Twin sweater sets (pullover and cardigan) in cashmere were popular for campus and dressy sports wear. Cowl-necked sweaters and bulky-knit turtlenecks or coat-sweaters with collars were also in fashion.

For active sports, the styles of the preceding decade were still in evidence, with new variations showing up constantly. There were matching or coordinated sets of shorts, shirts, halter tops, and button-on skirts (Figure 48). There were one-piece sunback playsuits with straight shorts or romper panties. Slack suits often had jackets or vests combined with shirtwaists. Pants for playtime wear came in all lengths, from the shortest shorts to ankle-length tapered slacks—including Bermuda shorts, culottes (divided skirts), pedal pushers, cabin-boy breeches, clam-diggers, blue jeans, loose judo pants tied with a drawstring, and toreador pants (Figures 27, 48, 49, 50, 51). Bathing suits were growing briefer and briefer (Figure 52). One-piece models were cut away to reveal sections of the torso, and the bikini arrived on the scene—the merest wisp of abbreviated bra and G-string panties (Figure 53).

> The big trend in beachwear fashion is the take it off, put it on fashion. Modest jackets that suddenly reveal the barest bikinis. As a result, the resort shows were one stylish strip marathon from hotel to showroom. For the benefit of their retail audiences, models untied, unbuttoned, slipped in and out of beach jackets, sweaters to display the body beautiful barely touched by fashion artistry.[10]

Cover-up garments for the beach included ponchos, capes, loose slip-on tunics with boat necks and flaring bell sleeves, and short ruffled muumuus like baby-doll pajama tops.

Coats and Wraps

Early in the fifties coats might still have the well-fitted princesse lines typical of Dior's Cossack coat, with wide flaring skirts and often with large capelike collars. However, the coats of the middle and late fifties were more likely to be loose and widely flaring, or rounded cocoons, full under the arms and tapering to a slender hemline. The coats designed by Balenciaga were wide-necked and loose, with three-quarter-length sleeves (Figure 35). The wrapped coat of the twenties with a big fur collar reappeared late in the decade. Coat styles followed the trend toward Empire waistlines in 1958, with results that were not always flattering to the wearer. A bulky wool fabric gathered on a high-busted yoke made the slenderest figure look bunchy or pregnant. Fur coats were lavish and voluminous in this era. Luxurious all-enveloping wraps resembling mink bathrobes were carelessly lapped and belted. Fur-lined coats and jackets were popular. An evening wrap or cape might be made of white satin and lined with black sable. New on the scene were fake-fur acrylic fabrics, a creditable imitation of real fur. Coats and jackets made of these materials had a luxury of their own. One style in coats had a semifitted front and more fullness in back, belted in with a half-belt. Short jackets were very popular, in fabric, fake fur, or real fur; they might be straight, flared, or cocoon-shaped. The car coat, or suburban coat, was worn by women as well as by men (Figure 56). There were summer coats of sheer fabrics, more decorative than functional, and evening coats of satin or brocade. Raincoats were very attractive, available in waterproofed silk or synthetics, patterned as well as plain, and wearable in any weather. Vinyl coats and jackets had a shiny surface reminiscent of the oilcloth slickers of the twenties. Clear plastics were also being utilized for rainwear.

Shoe styles through the middle fifties continued in the fashions of the New Look era. Toes were rounded, and open-toed models were still in evidence. Ankle-strap sandals for evening were worn with bouffant-skirted formal gowns. In 1958 the styles began to change to elongated, pointed toes and very slender, needle-like heels. The open-toed and high ankle-strap models disappeared. The pointed-toe styles had low-cut vamps and often had instep straps, sometimes quite low on the instep. Evening shoes were most often pumps with very pointed toes and high spike heels, or they might have lower heels (underslung and curved to a dime-sized heel cap, called "little heels") and perhaps ankle straps. Shoes for street wear had little heels or "stacked heels" of layered wood or leather in Cuban height. Bright colors were popular — red, blue, violet, green, yellow — in calf, alligator, or fabric. Boots for women as well as men came into fashion late in the fifties. Slippers for lounging appeared in the ankle-high, pointed-toe styles of the medieval era. Boots for leisure wear came in ankle-high suede models with low heels.

Footwear

Hosiery took on added glamor and importance as legs began to show more and more. In the mid-fifties nylon hose became available in colors such as pink, mauve, and pastel greens and blues.

Jewelry in the early fifties continued in the New Look spirit, with dog-collar and bib necklaces in rhinestones, pearls, or colored stones in favor. Late in the decade there was a trend toward long strands of beads, waist-length or hip-length, as in the twenties. They might be wound around the neck once or twice, or worn in multiple strands. Metal chains were also popular. Earrings became more exotic — long, dangling chandeliers with mobile structures. Bracelets might be wide and bold — bangles, charm bracelets, or multiple strands of beads, pearls, or stones. Jewelry appeared in the colorful new plastics as well as in metal, pearls, and jewels. Hair ornaments were once more in fashion for evening dress — rhinestone clips or combs tucked into the evening coiffure, or jeweled headbands or tiaras added to the elevated locks. Wristwatches were now being made in waterproof and shockproof models. Gloves were frequently gauntlet- or elbow-length to accommodate the three-quarter-length sleeves of coats and suits. Wrist-length gloves were also popular; opera-length gloves were worn for formal occasions. The patterned gloves and matching printed accessories of the forties had disappeared — plain colors were now in

Accessories

fashion. Purses continued in the styles of the preceding era, but were often quite large (briefcase or satchel size). Clutch bags and box-shaped purses were still in fashion. Novelty styles were made in tapestry or needlepoint fabric, in short-haired fur, and in vinyl. Muffs were carried occasionally, sometimes matching a fur hat or fur-collared coat or jacket. Umbrellas were pencil-slim, with elongated tips and handles.

CHILDREN'S FASHIONS

Children's fashions during the fifties did not change materially from those of the preceding decade. Little boys might wear short pants until the age of six or eight, but might also wear long trousers at any age — coveralls, overalls, or slacks. Dress suits for small boys might have collarless Eton jackets. The jackets of suits for grammar-school and high-school boys reflected the natural shoulder and slender lapels of their fathers' Ivy League styles. A suit with matching jacket and trousers was worn infrequently — perhaps for Sunday School or for high school dances. School wear was informal: sport shirts and slacks worn with pullover sweater-vests, long-sleeved pullover or cardigan sweaters, sports jackets, or windbreakers. Car coats, or suburban coats, with Orlon fleece linings and detachable lined hoods for winter were worn by boys and girls as well as by their mothers and fathers.

Girls' dresses continued to have fitted bodices and full gathered or flared skirts in the early and mid-fifties. Late in the decade a Kate Greenaway style appeared, a flaring tent gathered on a neckline yoke, which resembled the trapeze style for adults. As waistlines began to fluctuate at the end of the decade, there appeared a girls' style with dropped waistline and short pleated skirt, reminiscent of little girls' styles in the twenties. A tent-shaped coat for girls also appeared. Matching coats and slacks or leggings might be worn in cold weather. Girls wore trousers more than they ever had in preceding decades — shorts, rompers, pedal-pushers, clam-diggers, blue jeans, stretch pants, and tapered slacks (Figure 57). Playclothes for little girls resembled the range of garments worn by their mothers.

TYPICAL MATERIALS, COLORS, MOTIFS, AND TRIMMINGS

During the fifties the manufacturers of synthetic fabrics continued to bring new textiles to the market. Dacron had proved to be excellent for contributing wash-and-wear properties to cotton, wool, and rayon fibers. A typical drip-dry blend was 35 percent cotton and 65 percent Dacron. Wool-and-Dacron blends were fine for wrinkle-resistant, washable suits and coats. Knitted Orlon made wonderful sweaters that looked like fine wool, washed easily, and needed no blocking. Banlon, a new fiber similar to Orlon with a slight nap, was excellent for sweaters, two-piece suits, and dresses; it was absolutely wrinkle-free and needed no pressing—perfect for traveling. Fake-fur fabrics were new on the market, made of deep-pile Dynel. These imitations were remarkable copies of real fur, with long and short hair, curled, straight or shaggy, patterned or plain; they came in zebra and tiger stripes, leopard and calfskin spots, Persian lamb curls and monkey-fur shagginess. Novelty fabrics with loops and raised textures appeared— hairlike loops added texture to the surface of a patterned print; "eyelash" fabric with a glittering nap of metallic or iridescent colored Mylar threads made an effective evening gown or theatrical costume. Stretch fabrics became available for hosiery, tights, leotards, and stretch pants. Tubular jerseys, which might easily be made into sheaths or chemise dresses, appeared on the market. Sequined jerseys were also available. Bold jerseys in brilliant horizontal stripes became very popular for shirts, tunics, and chemises as the decade ended. Bonded knits appeared; they had more body than ordinary jerseys, but did not survive dry cleaning very well. Cotton, silk, or nylon sheers might be machine-embroidered or printed with allover floral designs or with decorative borders for dressy gowns. During the early fifties, while circular skirts were in fashion, one might purchase fabrics printed in bordered circles of skirt size. Patterned fabrics were rather demure, soft in color, and tending toward small floral designs, polka dots, checks, stripes, or plaids. Polynesian prints in cotton or synthetic blends were popular for sportswear. Applied trim included ornamental buttons, lace, eyelet embroidery with ribbon inserts, braid, artificial flowers, jeweled clips, or pinned-on ornaments. Formal dresses might be trimmed with sequins, rhinestones, or beads.

SUGGESTIONS FOR COSTUMING PLAYS IN THE PERIOD

When the period of the fifties is presented on stage, well-dressed men should wear the Ivy League silhouette with natural shoulders, slender lapels, and tapered trousers. An older, poorer, or conservative character might still wear the wide, padded shoulders and full-cuffed trousers of the forties. If the costume wardrobe is limited to suits of older cut, trousers may be tapered with a seam down the side leg to a cuff of fourteen or sixteen inches. Coats should be single-breasted and should have notched rather than peaked lapels. Shoulders of old models might be relaxed by removing the shoulder pads. Jacket styles of the sixties are appropriate for the mid-fifties and following years. Teenagers might wear blue jeans or Levi's, T-shirts or sport shirts, bulky knit sweaters, or leather jackets. After 1955 they might wear sideburns and have longer hairstyles. They might wear boots or go barefooted. Beatniks, hippies, or other Bohemian characters might wear beards or mustaches.

In the early fifties, most women would probably still be wearing the New Look, with indented waistlines, closely fitted bodices, and full skirts. With these styles a waist-cinching girdle should be worn, and usually a bouffant petticoat is required to extend the skirt. Strapless styles would call for a boned, strapless brassiere. Beyond 1957 the chemise, trapeze, or bubble styles might be worn generally. An unfitted sack dress may be very shapeless and unbecoming. It is well to work from a good pattern for a chemise or shift that has darts to give shape to the garment. Dresses in these styles from the fifties are available in the thrift shops, and patterns are easily found for making them. The principal concern for the costumer should be to choose a style that reflects the temperament and personality of the character to be portrayed.

TITLE	AUTHOR	PERIOD
Advise and Consent	Loring Mandel	1960
The Bad Seed	Maxwell Anderson	1954
Bells Are Ringing (M)	B. Comden, A. Green, J. Styne	1956
The Best Man	Gore Vidal	1960
The Birthday Party	Harold Pinter	1957
Bus Stop	William Inge	1955
Bye Bye Birdie (M)	Michael Stewart, Charles Strouse, Lee Adams	1960
Camino Real	Tennessee Williams	1953
Cat on a Hot Tin Roof	Tennessee Williams	1955
The Cave Dwellers	William Saroyan	1957
The Chalk Garden	Enid Bagnold	1955
Clara's Ole Man	Ed Bullins	mid-1950s
Coco (M)	Alan Jay Lerner, Andre Previn	1953-54
The Desk Set	William Marchant	1955
Damn Yankees (M)	Richard Adler, Jerry Ross	1955
Fantasticks (M)	Tom Jones, Harvey Schmidt	1960
Flower Drum Song (M)	Richard Rodgers, Oscar Hammerstein	1958
A Gift of Time	Garson Kanin	1954
Grease (M)	Jim Jacobs, Warren Casey	1950s
The Hostage	Brendan Behan	1960
L'il Abner (M)	Johnny Mercer, Gene de Paul	1956
Look Back in Anger	John Osborne	1957
The Mousetrap	Agatha Christie	1955
Pajama Game (M)	Richard Adler, Jerry Ross	1954
Picnic	William Inge	1953
The Pleasure of His Company	Samuel Taylor, Cornelia Otis Skinner	1958
The Rimers of Eldritch	Lanford Wilson	1950s
Romanoff and Juliet	Peter Ustinov	1957
The Solid Gold Cadillac	Howard Teichmann, George Kaufman	1953
Sweet Bird of Youth	Tennessee Williams	1959
Sty of the Blind Pig	Phillip Hayes Dean	1950s
A Taste of Honey	Shelagh Delaney	1958
Tea and Sympathy	Robert Anderson	1953
Toys in the Attic	Lillian Hellman	1960
Two for the Seesaw	William Gibson	1958
A View from the Bridge	Arthur Miller	1955
West Side Story (M)	Bernstein, Laurents, Sondheim	1958
Will Success Spoil Rock Hunter?	George Axelrod	1955
Witness for the Prosecution	Agatha Christie	1954

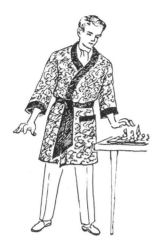

1. Leisure kimono in metallic brocade. 1958.

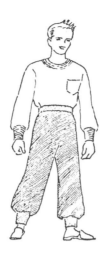

2. Ski-type, cotton knit pajamas in maroon and gray. 1959.

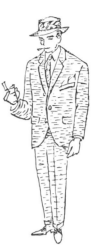

3. Tropical-weight light gray suit of Italian Dupioni silk. 1957.

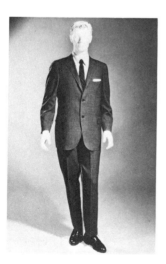

4. Two-piece gray suit: single-breasted, two-button jacket; cuffed trousers. Worn in Denver, Colorado. About 1958 – 62. (Division of Costume, Smithsonian Institution.)

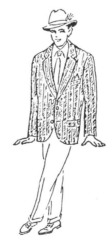

5. Ivy League sport coat with natural shoulders and narrow lapels; tapered slacks. 1956.

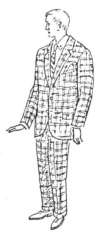

6. Ivy League business suit: Glen plaid in Dacron-worsted blend. 1956.

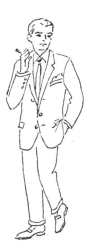

7. Tailored summer business suit in washable Tycora. 1959.

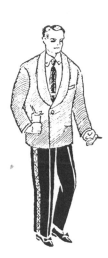

8. Red flannel dinner jacket; black trousers with red tartan braid. 1955.

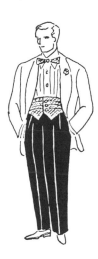

9. Cummervest and tie for evening of red-and-gray checked Shantung. 1954.

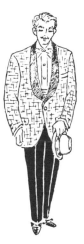

10. Bermuda blue dinner jacket of Dupioni silk; black silk trousers. 1957.

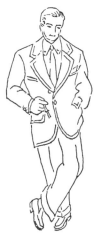

11. Sports jacket and slacks of spun rayon and cotton. 1954.

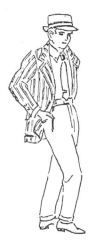

12. Maroon and navy striped blazer in lightweight worsted. 1959.

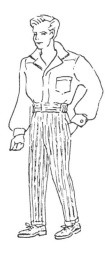

13. Blouson and slacks of wash-and-wear cotton with Velcro closing. 1959.

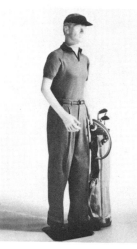

14. Golfing outfit: blue-gray cuffed trousers with belt; short-sleeved blue knit shirt. Worn in Lancaster, Pennsylvania, 1953–55. (Division of Costume, Smithsonian Institution.)

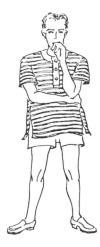

15. Striped cotton shirt; khaki beach trunks. 1954.

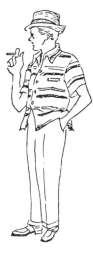

16. Chromspun-and-cotton striped shirt; polished cotton slacks. 1957.

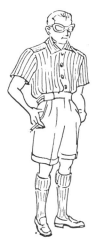

17. Printed striped cotton shirt; khaki walking shorts. 1954.

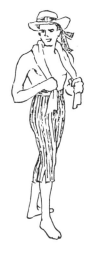

18. Calypso-stripe clam-digger pants. 1957.

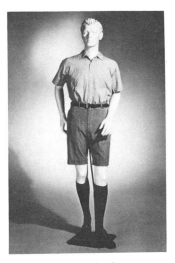

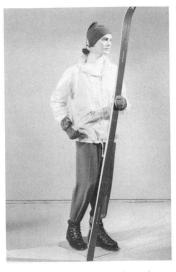

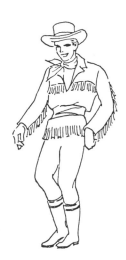

19. Gray Bermuda shorts;
blue-and-white checked gingham
short-sleeved shirt. Worn in
Delray Beach, Florida, 1954 – 56.
(Division of Costume,
Smithsonian Institution.)

20. Ski costume in wool, cotton,
and nylon. Jacket, American.
Shirt and trousers, Swiss, by
Kaltenbrinner-Davos, 1958 – 60.
(The Costume Institute of The
Metropolitan Museum of Art.
Gift of Mr. and Mrs. Burton
Tremaine.)

21. Western outfit: fringed tan
suede shirt; brown suede pants;
gray hat. 1953.

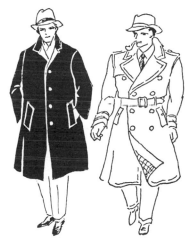

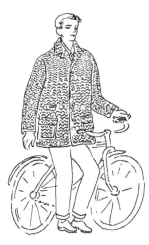

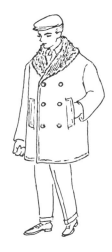

22, 23. Reversible raincoat, tan
and black, for day or evening
wear. 1956. Military-style poplin
raincoat, lined in plaid. 1953.

24. Four-button suburban coat
of brushed tweed with Orlon
fleece lining. 1956.

25. Coat of heavy tan cotton
with raccoon collar and Orlon
pile lining. 1957.

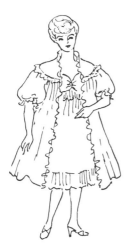

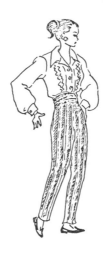

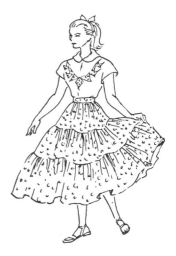

26. Waltz-length nightgown and peignoir in paprika pink chiffon. 1959.

27. White ruffled shirt; tapered slacks in Topsail cotton stripes. 1955.

28. "Broomstick" dress, of crinkled calico, for square dancing. 1953.

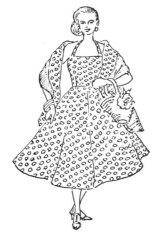

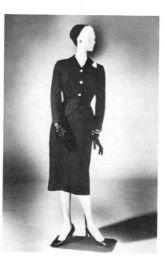

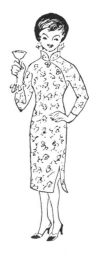

29. Sundress and stole in turquoise-and-white polished cotton. 1956.

30. Two-piece suit of brown wool: fitted jacket with detached belt, rhinestone buttons, straight skirt with side zipper and back pleat. By Maurice Rentner, 1956. (Division of Costume, Smithsonian Institution.)

31. Chinese cheongsam, sheath with slit skirt, in white silk brocade. 1960.

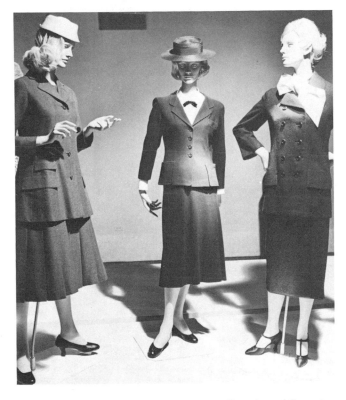

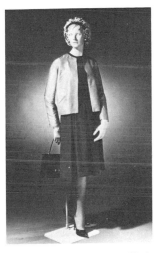

33. "Jackie Kennedy look": box jacket suit; pillbox hat; pumps. 1960.

32. Left, "A-line" suit for spring in gray silk-and-wool flannel: hip-length overblouse; semifitted jacket, narrow at top, flared below waist; full pleated skirt; Baku straw hat. By Christian Dior, 1955. Center, daytime suit of navy blue wool jersey with tucked white cotton blouse; navy blue straw sailor hat. By Chanel, 1954. Right, "H-line" dress and long-torso jacket of black wool flannel, in the sheathed silhouette. By Christian Dior, 1954. (The Costume Institute of The Metropolitan Museum of Art. Gifts of Christian Dior and Bettina Ballard.)

34. Sleeveless orange silk dress with box-pleated skirt; gold-colored silk box jacket. By Donald Brooks, 1959. (Division of Costume, Smithsonian Institution.)

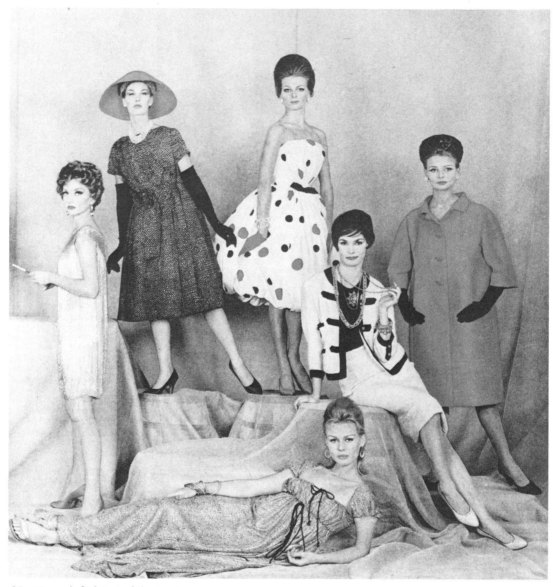

35. Women's fashions of the 1950s.
  Left to right: Beaded chemise in pearl gray. By Norman Norell,
1957. "Trapeze" dress in black-and-white houndstooth check print.
By Yves St. Laurent. Black gloves and shoes, red hat.
1958. "Bubble" dress in white with black and red polka dots. By
Arnold Scaasi, 1959. Cardigan knit suit in navy and white. By
Chanel, 1960. Coat in bright coral wool. By Balenciaga. Black hat,
shoes, and gloves. 1960. Reclining, evening gown in gold lamé with
Empire waistline. By Claire McCardell, 1956. (The Costume Institute
of The Metropolitan Museum of Art, and The Brooklyn Museum.
Photograph by Milton H. Greene.)

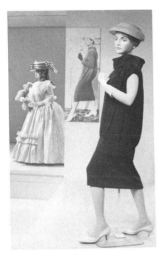

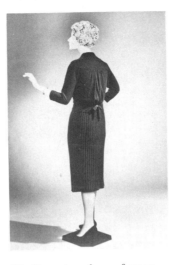

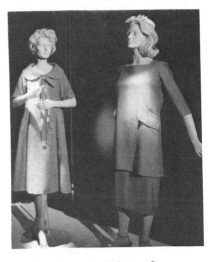

36. Day dress of wool jersey. French, by Cristobal Balenciaga, 1955. Fashion plate: day dress of wool by Balenciaga. (*Vogue*, New York, September 1, 1955, p. 189.) (The Costume Institute of The Metropolitan Museum of Art. Gift of Muriel Rand.)

37. Two-piece dress of green knit: rib-knit straight skirt; top with rib-knit ornamentation, three-quarter-length sleeves, bloused back with bow accent at center back waist. Worn in Waukesha, Wisconsin. Made by Softies by Lawrence, 1957. (Division of Costume, Smithsonian Institution.)

38. Left,"trapeze" dress of gray bouclé wool, narrowed and lightly fitted at top, flaring to the hemline. By Yves St. Laurent, 1958. Right, chemise tunic, belted across the back, and slim skirt of bright red linen; white organdy pillbox hat. French, by Balenciaga, 1955. (The Costume Institute of The Metropolitan Museum of Art. Gifts of Imogene Schubert and Balenciaga.)

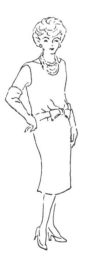

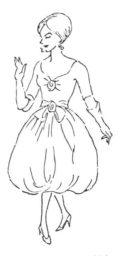

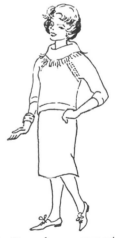

39. Dior chemise in light gray crepe, with pearl-and-rhinestone beading. 1957.

40. "Bubble" dress of blue-violet barathea silk; puff skirt. 1958.

41. Givenchy sweater with fringed cowl collar, in Orlon; tweed skirt. 1958.

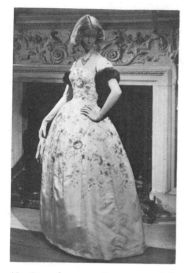

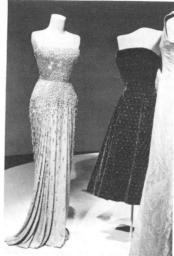

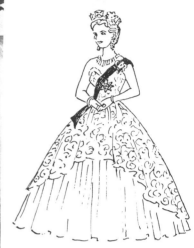

42. Strapless evening gown with matching gloves of pale blue ribbed silk; tiny mink-trimmed jacket. By Christian Dior, 1954. (The Costume Institute of The Metropolitan Museum of Art. Gift of Mrs. Byron C. Foy.)

43. Left, evening gown, called "Aurora Borealis": gold lamé encrusted with iridescent beading. By James Galanos, 1959. Right, short evening gown of ruby-red velvet with jet bead embroidery; fitted princesse line with strapless bodice and full mid-calf-length skirt. By Christian Dior, 1955. (The Costume Institute of The Metropolitan Museum of Art. Gifts of James Galanos and Mrs. Byron C. Foy.)

44. Coronation gown of Queen Elizabeth II, of white tulle and lace. 1953.

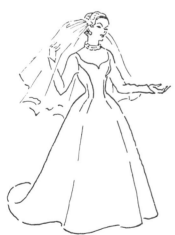

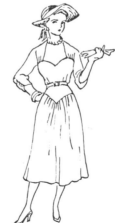

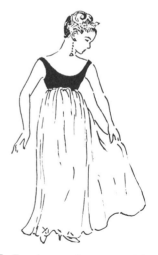

45. Princesse bridal gown of pure silk ivory satin. 1954.

46. Dinner dress of soft silk crepe. 1953.

47. Empire evening gown with black velvet bodice and white chiffon skirt. 1958.

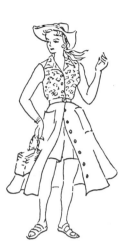

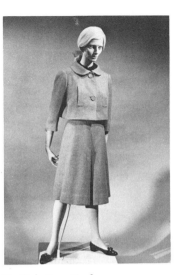

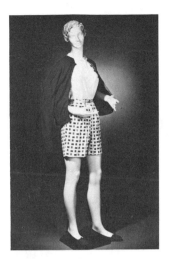

48. Three-piece playsuit: shorts, shirt, and button-on skirt. 1955.

49. Culotte suit of pomegranate-red wool tweed. By Norman Norell, 1960. (The Costume Institute of The Metropolitan Museum of Art. Gift of Mrs. Beatrice Simpson.)

50. Bermuda shorts in printed red-and-blue flag motif; side zipper; belt. White sleeveless blouse with four flags embroidered on left front. Red cardigan sweater. By Aansworth Ltd., 1958 – 60. (Division of Costume, Smithsonian Institution.)

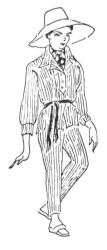

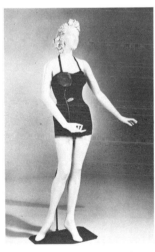

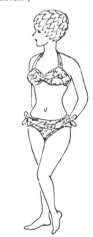

51. Arnel flannel slack suit. 1959.

52. Black "stretch taffeta" bathing suit with red taffeta rose on right breast; suit shirred under vertical green stem of rose; strapless with hook-on strap. Worn in Akron, Ohio. By Catalina, 1954. (Division of Costume, Smithsonian Institution.)

53. Bikini swimsuit. 1960.

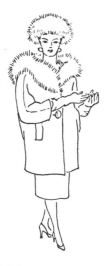

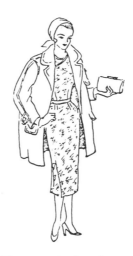

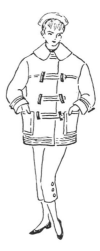

54. Walking suit in russet tweed, with badger collar and hat. 1958.

55. Three-quarter-length coat over mandarin print sheath dress. 1955.

56. White corduroy car coat with wood toggles; pedal-pushers. 1956.

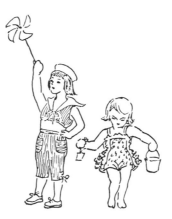

57. Children's playsuits. Left, two-piece pants and top. Right, ruffled romper suit. 1955.

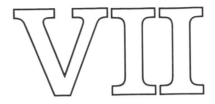

The Sixties: Unisex and Mini-Skirts
(1961-1970)

FASHIONS IN THE sixties veered toward some startling fluctuations and innovations. The nation seemed to be undergoing violent efforts to assimilate the series of shocks that the twentieth century had dealt it. As the rest of the world came closer, through swift travel and communication, an intense interest in the culture of other countries was reflected in the clothing styles of Americans — the furs and boots of Russia; the sheaths, feminine trousers, acceptable nudity of the Orient; the brilliant colors, heavy embroideries, and flowing garments of the Middle East; the bizarre prints and beads of South Africa; the Nehru jackets and saris of India. On another continuum, styles were gyrating backward and forward in time, going in quick succession from the silhouettes of the Victorian era, to the twenties, thirties, and forties, to the medieval era, to the prehistoric undress of cave dwellers, and to a futuristic "Star Trek" mode suggestive of space travel. These phenomena might have been a sign of severe disorientation or a search for security in old, familiar fashions. On the other hand, such eclectic styles might simply have been the result of a lively curiosity and widened perceptions.

CONCERNING THE PERIOD

The human race forsook its firm foothold on the planet Earth during the decade of the 1960s and thereby changed its perspective for all time. The thrust into space that began with the launching of Sputnik in 1957 reached another milestone with the landing of men on the moon in 1969. The nation thrilled as Neil Armstrong took his first "giant step for mankind" on the rocky lunar surface. This shift in focus enabled earth dwellers to see the planet as a whole; suddenly the world seemed more finite and its resources limited. A new interest in ecology and conservation of natural resources was the logical result.

The war in Vietnam involved the United States in 1964 and dragged on through the sixties — the most expensive and least-popular conflict in American history. An unpleasant aura of fascism and dictatorship hung over the White House, as President Richard Nixon, who inherited this problem when he came to office in 1969, joined forces with the Pentagon to pour billions of dollars into the destruction of Southeast Asia with no formal declaration of war. On campuses across the country and in the ranks of young rebels, there were peace demonstrations; disillusionment with the sham of American democracy turned to contempt. This sentiment was reflected in the fashion labeled "flag-spoofing" — crazy combinations of red-white-and-blue stars and stripes in clothing. It was touched off by the hit musical *Hair*, which embodied the "hippie" criticism of the "Establishment." In May 1970, when without warning President Nixon expanded the war in Asia and ordered United States troops to invade Cambodia, colleges and universities throughout the land were closed by student strikes and riots. This situation erupted after the death of four protesting students, when peace demonstrators were fired upon by the National Guard at Kent State University in Ohio. Gone forever was the patriotic fervor of World War I — the simple faith in a righteous Uncle Sam and Miss Liberty that had prevailed at the Victory parades after the Armistice of November 1918 had "ended war for all time."

During the decade the advancement of the Black cause continued, and in 1964 Congress passed the Civil Rights Act. Several large cities with Black populations in the majority elected Black mayors — Cleveland, Newark, Gary. On the West Coast, the Spanish-American minorities were also agitating to improve their condition and gain their rights as citizens.

The decade was marred by a sharp increase in crime and a series of political assassinations: President John F. Kennedy was shot in 1963, and Lyndon B. Johnson became President; the martyred President's brother, Senator Robert Kennedy, was killed in 1968; the Black leader, Rev. Martin Luther King, Jr., fell to an assassin's bullet in 1967. An alarming increase in the use of marijuana and hard drugs was correlated with an upsurge of violence and burglaries in the big cities. And a new form of piracy developed, the hijacking of jet airplanes.

Sexual behavior was characterized by unprecedented freedom, possibly as a result of the advent of "the Pill" (oral contraceptive) in 1961. This casting off of inhibitions spawned a parallel trend in literature, in motion pictures, and on the legitimate stage of frank sexual expression — nudity and explicit erotic scenes. There may have been some connection between this "release from the consequences" of normal sex relations plus a new trend toward equality of the sexes and a move toward "Unisex" in fashion. A strong Women's Liberation movement sprang up; at the same time there was a movement to gain equality for homosexuals (Gay Liberation). Females became militant, demanded equal rights with men, and went wholesale into "pants suits." Both sexes seemed to strive consciously to look like the other; one expression of this trend was a fad in which couples, married or unmarried, dressed identically.

The arts of the sixties (including costume design) seemed to glorify vulgarity and ugliness, embodied the nightmare qualities of the atomic age, and adopted the underlying theme of self-destruction and debauchery epitomized by the presence of the A-bomb and the H-bomb. A walk through an art museum during the sixties might bring the startled viewer face to face with a crumpled automobile fender or a broken-down toilet seat enshrined on a pedestal. These works satirized the state of American culture, saying, in effect, "We have come to this!" The Pop and Op artists were still in full swing. Roy Lichtenstein's comic-strip paintings and Andy Warhol's soup cans began to replace the abstract patterns of Kandinsky and Mondrian on apartment walls. Electronic sculptures moved across the floor at the touch of a button. Mobiles suspended on strings from the ceiling added a new touch to interior decoration. Another form of expression somewhere between art and theatre, launched by the Pop art school, were the "Happenings," or surrealist improvisations, in which living actors served as ingredients in a mobile collage. Distorted eroticism and destruction were seemingly the most oft-repeated elements in this brand of "kinetic art" — if it may be called art. The young artists were "skeptical, irreverent and extremely curious about the real nature and function of art in an existentially absurd era — the era of the Bomb."[1]

Interior decoration in the sixties evidenced a tongue-in-cheek approach (labeled "camp" in some cases), which seemed to be a studied effort to be garish, ugly, and in poor taste, through the use of jarring color, overdone ornamentation, cheap and vulgar motifs, and a nerve-wracking jumble of line and detail. This whole reactionary movement was, in a sense, an overcompensation for and deliberate negation of the machinelike precision of the functional modern style that had prevailed for several years. In the early sixties there was a return to the Art Nouveau styles of the early 1900s. There was a craze for decorating the walls of hippie "pads" and Mod apartments with posters in this voluptuous and florid style. In 1964 there was a mannered rediscovery of the ornate clutter of the Victorian era, complete with old-fashioned rocking chairs, stained-glass lampshades, and clusters of multiple gilt-framed paintings. New furniture pieces to appear on the scene were huge puffs for sitting on the floor, bean-bag chairs and hassocks, inflated plastic chairs (sometimes transparent), water beds, and king- and queen-sized beds. The "conversation pit" was an architectural novelty, a submerged area below the living room floor level, sometimes adjacent to a fireplace, thickly carpeted and arranged for intimate groupings. Cocktail tables with heavy plate glass tops on aluminum frames were very popular. Black-and-white television sets had given way to color television.

The rock 'n' roll music of the fifties continued to hold sway in the sixties. There was a spineless droop to the dancing that went with this music — the eyelids and mouths of the singers and dancers drooped, the shoulders and backbones sagged, the knees were bent, and the heads and hips were carried forward. The rhythms of the dance were staccato and rather spastic, which caused the head to jerk and the loosely held arms to flop at the sides; the hips swiveled. Although the dancers had partners, they danced separately and at some distance from one another, rather than embracing. The rock 'n' roll rhythms led to a variety of dances whose names were descriptive of the special gyrations of each. In the early sixties, as teen-age discothèques sprang up to accommodate the new music and dancing, new dances were invented weekly or nightly, based on the original "Twist" of 1960 — frequently with arm and hand motions attached to them — the Frug, the Slop, the Wobble, the Mashed Potato, the Shimmy, the Hitch-hike, the Swim, the Surf, and the Jerk, the Hully-Gully, the Monkey, and the Boogaloo. All these dances were accompanied by a volume of sound that was deafening to the uninitiated. The electric guitar was the central instrument of this era, as the saxophone had been of the 1920s; its sounds were amplified to a decibel count that assaulted the eardrums and left many of the younger generation with impaired hearing. The decade of the sixties was an era of jangled nerves, and its costume styles (often freakish and bizarre) reflected this condition faithfully.

GENERAL CHARACTERISTICS OF COSTUME

Fashions during the sixties were increasingly colorful, heterogeneous, varied, and individualized, often to the point of wildness. Hemlines for women crept steadily upward until they reached an all-time high about 1967; the mini-skirted garments hardly qualified as dresses any longer, but were rather long shirts or hip-length tunics. In 1969 there was a countertrend toward longer skirts. The midi-skirt or calf-length hem was adopted by more-mature women, while the very young continued to wear the mini-skirt. Another favored length was the "maxi," or ankle-length, skirt, particularly in outerwear — overcoats and long, sleeveless jackets. Styles were borrowed freely from national garments around the world, particularly from Russia, India, Hawaii, Morocco,

Spain, and Africa. Elements from America's own past were sought out and adopted, too; there was a quick recapitulation of styles from the twenties, thirties, and forties, as well as those from the Victorian era; American Indian styles also appeared. Toward the end of the decade, in "the costume look" everyone dressed to suit himself, and party clothes and even street wear began to look as if the wearers were ready for a fancy-dress ball. Pants suits for women became more and more popular, until by the end of the sixties they were an almost universal uniform, accepted for business and professional wear as well as for home and street garb (Figures 69, 70, 71, 82, 84). Airline hostesses wore them, and so did their passengers. Nurses appeared in white pants uniforms; female professors as well as students adopted trousers for classroom wear; secretaries and women executives showed up at their offices in pants. In the academic and business worlds this changeover elicited some remonstrance from conservative administrators, but the wearers of pants eventually won the battle.

Among the "hippie" group of young liberals, radicals, and dropouts, long hair for boys and girls and luxurious beards and mustaches for the young men were a badge of membership. They wore multiple strings of beads, pendants with peace symbols and fertility symbols, and lapel buttons championing various causes. Face and body painting originated with the hippies and was adopted as a fad for Mod partygoers — makeup was applied in exotic patterns and colors, particularly around the eyes. In the late sixties, the best-dressed beauties were made up to look like zombies, with cavernous eyes, heavily lashed and mascaraed, and the pale complexion of advanced illness or death. In the long shadow cast by Hiroshima — through some quirk of the guilty mass subconscious — it had become high fashion to look like the victims of atomic fallout.

Fashions for men broke away from the traditional rather quiet and conservative styles that had prevailed since the middle of the nineteenth century. There was a sudden new daring in male dress and a resurgence of sartorial splendor, unheard of since the days of Louis XVI or Napoleon. Men began to wear shirts (and sometimes slacks) in colorful floral prints, shirts with full gathered sleeves in lace or sheer fabrics, and evening shirts with ruffled fronts and cuffs. Suits departed from the century-old styles of correct coat, vest, and trousers and began to appear in sleeveless jerkin or vest styles, one-piece jump suits, or slacks with tunic tops. Evening suits and lounging outfits were made in elegant fabrics — crushed velvet or brocade, in brilliant colors and bold prints. In 1968 the Nehru jacket appeared, with the standing collar of Hindu coats. Some nonconformist men began to wear elegant white turtleneck sweaters in place of pleated evening shirts. Instead of ties, necklaces were worn to complete the Nehru or turtleneck outfit.

Men's fashions also recapitulated styles from the nineteenth and earlier in the twentieth century, with Edwardian suits, "gangster" pinstripes of the 1930s and 40s, and Wild West fashions. By the end of the decade, some men had adopted the new longer coat lengths; overcoats were appearing in the "midi" calf-length and the "maxi" ankle-length. Men also returned to wearing fur coats and hats, in seal, mink, raccoon, and kangaroo skins.

There was a strong trend throughout the decade toward a "Unisex" look. As the women took to wearing pants on a grand scale, it became increasingly hard to tell the boys from the girls. The following quotation sums up the quandary many found themselves facing:

"Well, it finally happened," Michael Murphy of California's Esalen Institute recently said. "A young person came up to talk with me, and I couldn't tell if this person was a man or a woman. Now, I've seen plenty of young people of both sexes dressed in slacks, sweater and long hair, but I'd always been able to find *some* sexually distinguishing clue. This time there was *no way for me to tell*. I admit it shook me up. I didn't know exactly how to relate. I felt it would take a new kind of relating, no matter if it were a boy or girl."[2]

By the late sixties, nudity seemed to be gaining public acceptance, with topless bathing suits on the beaches, topless waitresses and dancers at night clubs, and scenes in avant-garde theatre productions in which performers of both sexes might appear nude or disrobe on stage.

MEN'S FASHIONS

The "peacock revolution" in men's fashions during the sixties, with its return to brilliant colors, luxurious fabrics, frills, and jewelry, which had been absent from male costume since the late eighteenth century, brought about some changes in the fashion industry. Couturiers who were well known as high-fashion designers of women's clothing now turned their attention to designing for men as well, such noteworthy figures as Pierre Cardin, Norman Hartnell, Oleg Cassini, Oscar de la Renta, and Bill Blass. For the first time in 1969 the American fashion world issued a list of "ten best-dressed men" to join the ranks of the long-established annual lists of "ten best-dressed women." Carnaby Street in London became a center for "Mod" fashions, and Cardin took the lead in promoting this mode in Paris (Figures 4, 12).

Hair Styles and Grooming

Men wore their hair longer in this decade than it had been since the Romantic era of the nineteenth century. The hippies and rebellious members of the younger set in particular let their hair grow to shoulder- or waist-length, sometimes with shaggy bangs over the eyebrows, in a style reminiscent of Prince Valiant, peasants of the Middle Ages, or biblical patriarchs. This gesture of defiance was a source of much emotional conflict between conventional parents and teen-age adolescents. The mood was reflected in the title song from the hit musical *Hair* — they let it grow "down to here, down to there, down to where it stops by itself." Long hair was sometimes responsible for expulsion from high school or the loss of a job. However, by the end of the sixties the Establishment had succumbed to this trend, and even conservative men were adopting the shaggier look, letting their hair curl softly on the neck and grow a little fuller over the ears, and affecting more luxurious sideburns. Beards and mustaches were flowing in the hippie ranks, but appeared in more-clipped and controlled fashion with increasing frequency on the faces of members of the Establishment. Barbers of the old school specializing in short haircuts found themselves almost out of business, but men's barber salons rivaling the women's beauty shops became a thriving new field of enterprise. An advertisement of a typical salon offered "mod cuts, shag cuts, long hair and beard cutting and styling, hair tinting and dyeing, waving and straightening, long and short hair pieces and wigs, manicures and pedicures." Men were following the example of the women, improving on nature and recapturing their youth with the aid of hair coloring to cover gray, waving and straightening to modify the natural state of their locks, and the addition of hairpieces and wigs for added length — sometimes just for state occasions. Young men who preferred long hair but found themselves at odds with an Army ruling for short haircuts often solved their dilemma by tucking their long locks under a short-cropped wig. Negroes adopted an "Afro" hairstyle as one expression of their drive to assert that "Black is Beautiful." The Afro was an exaggerated extended bubble of kinky, frizzy hair (Figure 1). Many young white people wore their hair in similar fashion to express sympathy for the Blacks.

For general body toning, there were massage parlors, saunas, and whirlpool baths. An ever-increasing list of grooming aids for men appeared on the market — deodorants, lotions, hair sprays, and perfumes with virile names such as "Russian Leather" and "Hai Karate."

Hat Styles

Men's hats retained all the old faithful models — the fedora and the homburg, and a variety of straws. The high silk hat for formal wear almost disappeared from the scene. Brims on felt and straw hats ranged from narrow to wide. In the late sixties, when double-breasted "gangster suits" were rediscovered, the wide-brimmed hats of the 1940s were also resurrected. There was a reappearance of fur hats and caps (some resembling fez shapes) in astrakhan, seal, and mink early in the decade. Fedoras in luxurious velour were worn with fur coats, which had attained new popularity. The "Mod" fashions brought a flurry of billed caps for both men and women. Hats worn by Blacks included knitted caps in many styles, some with bills, some with pompoms. The motorcycle crowd known as "Hell's Angels" elected to wear old Nazi helmets instead of prescribed cycling headgear. Headbands in leather or American Indian beadwork and Black Bart broadbrimmed black felt hats reminiscent of the Wild West were popular.

Underwear, Loungewear, and Sleepwear

Underwear for men in this decade was pretty well limited to boxer shorts and briefs. Bare chests were very much in vogue, and men went without shirts much more frequently than in any other decade of the century. Whereas such attire had heretofore only been seen on beaches or in bedrooms, now one might well come upon a man working in his backyard or lounging about the house, or even wandering across campus or down Main Street, clad only in a pair of slacks, barefoot, and naked from the waist up. Shopkeepers and restaurant owners, striving to maintain a certain decorum, began to post signs on their front doors saying "Shirts and shoes required."

Lounging attire followed the general trend toward brilliance and a new carefree look. For a decade or two men had been wearing Japanese-style kimonos for dressing gowns. They were still in vogue, but in addition there were a variety of robes showing foreign influences — "dashikis" from Africa (Figure 1) and caftans from the Middle East in long and short versions (Figure 2). Smoking jackets appeared in luxurious crushed or cut velvets, brocades, batiks, and bold prints. They were by no means confined to evenings at home but might be worn to enliven an informal gala affair. One-piece jump suits and two-piece tunic outfits or shirt-suits also belonged in this multipurpose category, used for lounging at home, lolling on the beach, or casual evening dress (Figures 25, 26, 27).

For sleeping, pajamas continued in favor. For summer, they might have short sleeves and above-the-knee pants (Figure 3).

Neckwear

Men's shirts during the sixties abandoned the small, neat, button-down collar and veered toward a wider collar with long, spreading points and a higher neckline. The "body shirt," tapered to the waistline and fitted snugly to the contour of the body, was often combined with the wider, long-pointed collar and fuller sleeves with deep cuffs (Figure 4). Daring or "Mod" versions of the body shirt appeared in lace, sheer, or "see-through" fabrics (Figure 5). Bright floral prints, bold stripes, polka dots, batiks, and Op-art motifs were all made up into shirts. Brilliant colors were in vogue for shirts and ties and were coordinated in plain and patterned combinations, in such colors as burnt orange, deep peach, wine red, royal blue, or deep lavender. For evening wear the traditional white dress shirt was enlivened with ruffles down the front and on the cuffs (Figures 17, 19). Dress shirts also appeared in vivid colors. For example, a cerise, hot pink, or French blue ruffled shirt might be worn with an elegant black velvet evening jacket.

Four-in-hands, which had been slim throughout the Ivy League phase of the fifties and early sixties (a demure one and a half or two inches), now expanded to three or four inches — a width that had been popular in the thirties and forties (Figure 6). Patterns and colors were often bold and bright. The fad for combining patterned motifs sometimes reached excessive proportions — checked shirts with striped ties, polka dot shirts with floral ties, striped shirts with Op-art ties. Many men discarded ties entirely, and filled in the neckline of an open collar with a knotted scarf or ascot. Turtleneck sweaters and knit shirts attained a new popularity, not only for sports wear but for informal dress occasions. In 1967 and 1968 there was a brief fad for wearing very elegant turtleneck evening shirts of silk or nylon knit, especially made with French cuffs, for formal dress affairs (Figure 20). Bow ties were still in fashion — black for informal evening wear, white for formal evening dress.

Day Wear

The Ivy League silhouette that had prevailed through the late fifties was modified somewhat in the sixties by several different trends. Early in the decade President John F. Kennedy adopted a two-button suit that had somewhat more breadth in the shoulder, longer lapels, and more chest room and exposed more shirt and tie (Figure 7). This comfortable, trim, and easy fashion gained immediate acceptance as an adoring public followed the popular President's lead. Another influence came from England, with an upsurge in Edwardian styles when the Beatles toured America in 1964. Their clothes were designed by Pierre Cardin and featured slim, well-fitted suits, coats buttoned high (with four buttons), nipped-in waists, longer flared coattails, narrow trousers sometimes belled at the bottom, bright shirts, and wider ties (Figure 10). With these outfits they wore longer hair, bangs, sideburns, mustaches, and trainmen caps with visors.

In 1966 American designer Bill Blass rediscovered and promoted the "gangster suit" of the forties — double-breasted and broad-shouldered, with bold pinstripes (Figure 13). The silhouette was even more exaggerated than in the forties, more trimly fitted at the waistline, and sometimes worn with narrower trousers. This style was adopted by business men and bankers. The true gangsters of the era, the Mafia, clung to the conservative Ivy League look.

In 1968 the Nehru jacket, also known as the "Mao" or "cadet" jacket, made its appearance. It was a break from the traditional suit jacket with turnover collar and lapels. The Nehru had a standing collar, was buttoned up the front to the neckline, and was well fitted at the waistline (Figure 14). It proved to be a short-lived fad and disappeared after a year or two.

The young rebel group, bent on defying the "Establishment" by their unconventional dress, adopted blue jeans and sometimes bizarre or off-beat tops. Frequently they might have bare chests and bare feet, and usually they wore their hair long and flowing (Figure 15). *McCall's* presented this graphic picture of the hippie scene:

> Hippie garb follows a prescribed exotic pattern, and the males of the species, like birds, are infinitely more colorful than the females. They wear boots decorated with small brass bells, turtleneck jerseys, miscellaneous vests, opera cloaks, buckskin tunics, ponchos, tattered bits of fur. Triple and quadruple strands of seed beads, glass beads, wooden or plastic beads are a must and often hang entangled with amulets, crosses, Egyptian ankhs, religious medals or copper pendants. Tin buttons (the kind now familiar across the country) lauding peace, love and LSD are worn by everyone. A blanket, wrapped Geronimo style, or a long, hooded cloak may be added for warmth. Hippie tresses are often parted in the center in a style that sometimes looks like a Renaissance Jesus and sometimes, when a headband is worn across the brow, like Sitting Bull. An eighteen- or twenty-year-old hippie in full fig, glittering and jingling with the symbols of his faith, fingering a recorder or a guitar or holding a stick of burning incense in front of him as he walks solemnly toward you, is hard to believe.[3]

The following description comes from a news commentator visiting the Haight-Ashbury district in San Francisco:

> The best show on Haight Street is usually on the sidewalk in front of the Drog Store, a new coffee bar at the corner of Masonic Street, [which] features an all-hippy revue that runs day and night. . . . There will always be at least one man with long hair and sunglasses playing a wooden pipe of some kind. He will be wearing either a Dracula cape, a long Buddhist robe, or a Sioux Indian costume. There will also be a hairy blond fellow wearing a Black Bart cowboy hat and a spangled jacket that originally belonged to a drum major in the 1949 Rose Bowl parade. He will be playing the bongo drums. Next to the drummer will be a dazed-looking girl wearing a blouse (but no bra) and a plastic mini-skirt, slapping her thighs to the rhythm of it all.[4]

The gangs of motorcycle riders known as "Hell's Angels" appeared in the early sixties. They were tough, fast, and sadistic and traveled in packs. Their uniform was blue denim (Figure 16).

> The girls, with their chalk-white faces and dark glasses, wore Levis and boots and sawed-off jackets. The men wore the same carefully ratty uniform, but with decorations: wings, swastikas, Luftwaffe insignia, cloth

patches of a skull wearing a winged helmet, patches with the number '13' . . . the whole place had the ludicrous air of a costume party. . . . Nazi uniforms were worn [by some] only because they have become identified . . . with the license to band together, to push people around, to be somebody. . . . "When you walk into a place where people can see you, you want to look as repulsive as possible," said one Angel. . . . [5]

Evening Wear

Although a certain sector of the population clung to the traditional black-and-white formal wear that had been standard for dress occasions for more than a century, many men began to break away and express themselves in highly colorful evening attire (Figure 17). Red dinner jackets were popular; crushed velvet jackets appeared in jewel tones, such as burgundy, gold, and royal blue. Informal evening jackets might be made of batik or Mod prints or patterned cut velvet (Figure 18). They were usually worn with black evening trousers. Brilliantly colored formal dress shirts might be worn with a black dinner jacket. Shirts might also have ruffled fronts and cuffs. One novel style was the jump-suit combination for evening designed by Oscar de la Renta — a vest and trousers in one piece worn with a formal jacket (Figure 19). The Nehru jacket, with standing collar, also appeared for formal wear in white piqué or patterned fabrics. In 1968 fine white or black turtleneck sweaters with French cuffs were worn in place of the usual dress shirt (Figure 20). This rather radical departure from custom did not last very long and was flaunted only by the daring, but it created quite a furore while it was in vogue.

> While the girls were drawing attention to the legs, the men were getting it where they always get it in matters of fashion — in the neck. The turtleneck, long accepted by sailors and skiers and Dartmouth men, to say nothing of turtles, has arrived in urban night life. Led by a few nonconformists — chiefly actors, Picasso fans, people who don't have to deal with the chairman of the board and people who are chairman of the board — white turtlenecks have invaded the theater, nightclubs and other cultural areas, swathing in cotton or silk Adam's apples that would otherwise have chafed against black ties. . . . But they may be doomed by that reactionary, the *maitre d'*. A tie is still de rigueur at "21" and downstairs at Sardi's. And when Richard Harris, star of the film Camelot, tried to wear one in the Plaza's Oak Room, they wouldn't let him in.[6]

The relatively plain necklines of the Nehru jackets and the turtleneck sweaters led to the wearing of gold necklaces or chains and pendants (Figure 14). Other innovations in the evening scene were all-velvet suits, or suits in light colors, such as white, light blue, or yellow.

Sportswear

For active sports during the sixties, men wore much the same kind of clothes that had been in fashion for the preceding decade. Slacks, sport shirts, and sweaters were most commonly worn. Slacks were trim and not pleated at the waistline. Waistlines were relatively low-slung, "Western cut" or "hip-hugger" in style (Figures 4, 21). Blue jeans or Levi's were favored, particularly by the young, for work or all-purpose wear (Figure 22). Shirts were bright and colorful, often in bold stripes, plaids, checks, or prints. Wash-and-wear fabrics made laundry simple and easy. Many shirts now could be washed, hung up to drip dry, and worn without ironing. Knit shirts were popular and frequently came in slipover styles. Shorts for active sports came in varying lengths — quite short for tennis; medium-length, or "walking shorts," for dressier or spectator wear. Beach trunks came in many styles, trim and brief, of terry cloth, cotton madras, or jersey. A passion developed among the younger set for surfboarding, and its devotees formed a cult of the sun. The uniform for this sport was a pair of short beach trunks with a contrasting color for the waistband and cuffs (Figure 23). Swimming trunks might have matching shirts, and sometimes also cover-up robes, in "cabana sets" (Figure 24). Beach robes became more and more colorful, in brilliant prints and stripes, and appeared in various styles, including caftans, ponchos, and kimonos. Leisure suits for resort and beach wear featured loose, comfortable shirt-jackets with matching slacks, often in a bold and bright print (Figure 25).

For casual wear and leisure, some new styles appeared. One was the jump suit, a one-piece coverall neatly tailored in denim or finer fabrics (such as lightweight wool), buttoned or zipped up the front (Figure 26). Another casual style was the sleeveless belted jacket or jerkin, worn over a full-sleeved shirt (Figure 27).

The unlined blazer jacket was popular throughout the decade, in two- and three-button styles, lightweight and casual; it came in bright colors and in checks, plaids, and stripes. Sweaters were worn in profusion, patterned for country wear and skiing, in trim slipover models for more conservative wear (Figure 28), bulky knit varieties (Figure 29), and the perennially popular turtleneck for all occasions. The "layered look" was fashionable and was sometimes achieved by the addition of a turtleneck bib under the V-neck of a slipover sweater.

Coats and Wraps

For evening, the black Chesterfield was still the most-conservative and elegant coat. However, many men were substituting a good, dark overcoat or an unbelted, well-tailored black all-weather coat for this purpose. Men had rediscovered fur coats, and along with their turn toward opulence and luxury in other garments, were sporting coats of seal, mink, raccoon, Persian lamb, and chinchilla (Figure 30). Early in the decade, topcoats were still short and classic in cut; raglan tweeds and camel's hair were popular. In the mid-sixties, a vogue appeared for coats in black-and-white houndstooth check or herringbone tweed. As the Mod styles caught on, topcoats appeared with increasing flare and shaping. Late in the decade, Bill Blass introduced the longer top-coat in a mid-calf length (Figure 32), and as women adopted maxi-length coats, some men followed the trend with coats to the ankle.

Capes gained a new popularity, and some Mod outfits included a matching cape (Figure 11). The hippie crowd might wear opera capes or floor-length capes as part of their regalia.

For sports wear and country wear there were a great variety of short coats and jackets. The three-quarter-length car coat, or "subur-ban coat," was a favorite of the commuting crowd. A "ski look" was popular for country clothes, and many jackets had parka hoods or toggle closings (Figure 33). Some had fur collars or fur linings, while less-expensive models might have acrylic pile linings and collars. Sporty outer jackets of short-haired fur were also on the scene; one new model imported from Australia was made of kangaroo fur. Suede jackets were increasingly popular. All-weather coats and jackets were often made with zip-in linings for heavy weather.

Footwear

Footwear for men continued to include old favorites such as oxfords, ankle-high chukkas, and suede desert boots (Figure 33). Slip-ons gained in popularity and appeared in high-rise models that covered the instep. They might be trimmed with a chain decoration or a buck-led strap across the instep. Higher heels came into favor, and British designer Hardie Amies introduced an ankle-high boot with a heel that was underslung or pitched forward. In the middle of the decade, as sports coats and shirts burst forth in bright colors, suede shoes ap-peared in Easter egg shades, such as yellow, blue, and green. Boots were worn more and more frequently, not only for country and sports activities such as horseback and motorcycle riding, but in town. They were available in smooth leather, suede, or vinyl and came in assorted lengths — ankle-high, mid-calf, knee-high, or above the knee. Zipper closings made it possible to have them snugly fitted. The young Mods adopted boots, and so did the hippies when they weren't going barefoot. The rebel groups sometimes wore suede moccasins or soft suede knee-high boots with fringed cuffs. Late in the decade, shoes for both men and women went square-toed, heavy-soled and -heeled, and generally "clunky." Two-toned oxfords in black and white were still seen on the golf links or elsewhere. Tennis shoes went fanciful in color, sometimes multicolored. Red-white-and-blue shoes were popular as the "flag-spoofing" craze developed. Shoes were also made of Corfam, a new man-made material brought out by Du Pont that was shiny and similar to patent leather.

Jewelry for men was the most conspicuously expanded accessory of this decade. Hippies and college youths were the first to adopt the wearing of beads around the neck, which might be Indian beads, seed beads, chains, or leather thongs with pendants — peace symbols, Egyptian ankhs, amulets (often handmade) of metal or ceramic (Figures 14, 15). Late in the decade, when evening styles turned to turtleneck sweaters and Nehru jackets, the more-daring members of the Establishment also took to wearing gold neck chains and pendants, or chokers (Figure 20). Cuff links and tie tacks in novel styles were worn, some in brilliantly colored stones. Hippies festooned their lapels and chests with buttons asserting political views, such as "Make love, not war" and "Ban the bomb." They wore headbands of leather thongs or Indian beadwork. Macramé was a popular new hobby, and some adorned themselves with bibs or ponchos made of this knotted network of rope or leather thongs and wooden or ceramic beads.

Wristwatches, which had been small and self-effacing for many years (about one inch in diameter with a half-inch strap), now appeared in flamboyant styles, sometimes with colored faces, in bolder sizes and mounted on decorative leather or bright-colored plastic wristbands two or three inches wide. Sunglasses were worn as an exotic decoration as well as for protection. Frames were often quite heavy and innovative in shape — squares, hexagons, or extended ovals (Figure 25). There was also a return to old-fashioned thin gold metal frames for eyeglasses, reminiscent of the late nineteenth century.

Handkerchiefs worn in the breast pocket of a suit coat might be of dark patterned silk and coordinated with the color of the necktie. In the sixties the favored fold for the breast-pocket handkerchief showed no points but a billowing puff from the pocket. Silk scarves in colorful prints were frequently worn with an open collar on a sport shirt.

Wallets, money belts, and key cases of leather were carried in the hip pockets. Members of certain groups dedicated to "sharp dressing" might carry a clutch purse or a shoulder bag when their tight pants had no pockets (Figure 4). Men's belts also went innovative and might be as wide as four inches; or might be made of metal links or patterned fabric, trimmed with metal studs or beads; or might sport decorative buckles.

Gloves continued in perennial styles, worn now only for protection from cold weather. In addition to the usual knitted wool or leather models, some were made of synthetic materials, such as vinyl lined with acrylic pile.

In the sixties some men smoked small cigars or cigarillos instead of cigarettes.

The look for the women of the sixties might be variously characterized as "leggy," "mannish," "total" (meaning coordinated pattern and color from head to toe), "little girl," "costume," or "Unisex." Perhaps the designer who best expressed the spirit of the decade was Courrèges, with his glorification of the very young—his brief skirts, sculptured wools and knits, bold stripes, and dashing boots. The British model Twiggy embodied the Mod look and became the idol of fashion-conscious teen-agers with her boyish haircut, big eyes rimmed with painted-on eyelashes, exceedingly slender and flat-chested figure, and gangling grammar-school legs.

It was a decade of tremendous variety in clothing, running the gamut from ultrafeminine to starkly masculine, from Victorian demureness to daring near-nudity. It reached a point where life seemed to be one long costume party, with every woman for herself, and no wild getup was considered too startling or outrageous to be worn on the street. The younger set started haunting thrift shops and second-hand stores, pouncing with glee on quaint gowns from the twenties, thirties, and forties.

Hair Styles and Makeup

One of the most-typical coiffures for women in the sixties was hair worn long, straight, and flowing, undressed and untrammeled, and often uncombed (Figures 40, 47). Hair streamed out behind a girl running for a bus, or bounced and swung as she danced the Boogaloo. Often she peered out from behind a fringe of bangs or squinted with one eye as a long lock fell across the other. Straight hair was prized above curls, and if a girl's hair was naturally curly, she might use a straightener to correct that condition, or might lay her head on an ironing board and run a warm iron over her tresses to remove unwanted waves. Permanent waves no longer imparted a tight curl to the hair, but simply added "body" or made the hair more tractable and easier to set in huge, sculptured swirls or puffed-out bouffant styles. The hair was often back-combed ("ratted" or "teased") to give it added fullness. The bubble and beehive styles of the late fifties were still in evidence (Figures 38, 54, 57).

Wigs were worn increasingly and finally almost replaced hats. A good wig of human hair was still quite expensive, and might cost as much as $200, but wigs made of synthetic materials such as Dynel or modacrylic were available for the multitudes for as little as $5. Wigs came in all lengths, colors, and styles, from a short cap of ready-to-wear loose curls to a shoulder-length or longer hairpiece. The styling and dressing of wigs was a new and lucrative addition to the duties of the beauty operators. A variety of partial hairpieces might also be worn — wiglets, crowns of curls, braids, or chignons. New in the sixties was the "fall," a partial wig consisting of long locks matching one's own hair. It might be attached to the back of the head with a comb or tucked under a headband to give a shoulder-length or longer bob, or it could be piled up in ornamental curls on top of the head. With the rise to popularity of the French actress Brigitte Bardot, a tousled, uncombed, flyaway long bob became fashionable, particularly with teen-agers. In the same spirit was a hair-do that appeared late in the decade, "the washerwoman," wherein the hair was carelessly piled on top of the head, twisted into a bun on the crown, and left with curls escaping at the neckline.(Figure 45). *Vogue* described it thus, mentioning various other labels:

> Still adored in London, Paris, New York, is the *concièrge* hairdo also called the Brigitte Bardot, La Goulue, the Gibson Girl. Badly done, it is messy; properly done, enchanting — the hair pulled up cleanly off the face and nape of the neck with plenty of sag in back, the top-knot symmetrical, little tendrils escaping. . . . [7]

For evening, coiffures often rivaled some of the outlandish build-ups achieved in the eighteenth-century French court. One of the nuisances of theatre-going was the possibility of being seated behind one of these towering extravagances. Interesting effects were achieved with braids of all sizes, from very fat to very skinny, looped and entwined in novel coils and patterns (Figures 37, 61).

In mid-decade, hair styles by Vidal Sassoon caught the fancy of the young. They were short, exotic, geometric cuts in straight lines and angles, which seemed to go well with Mod fashions, mini-skirts, and boots (Figure 62). As the sixties ended, small heads were again in fashion, with hair skimmed back smoothly from the face and rolled into a neat bun at the back of the head. Also popular were short "porcupine" haircuts, layered cuts, or "blow" cuts that could be styled with a hand hair-dryer, and the very short clipped "little-boy" cuts (Figures 60, 82).

Makeup in the sixties continued in the subdued, "no makeup" look of the late fifties. Little rouge was worn, and lips were pale to the point of ghostliness, touched with soft, light pastel color or sometimes whitened. Eyes, however, might be quite heavily made-up. Eye shadows came in a wide range of colors — browns, blues, greens, or iridescent tones, also gold, silver, and copper. Eyes might be lined in a fashion reminiscent of ancient Egypt. The effect of pale lips and great, bruised eyes ringed with kohl achieved a somewhat dissipated, unhealthy look for the women of the decade, as though the poor creatures had been on a prolonged binge or a starvation diet. Evening makeup might be quite exotic, with sequins and iridescent eye shadow and nail polish, perhaps in gold, mauve, or olive green (the color of decay). The hippies and discothèque dancers also affected body paint as ornament. The fad is described in *Look*:

> The passion for painting faces and bodies has come straight out of psychedelia into the parlor. Hippies and their friends kicked it off by decorating feet, hands and faces with the kind of patterns they saw on psychedelic trips. They used ball-point or felt-tip pens plus what looks like a lot of barn paint to get sufficiently groovy effects. Then, last summer, the paste-on tattoo fad swept the beaches. At a few very nice parties . . . the society version of paint-ons appeared, with butterflies and flowers pointing up a pretty cheek or décolletage. And in the east Village, face-painting flashed to success at the Electric Circus, New York's most frenetic discothèque to date. If you're not switched on by the pulsating strobe lights, a monster ultra media light show on stretch-nylon ceilings and walls, cacophonic electronic music, rock 'n' roll groups, circus acts and dancers, you will be when you're painted for free by a gentle, dark-haired girl named Lydia. . . . [8]

Rhinestones might be applied in patterns with surgical adhesive; white paste-on flowers might adorn the body to go with a clown-white face and black-and-white fingernails.

Hat Styles

During the sixties, women tended to go hatless more often than not. As the wearing of wigs increased, hats seemed unnecessary, or simply would have demolished the elaborately styled and dressed coiffures. In 1970 the musical comedy star of *Company* inquired quizzically of the audience, "Does anybody still wear a hat?" The hats that did appear belonged to certain kinds of outfits. In the early sixties, the Jackie Kennedy pillbox was worn with a boxy suit. The sou'wester, with a swooping brim in back, was worn with a flaring coat (Figure 81). The cloche of the 1920s was resurrected to go with the drop-waisted twenties styles (Figure 59). The beret reappeared, ranging from a small "beanie" to a voluminous draped model (Figure 48). Hats of real or fake fur came in all shapes, sizes, and prices (Figure 85). The high derbies of the late fifties were still being worn. Billed caps topped off the Mod mini-skirt outfits, and might be made of fabric, fur, or vinyl (Figures 71, 83). The dashing big-brimmed hats reminiscent of Greta Garbo showed up once in a while, sometimes with brims turned back on the forehead. Straight-brimmed gaucho hats were worn with Latin fashions (Figure 72). Late in the decade, helmets like ski caps became popular, swathing the small, sleek heads and the necks, and leaving an opening for the face. Crocheted and knitted caps and berets also gained favor with the smaller head-treatments.

For evening wear, headbands were popular throughout the decade; they might be jeweled or beaded. Small ornamental hats were sometimes worn for evening — feathered caps, golden hoods or snoods, turbans or fez shapes.

Underwear, Loungewear, and Sleepwear

Two major shifts in styles for underclothing occurred during the sixties. The first was the discarding of brassieres. The "bra-less look" emerged with the Women's Liberation movement. Bras were burned in public demonstrations to symbolize women's new emancipation from old bonds and restrictions. For the slim and svelte figures this gesture of defiance sometimes enhanced their silhouettes with a softly curvaceous effect. But for the buxom and those with drooping bust lines, a general air of sloppiness and bovine bulges went along with their "liberation." In any event, the manufacturers of undergarments took proper notice of the trend and produced bras in soft, natural lines. Some were simply knitted camisole tops of nylon jersey.

In 1964 the second breakaway from old styles in underclothing occurred — the changeover from garter belts and girdles to panty hose. These sheer tights, made of stretch nylon from waistline to toe, which replaced panties, garter belts, and hose, became necessary to "cover the situation" when skirts rose well above the knees, indeed, barely covered the hips. For the figures that still needed some corseting and shaping, there were "panty girdles," longer two-way stretch girdles with panty legs. Another innovation was the "body stocking," a stretch suit (combination of tights and leotard) that covered the body from neck to toe. In flesh tones, it provided a gesture toward demureness as a base for near-nude fashions or the briefest of mini-skirts. In dark shades, it might serve as a backdrop for torso jewelry.

Panties were briefer than ever. Bikini styles which were little more than a G-string appeared on the market. Diminutive half-slips were designed to be worn under the shorter skirts. Lingerie became wildly colorful for those whose tastes ran in that direction. Bras, panties, and slips came in leopard prints, brilliant floral prints, or deep colors such as cerise, orange, or coffee.

Sleepwear showed much variety, from the traditional floor-length gown to very brief bikini shorts worn with a flaring tunic top. "Baby-doll" pajamas combined short bloomer panties with a hip-length top (Figure 34). "Toreadoll" pajamas had mid-calf-length pants. Waltz-length gowns came just below the knee. Shorter nighties appeared in above-the-knee lengths. Combination sets of peignoir and nightgown were popular, either waltz-length or floor-length (Figure 35).

For lounging, there were robes in many styles. Some were fitted with a princesse line; some gathered in on a drawstring at an Empire waistline; some tent-shaped or flaring. Some buttoned up the front, and some had a long zippered front closing. There was a fad for making loose robes out of brightly colored fringed bath towels, long or short. The knee-length duster was popular, loose and flaring and buttoned up the front. Caftans and muumuus were worn for lounging as well as for informal hostess and evening wear (Figures 36, 37). Tapered capri slacks were popular for "at-home" wear early in the decade (Figure 38). Later in the sixties pants legs grew wider; "palazzo pajamas" as full as evening skirts became fashionable (Figure 39).

Day Wear

Hemlines during the sixties rose and fell; they stood just below the knee in 1961, hovered just at knee height in 1964, went soaring upward to break all previous records in brevity from 1966 through the end of the decade — mini-skirts and micro-mini-skirts were three to eight inches above the knee (Figures 40, 41, 42). In 1970, just as it appeared that skirts might vanish altogether, the trend reversed, with midi-skirts at mid-calf length (Figures 43, 44, 45) and maxi-skirts at ankle length (Figure 46). Early in the decade, the chemise or shift was still much in evidence (Figure 47). These models were loose and easy, but better fitted than the sack of the late fifties. The A-line, or skimmer, flared gently over the hips (Figure 49). Waistlines, when indicated, ranged from a high Empire to below the waist. Sometimes an Empire waistline in front dipped low in back and often was loosely belted in back. Pleated skirts and hip-length blouses recalled the flavor of the twenties. Suits with boxy jackets continued to be popular (Figure 50). There was a brief rediscovery of deep dolman, or "bat-wing," sleeves. Knitted fabrics were worn more and more frequently, since they needed no ironing. Knitted suits (Figure 44) or the perennial shirtwaist style made excellent traveling outfits. Knitted sweater-dresses and T-shirt dresses shaped like tubes were popular; they were frequently in bold horizontal stripes and had turtlenecks.

Evening Wear

Evening wear during the sixties reflected the great variety in styles that prevailed, running the gamut from mini- to floor-length and from the traditional (Figures 51, 52, 53) to the kookie. Early in the decade brocade theatre suits were popular, with straight, pencil-slim skirts slit up the side, front, or back (Figure 54). Full-length straight sheaths without jackets were also worn for evening. Some had an overdrape resembling a Roman toga, or a sheer caftan topping the sheath, or were worn with a matching floor-length coat (Figure 55). Another fashion was full and flowing, swinging free from the shoulders and similar to a Hawaiian muumuu (Figures 36, 56). The early sixties also saw Empire waistlines for formal gowns, with full skirts gathered in softly under a high, fitted bustline. About mid-decade "cage," or "tent," dresses in sheer or see-through fabrics or wide-meshed nets were very popular; they were worn over form-fitting narrow sheaths (Figure 57). Short formals, knee-length or mini-length, were favored for dinner and theatre (Figures 58, 59) as well as for discothèque dancing (Figures 60, 61, 62). In mid-decade, a recapitulation of thirties styles brought halter necklines and backs bared to the waist. One-shoulder styles appeared throughout the sixties (Figure 63). A new departure reflecting the temper of the sixties was the deep décolletage, with the front neckline plunging to the waist or lower, the breasts "barely covered." Other daring models for evening were sheer or see-through blouses or tunics that revealed the unclad form beneath. With the development of the "costume look," formal wear might draw inspiration from any part of the world — harem bloomers from the Near East (Figure 64), gypsy styles from Central Europe (Figure 46), Oriental cheongsams (Figure 38), or nostalgic demurely feminine ruffles and flounces from Victorian days (Figure 65). Even as pants suits and jump suits took over for day-time wear, they also appeared at elegant dinner parties and theatre openings, in fine fabrics such as satin, velvet, lamé, or sequined knits (Figures 66, 67, 68). Full and flowing "palazzo pajamas" or loose caftans might be worn to formal events as well as for entertaining at home (Figures 37, 39).

Sportswear   For sports wear, two-piece outfits predominated in the sixties. Sweaters, blouses, or shirts were worn with skirts, slacks, or blue jeans; and pants suits were frequently seen (Figures 69, 70, 71). About 1967 gaucho pants were worn in town as well as for country and sports (Figure 72). Slacks were made of stretch fabric and tapered to the ankle; later in the decade they might have wide legs or be belled at the bottom. In mid-decade skirts and slacks might have a low waistline that rode on the hips, called "hip-hugger" models (Figure 73). The one-piece jump suit was worn at any time of day in denim or corduroy for sports, or in satin, jersey, or crepe for lounging or evening wear (Figure 66). Shorts continued to be popular for active sports. Longer "walking shorts" seemed to be favored early in the decade. Late in 1970 a brief fad arrived for extremely brief shorts labeled "Hot Pants" (Figure 74). They were worn everywhere — even to formal parties. *Life* reported:

> An improbable fad arrived in midwinter. They're called Hot Pants, Short Shorts, Cool Pants, Shortcuts or simply Les Shorts — and in no time they have captured the fashion scene. Augmented by tights or body stockings and boots, hot pants are everywhere, winter winds or not. In Paris, London and New York, department stores can't stock them fast enough. And their eager acceptance by designers from the smallest boutique to the

highest couture means that hot pants will be around for a while. "They are the sort of fad," said a European fashion observer, "that topples institutions."[9]

As skirts descended to midi-length or maxi-length, late in the era, midi-skirts and maxi-coats might be worn partially unbuttoned to reveal short shorts or mini-skirts beneath.

Blue jeans were typical garments of the sixties. They became the uniform of college youth and hippies of both sexes. The preferred jeans were made of worn and faded blue denim, not new and shiny (Figure 75). Ragged hems were admired. Thrift shops were scoured for properly aged blue jeans, and old ones were prized more than new models. Long jeans might be cut off to short lengths, with the hemlines left fringed or tattered.

For beach wear and swimming, the microscopic bikini was still favored (Figures 76, 77). These two-piece suits consisted of the briefest of bras and panties that were little more than a G-string. The navel, long hidden, came out of seclusion and saw the sunlight along with the rest of the body. Rudi Gernreich, designer for the young and daring, came out with a topless bathing suit in 1966; it was a one-piece suit with thin shoulder straps that left the bosom exposed. The fad received much publicity and created a sensation, but was actually rarely worn. One-piece cutaway suits added novelty to the beach scene and appeared more often (Figures 78, 79). Beach cover-ups came in a great variety of tunics, wrap-around robes, shifts, ponchos, and caftans. High fashion for the ski lodge is shown in Figure 80.

Coats and Wraps

Coats in general followed the lines in dresses and showed much variety. The free-swinging, often voluminous tent coat was popular throughout the decade (Figure 81). Another model was the semifitted coat, fuller and loosely belted in back. There were three-quarter- or seven-eighths-length coats, fitted or A-line, often worn over matching skirts or dresses. Early in the decade, coat sleeves might be bell-shaped, somewhat short or three-quarter-length, and were worn with gloves. Some coats were shaped like cocoons and had deep dolman sleeves. Short car coats were worn with slacks in the suburbs and country and for traveling. As skirts lengthened at the end of the decade, the maxi-coat gained immediate popularity, particularly with the very young and the Mod dressers (Figure 82). Raincoats and all-weather coats came out in exotic and bold patterns and were worn for all occasions (Figures 83, 84). When the motion picture *Dr. Zhivago* appeared in 1968, there was a flurry of Russian Cossack coats on the scene, midi-skirted and fur-trimmed (Figure 85). There were military coats with epaulettes and brass buttons. There was a belted coat in a "safari" style with four big pockets, similar to a trench coat. Fur coats and fake-fur coats were more popular than ever. The new awareness of ecology and conservation led some women to substitute fake furs for real fur as a matter of principle.

Footwear

In the early sixties, shoes were elongated and slender, with toes sharply pointed and heels that were needle thin, ranging in height from one to four inches. Women wearing these absurd stiletto heels teetered and tottered on insufficient support and frequently got their heels caught in the sidewalk gratings or floor vents.

As skirts went up above the knees, shoe styles shifted radically to flatter heels. Footwear soon took on a grammar-school look, with sturdy low heels and rounded or squared-off toes. Even party and formal shoes came with lower, sturdier heels. Patent leather Mary Janes with straps came out of the nursery to be worn by older girls. Low-heeled slip-ons with high tongues appeared, sometimes with a chain or a buckled strap across the instep. Later in the decade, pants suits called for another kind of shoe — sturdier, heavier, and low, with square toes and clunky heels.

Boots were the biggest news of the decade in women's footwear. Legs gained a place in the spotlight with the advent of mini-skirts, and boots began to be adopted for street wear or for any and all occasions (Figures 71, 73, 74, 83, 85). They came in all styles, from ankle-high to mid-calf, knee-high, or hip-high, with low heels or Cuban heels, in slip-on models or closely fitted with laces or zippered closings. The emerging sexless "pageboy" look for boys and girls — tights, tunic, and high boots — seemed to go well with the new Space Age. A popular song of the era stated, "These boots are made for walkin' and that's just what they'll do." The stance for this period was masculine and leggy, with feet planted firmly and wide apart and hands on hips.

Hosiery also gained a new importance in this era, which was focused on legs. New stretch fibers made hosiery, tights, and panty hose adjustable to a range of sizes. Mini-skirts led to the wearing of knee-high hose in vivid colors or patterns. Tights also came in patterns and high colors. About mid-decade there was a fad for complete coordination — "the total look" — where the same bold pattern might be carried throughout the costume, in sweater or tunic, tights or knee-hose, boots, and cap (Figure 86). Hosiery or panty hose appeared in printed or woven patterns, in lace, with ornamental clocks, multicolored, jeweled, or of metallic silver or gold thread for evening wear.

Accessories

Jewelry went wild, along with the other facets of style. Necklaces and earrings were exceedingly long and extravagant. Ropes of pearls or beads were sometimes long enough to be wound around the neck several times. At mid-decade elaborate bibs made of pearls or metal loops might cover the bosom. About 1967 there was a fad for "body jewelry," a network of ornaments worn over a body suit, leotard, or turtleneck sweater (Figure 61). Several costume rings might be worn at the same time on various fingers. Bracelets were exotic and large; serpent bracelets were popular. Toes might be ornamented with jeweled sandals or rings. At the end of the decade the "dog collar" was back in fashion, an ornamental choker that fit snugly around the neck.

The wrist-length gloves of the fifties lengthened to six- or eight-button lengths to be worn with the three-quarter-length coat sleeves of the early sixties. Purses tended to be larger than in preceding years. Handbags were frequently made of plastic, particularly a shiny soft vinyl with "the wet look." Shoulder-bags gained a new popularity; the bag rested high under the arm early in the decade, but with longer straps it hung almost to the mini-skirt hemline late in the era. Colorful snake and lizard bags were designed to match shoes. Tapestry prints and bright-colored kid were also in evidence.

Belts became very ornamental during this period. Buckles might be large and decorative, or the belt might be made of colorful leather or plastic; or it might be metal-studded, jeweled, or beaded. Chain belts became popular; and when body jewelry came into vogue, it was expanded into multichains to form a wide girdle about the waistline or hip (Figures 46, 66, 67).

Scarves were another bright and colorful accessory for the sixties. They might be squares, triangles, or long rectangles of various sizes. They might be tied around the neckline, waist, or hip or worn as a bandeau to confine fly-away hair. Macramé, the art of knot-tying, appeared in decorative belts, vests, and chokers. Sunglasses were often exotic, with heavy, bold frames in geometric shapes, sometimes jeweled, often in high colors. Women's wristwatches also attained exaggerated size, often with wide bands.

CHILDREN'S FASHIONS

Clothes for children during the sixties reflected the trends in adult styles. Little girls wore straight shifts or chemise dresses; but they also wore the perennial full gathered skirts attached to fitted bodices or shoulder yokes. Pinafores were more popular than ever (Figure 87). There were tent, or pyramid, dresses for little people as well as for their mothers. Sometimes the small tents were covered with flaring pyramid pinafores. The short skirts of tiny tots grew shorter than ever. As their legs showed more, they too adopted stretch tights in bright colors to replace short socks and bloomers. Danskin tights and leotards were no longer the special attire of ballet dancers, but became staples of the everyday wardrobe for young and old. For small girls, there was a vogue in mid-decade for party dresses made of black velvet with white lace trim. Quaint "granny dresses" in floral prints, with ruffled ankle-length hems, were worn for dressing up, at parties or playtime, by teen-agers as well as little tots. Jumpers were very popular throughout these years.

Little boys still wore Eton suits for dressing up (Figure 87). Blazer jackets in bright colors, plaids, or stripes were coordinated with slacks. Long pants for both boys and girls were worn increasingly, even by the preschool set. As fashions changed through the decade, pants styles varied from slim tapered slacks to straight line to bell bottoms. There were some low-slung hip-hugger models in skirts and pants. When the Nehru jackets arrived on the scene for adults late in the decade, these jackets with standing collars were also available in pants suits for boys and girls.

Boots were worn by both boys and girls — in ankle-high or knee-high models. White ankle boots were very fashionable for well-dressed little girls in Mod outfits. Knee-high hose were often brightly colored or patterned. The "total look," or coordinated patterns, in hose or tights and leotards or sweaters also appeared in children's clothing.

Long hair with bangs was a prevailing style for both boys and girls. Even in grammar school, it was increasingly hard to tell the boys from the girls.

TYPICAL MATERIALS, COLORS, MOTIFS, AND TRIMMINGS

New fabrics continued to appear throughout the sixties. Some of the old familiar materials, such as untreated cotton percale and linen, almost disappeared from the market. Denim, however, the old standby fabric for work and play clothing, took over as the preferred fabric of the decade. Most fabrics by now were at least partly synthetic and processed to be wrinkle-resistant or permanently pressed. Wools in the sixties appeared in very sheer weaves, and many had novel surface textures or were printed in brilliant patterns. Stretch fabrics were available in a great variety of textures and colors as well as striped, patterned, or plain. Double knits and bonded knits were much used for suits and coats, for men as well as women. In 1968 Du Pont came out with Qiana, a new silklike synthetic fabric, very soft and drapey. New novelty fabrics often had three-dimensional textured surfaces — ridged, puffed, or blistered. Cut velvet and crushed velvet provided interesting and handsome variety for formal wear. For evening there were very opulent glitter fabrics — metallic knits, sheer nylon brocades, gold and silver lamés in very soft and draping textures, jeweled chiffons, beaded or sequined crepes, and novelty laces. Late in the sixties wide-mesh nets became available, with half-inch or larger openings. These nets were popular for making cage, or tent, dresses; filmy chiffon and laces were also used for tent styles. Vinyl was much used for entire garments or for trim on coats, raincoats, skirts, caps, boots, and bags. Fur was everywhere, from coat linings to lounging pajamas. For the woman who had everything — and who could afford it — there was a mink jump suit. For the ecology-minded there was fake fur to help preserve the animal population. The imitation furs were such good copies that it was hard to tell a fake-fur coat from a real one. In addition to faithful reproductions of leopard, zebra, or lamb, the synthetic furs might be frankly "fake," appearing in exotic colors such as hot pink, orange, or purple, or might be printed in Op-art patterns. Suede and leather were used throughout the decade. Coats, vests, jackets, and skirts were made of suede or suede cloth as well as smooth soft leathers. Leather and suede were also used as trim in combination with wools or knits or finer fabrics such as crepe. The admired "bulky look" in suits, coats, and sweaters was achieved by such materials as mohair, heavy tweed, brushed wool, and bouclé. New stretch fibers made hosiery, tights, and panty hose adjustable to a range of sizes. In the sixties new styles and patterns in hose included brighter colors, lacy knits, wide-mesh knits, tights woven or printed in patterns matching tunics, knee-high hose in bulky knits or in patterns matching skirts or entire mini-skirted outfits.

Colors for the sixties were brilliant and often unexpected. Early in the decade patterns were going wild, veering toward high contrast, bold stripes, and geometric designs. Under an Art Nouveau influence fabrics became even wilder, with shocking color combinations, eye-jarring patterns in intricate curlicues, large-scale floral or abstract motifs, or Pop-art spot designs. Off-beat combinations of color were used, such as pink with brown, dark red with bright orange, dark green with pale blue, orange with pink. The parti-coloring of the medieval era reappeared, with two-tone treatments of divided sections of coats, dresses, tunics, or trousers. Red-white-and-blue combinations were popular for both men and women, with various arrangements of stars and stripes. Black and white was much used; so was black and yellow. Dresses were relatively simple in this era, depending more on beautiful fabric or combinations of fabric than on intricate cut or applied trimmings.

Big, bold, splashy prints were in evidence throughout the decade. The colors were wild, like something seen on a psychedelic trip or an Op-art design in jumpy geometric eye-tricking patterns. Stripes, checks, and plaids appeared in a "blown-up" and giant scale. When the "total look" was admired in mid-decade, identical prints might appear on a silk or cotton under-tunic, on a chiffon overblouse, on patterned tights, and on boots. Similarly, the same pattern might be applied to a vinyl raincoat, cap, and boots. Emillio Pucci, the Italian designer, came out with exotic floral or geometric prints in jewel-toned silks and synthetics, much used for palazzo pajamas and lounging attire. Multiple patterns were often combined, such as stripes and polka dots, or floral prints and plaid. Crazy-quilt patterns gained popularity at the end of the era, either printed or actually made of scraps sewn together in patchwork. There was a fad for tie-dyed patterns, in bleached-out blue jeans, in splotchy T-shirts, and even in crushed-velvet evening gowns.

Trimmings were elegant and voluptuous. A vogue for jeweled band trimming at necklines, cuffs, or hemlines prevailed in mid-decade. Bands of fur or ostrich plumes might edge a short formal hemline or a chiffon cape. Designs were applied to fabric surfaces with nailhead studs, sequins, beads, or paillettes. Fringe was rediscovered as a finishing touch for hemlines, sleeves, and ends of stoles.

SUGGESTIONS FOR COSTUMING PLAYS IN THE PERIOD

The word for costume in the sixties might be "anything goes." Several rock musicals from the period would require a hippie flavor for costuming. Hair styles for both men and women should be longer than in previous periods of the twentieth century. Men are quite likely to wear beards or mustaches. There should be an Edwardian flare to the suits of well-dressed men. Women of any age or station might appear in well-tailored pants suits on almost any occasion, particularly late in the decade. Patterns for these recently worn models are still available in yard goods shops or thrift shops. Boots and mini-skirts are the badge of the woman who is under thirty, dashing, or young in heart.

TITLE	AUTHOR	PERIOD
After the Fall	Arthur Miller	1940s; 1960s
Applause (M)	Comden, Green, Strouse, Adams	1970
Barefoot in the Park	Neil Simon	1963
Boys in the Band	Mart Crowley	1968
Butterflies Are Free	Leonard Gershe	1969
Ceremonies in Dark Old Men	Lonne Elder III	1969
Child's Play	Robert Marasco	1970
Come Blow Your Horn	Neil Simon	1961
Company (M)	Stephen Sondheim, George Furth	1970
A Delicate Balance	Edward Albee	1965
Do I Hear a Waltz?(M)	Richard Rodgers, Stephen Sondheim	1965
The Effect of Gamma Rays	Paul Zindel	1970
Godspell (M)	J. M. Tebelak, S. Schwartz	1971
Hair (M)	G. Ragni, J. Rado, G. MacDermot	1968
Hallelujah, Baby! (M)	Laurents, Styne, Comden, Green	1900–1960s
Happy Birthday, Wanda June	Kurt Vonnegut, Jr.	1970
The Homecoming	Harold Pinter	1967
The House of Blue Leaves	John Guare	1965
How to Succeed in Business (M)	Frank Loesser, Abe Burrows	1961
In the Matter of J. Robert Oppenheimer	Heinar Kipphardt, Ruth Speirs	1969
The Killing of Sister George	Frank Marcus	1966
Last of the Red Hot Lovers	Neil Simon	1969
Little Me (M)	Neil Simon, Carol Leigh, Cy Coleman	1962
Luv	Murray Schisgal	1964
Milk and Honey (M)	Jerry Herman, Don Appell	1961
No Strings (M)	Richard Rodgers, Samuel Taylor	1962
The Odd Couple	Neil Simon	1965
Oh Dad, Poor Dad	Arthur L. Kopit	1962
On a Clear Day You Can See Forever (M)	Alan Jay Lerner, Burton Lane	1965
Play It Again, Sam	Woody Allen	1969
Plaza Suite	Neil Simon	1968
Promises, Promises (M)	N. Simon, B. Bacharach, H. David	1969
Sleuth	Anthony Shaffer	1970
Slow Dance on the Killing Ground	William Hanley	1962
Sweet Charity (M)	D. Fields, C. Coleman, N. Simon	1966
A Thousand Clowns	Herb Gardner	1962
Tiny Alice	Edward Albee	1965
Vanities	Jack Heifner	1963, 1974
Wait Until Dark	Frederick Knott	1966
What the Butler Saw	Joe Orton	1970
When You Comin' Back, Red Ryder?	Mark Medoff	late 1960s
Who's Afraid of Virginia Woolf?	Edward Albee	1962

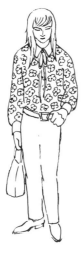

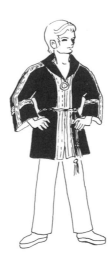

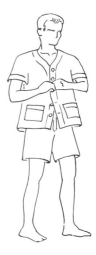

1. Africa: dashiki tunic in bright African print; Afro hair style. 1970.

2. Israel: short purple caftan with orange braid trim; orange slacks. 1969.

3. Knee-length pajamas of Dacron and cotton for summer wear. 1964.

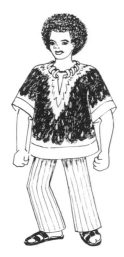

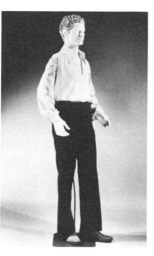

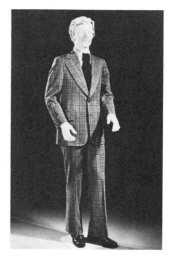

4. "Mod" British style from Carnaby Street: floral body shirt; Western-cut trousers; hand bag. 1966.

5. Purple and blue plaid trousers; white crepe "Tom Jones" shirt with lace sleeves and deep slit at front neckline; purple suede shoes. Worn in Washington, D.C., 1967. (Division of Costume, Smithsonian Institution.)

6. Two-piece suit of brown plaid polyester knit (fabric made of DuPont fiber); single-breasted, two-button jacket. By Phoenix Clothes, 1972. (Division of Costume, Smithsonian Institution.)

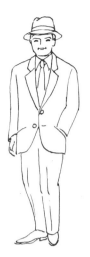

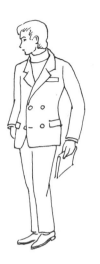

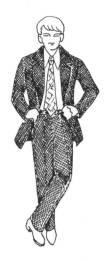

7. "J. F. Kennedy look":
two button suit; snap-brim hat.
1962.

8. Navy blue blazer jacket with
gold buttons; gray double-knit
slacks. 1964.

9. Printed corduroy suit in
red-and-black diagonal checks.
1969.

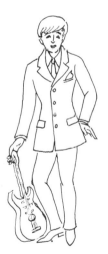

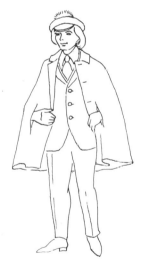

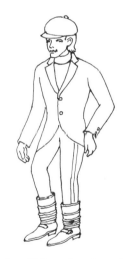

10. "Beatles" suit in fitted and
flared Edwardian style. By Pierre
Cardin, 1964.

11. Suit with matching cape;
vest; tapered trousers; billed cap.
1968.

12. "Mod" French style: suit,
cap, and boots by Pierre Cardin.
1966.

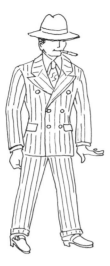

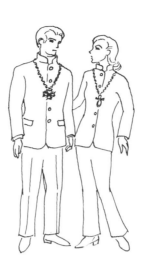

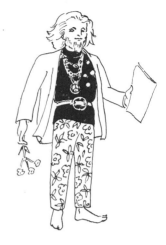

13. "Gangster suit" by Bill Blass: double-breasted, wide lapels, pinstripes. 1969.

14. His 'n her pants suits, unisex style: Nehru jackets; necklaces. 1968.

15. San Francisco "hippie" in floral print jeans; multiple beads and lapel buttons; long hair; beard. 1967.

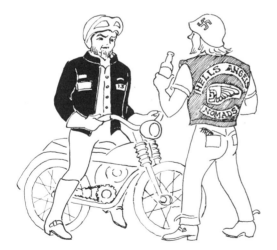

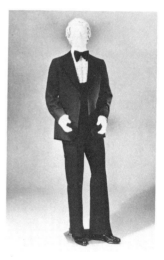

16. Left, motorcyclist in black leather jacket; boots. Right, "Hell's Angel" in denim jacket; Nazi helmet. 1965.

17. Three-piece formal suit: maroon trousers and jacket; black velvet vest; white ruffled shirt with maroon trim; large velvet bow tie. By After Six, 1974. (Division of Costume, Smithsonian Institution.)

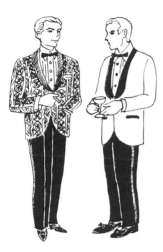

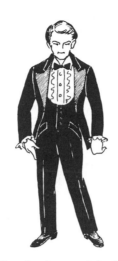

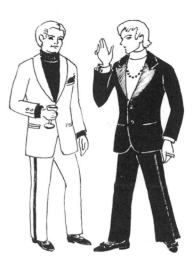

18. Left, batik dinner jacket for summer and resort wear. Right, host coat of gold velvet with black satin shawl collar. 1962.

19. Evening jump suit by Oscar de la Renta; ruffled evening shirt. 1970.

20. Turtleneck sweaters and shirts with French cuffs for evening wear. 1967 – 68.

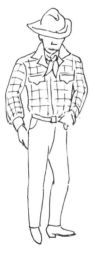

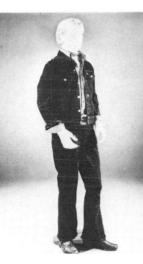

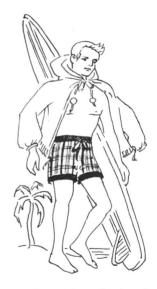

21. Western-style plaid shirt, jeans, and boots. 1965.

22. Levi's outfit: blue denim trousers and jacket; blue chambray workshirt. By Levi Strauss and Company, 1974. (Division of Costume, Smithsonian Institution.)

23. Surfer trunks; nylon beach parka with zippered front. 1964.

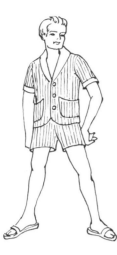

24. Cotton-Dacron shirt with matching trunks for poolside wear. 1961.

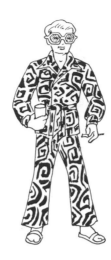

25. Slack suit with shaped body shirt, in cotton print for resort wear. 1970.

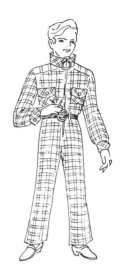

26. Jump suit in brown and tan checked wool with zipper front closing. 1968.

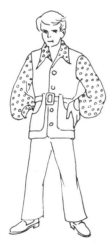

27. Polyster knit suit with sleeveless tunic; shirt of polka-dot voile. 1970.

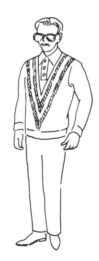

28. Italian pullover sweater in two-toned red, patterned weave. 1964.

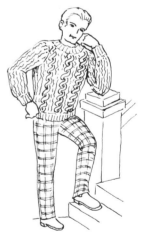

29. Bulky cable-knit sweater with crew neck, for sport and college wear. 1966.

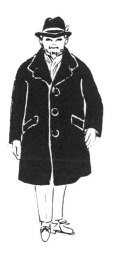

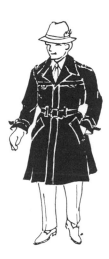

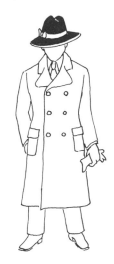

30. Fur coat of black Alaska seal with flap pockets; velour hat. 1962.

31. Raincoat of dark blue Dacron polyester with gold buckle trim. 1961.

32. Midi-length outer coat; matching slacks; black-and-white hat. 1970.

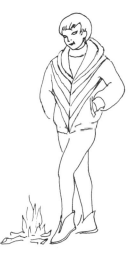

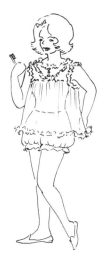

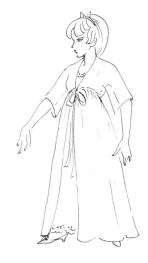

33. Reversible ski parka of nylon taffeta and Orlon pile; suede boots. 1963.

34. Sheer baby-doll pajamas with short bloomer panties and loose tunic top. 1961.

35. Negligee of printed nylon chiffon with Empire waistline. 1965.

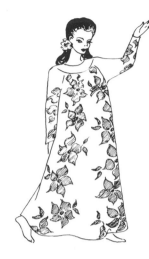

36. Hawaii: long muumuu of polished cotton in large floral print. 1962.

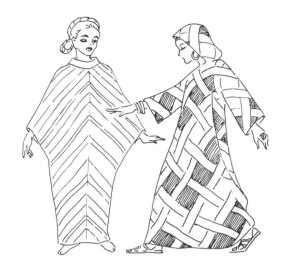

37. Flowing robes for lounging, beach, or evening from the Middle East. Left, caftan of striped rayon. Right, hooded djellaba, or burnoose, of bold print. 1967.

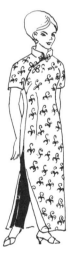

38. China: long brocade sheath with frog closings; slim, tapered slacks. 1964.

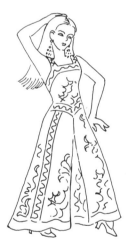

39. "Palazzo pajamas" for evening of exotic silk print. By Emilio Pucci, 1969.

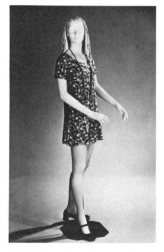

40. Multicolored printed acetate mini-skirt and overblouse with scoop neck and short sleeves. Worn in Washington, D. C., 1969. (Division of Costume, Smithsonian Institution.)

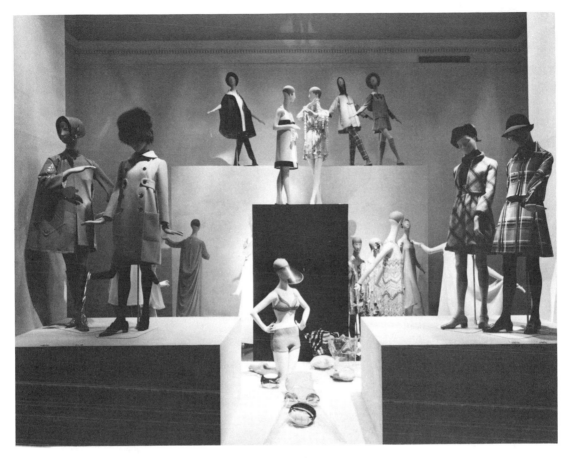

41. Women's Fashions of the 1960s (1967).

Lower level, left to right: Costume in red vinyl. By Anne Fogarty.   Red wool coat with black buttons. By Norman Norell.   Bikini of purple wool knit. By Thomas Brigance.   Long evening dress of sequined printed silk. By Mollie Parnis. Suit of red-and-blue blanket plaid; teal-blue jersey blouse. By Louis Clausen. Ensemble: dress, vest, and belt of bright-red plaid wool with large overcheck of navy blue, green, and yellow. By James Galanos.

Upper level, left to right: Short day ensemble: bright-red wool gabardine dress and black wool cape. By Don Simonelli.   Daytime dress: cerise and white double-knit wool with black velvet bands. By Bob Bugnand.   Mini-dress of Japanese printed silk; very long earrings. By Rudi Gernreich.   Sports costume: canvas coat with red-and-blue plaid wool lining; matching plaid wool slacks; hooded jersey blouse. By Bonnie Cashin.   Ensemble: mini-dress of black-and-gray checked jersey with matching accessories. By Rudi Gernreich.   Hat by Layne Nielson for Rudi Gernreich.

(The Costume Institute of The Metropolitan Museum of Art.)

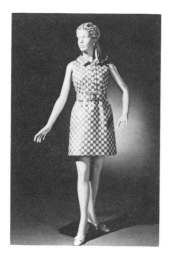

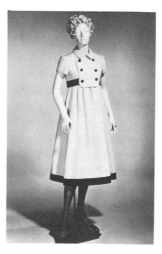

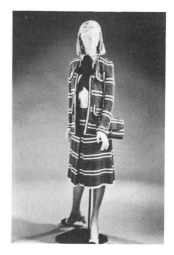

42. Sleeveless mini-dress of aqua-and-white polka-dot woven pattern; front-button closure; zipper closure in back; self-belt with buckle. Worn in Washington, D. C. By T. Jones, 1968 – 69. (Division of Costume, Smithsonian Institution.)

43. Midi-length dress of yellow piqué: raised waistline, bib front, black satin ribbon around waist and hem. By Geoffrey Beene, 1969. (Division of Costume, Smithsonian Institution.)

44. Two-piece suit of black-and-white wool knit trimmed with white-and-gold braid; inverted pleat in center front of skirt; elastic waist. By Adolfo, 1974. (Division of Costume, Smithsonian Institution.)

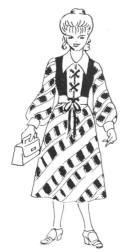

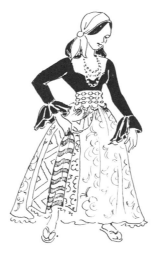

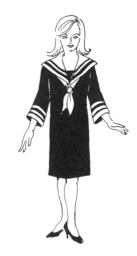

45. Midi-skirted peasant dress by Oscar de la Renta; "washerwoman" hairstyle. 1970.

46. Gypsy: multilayered brilliant skirt; purple blouse; coin-link girdle. 1970.

47. Shift middy dress of navy blue knit; white sailor collar and cuffs. 1964.

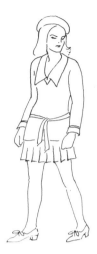

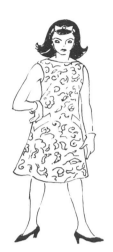

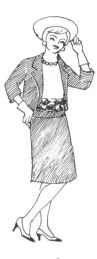

48. "Gangster moll" style: 1930s revival adapted to mini-skirts; beret. 1968.

49. A-line town dress of floral-print linen; wrist-length gloves. 1962.

50. Jacket suit of spun rayon with linen texture; short-sleeved blouse. 1964.

51. Upper level: Left, long evening dress of lavender-gray and silver sequins. By George Halley, 1967. Center, long evening dress of brown-and-white guinea hen and beige ostrich feathers on beige chiffon. By Donald Brooks, 1967. Right, long evening dress of gray wool banded with rhinestones. By Geoffrey Beene, 1967. Lower level, oyster-white wool coat with brown branch pattern. By Bill Blass, 1967. Matching hood by Mr. John. (The Costume Institute of The Metropolitan Museum of Art.)

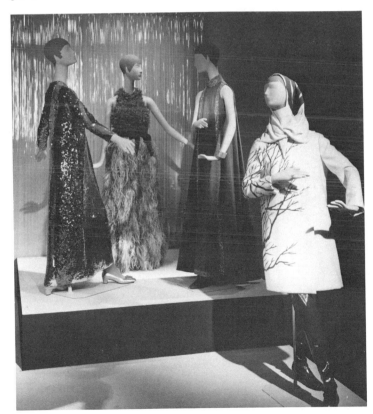

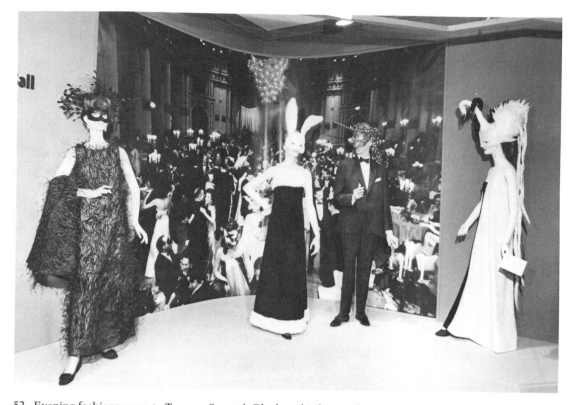

52. **Evening fashions worn to Truman Capote's Black-and-White Ball, New York, 1966.** Left, black organza gown and stole covered with black feathers; black feather headdress. By Halston of Bergdorf Goodman for Carol Bjorkman. Center, black velvet strapless gown edged in white mink; white mink bunny mask. By Halston of Bergdorf Goodman for Candice Bergen. Right, black-and-white wool jersey ball gown. By Galanos for Mrs. Frederick Eberstadt. Man's black evening suit by Brooks Brothers for Howard Olian; silver-and-black unicorn headdress by Gene Moore of Tiffany for William Baldwin. Background photo by Elliot Erwitt. (Museum of the City of New York. Gifts of Richard L. and John M. Burkman, Candice Bergen, Frederick Eberstadt, Howard Olian, and William Baldwin.)

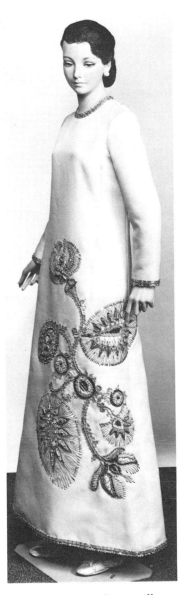

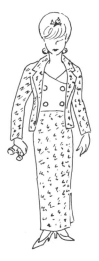

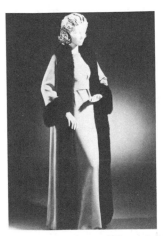

54. Brocade theatre suit with slit skirt; sleeveless satin blouse. 1965.

55. Evening dress of "hot pink" silk crepe in Empire style with self belt. Matching coat trimmed with mink. By Norman Norell, 1967. (Division of Costume, Smithsonian Institution.)

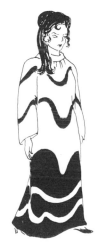

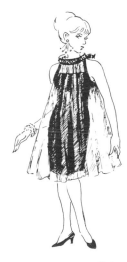

53. Dinner dress of ivory silk twill embroidered with gold and green beads, sequins, plastic, and silk floss. By Christian Dior, 1968. (Museum of the City of New York. Gift of the Duchess of Windsor.)

56. Black-and-white "op-art" print crepe evening dress by Bill Blass. 1967.

57. "Cage," or "tent," dance dress: sheer black chiffon over sheath; jeweled neckband. 1966.

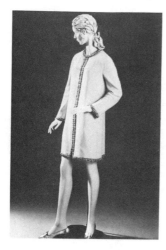

58. Short evening dress of yellow crepe in coat style with hidden front zipper. Trimmed with heavy beading of "turquoise" and rhinestones; front and back yokes and sleeves are cut in one piece. Worn in New York City. By Oscar de la Renta, 1966. (Division of Costume, Smithsonian Institution.)

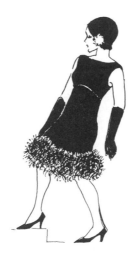

59. Dinner dress of black silk crepe with ostrich hem; cloche hat. 1961.

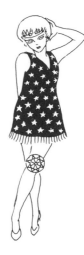

60. "Flag-spoofing" dance dress in dark blue with white stars; red tights. 1967.

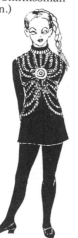

61. Silver body jewelry over black silk jersey shirt; wool mini-skirt. 1969.

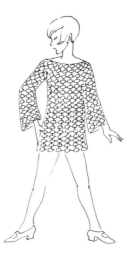

62. Plastic disc dress from "do-it-yourself" kit; Sassoon haircut. 1968.

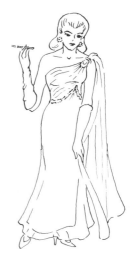

63. One-shoulder evening gown of silk chiffon with jeweled bodice trim. 1962.

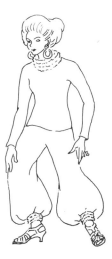

64. Harem pajamas of dark-green crepe with gold bead collar and pants cuffs. 1966.

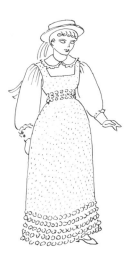

65. Victorian evening dress of yellow and white polka dots; sheer blouse. 1968.

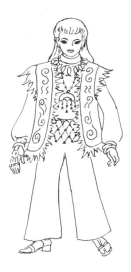

66. Afghanistan: goatskin jacket; silk jump suit; Middle East jewelry. 1968.

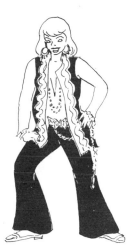

67. Black velvet evening pants suit: long bolero; metallic gauze blouse. 1968.

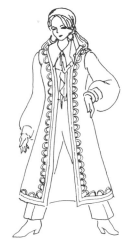

68. Arabia: pants and long bolero with gold braid trim; crepe blouse. 1969.

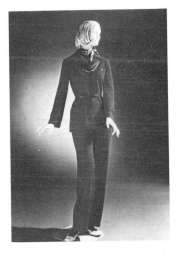

69. Two-piece pants suit of red knit; shirt-type jacket; red leather-like belt. By Kimberly, 1972. (Division of Costume, Smithsonian Institution.)

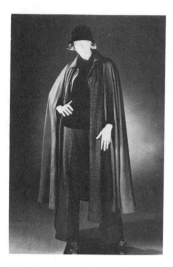

70. Sports ensemble: brown
wool tweed slacks; rust blouse;
green sweater-vest; full-length
circular beige and tweed
reversible rain cape. By Kasper
for J. L. Sport, 1974. (Division of
Costume, Smithsonian
Institution.)

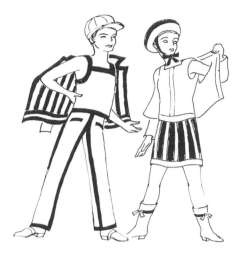

71. Left, Courrèges pants suit in black-and-white
knit; striped jacket lining. 1965. Right, Courrèges
dress, hat, jacket, and boots. 1965.

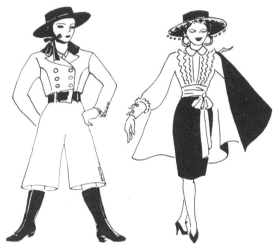

72. Spain. Left, gaucho pants suit; crepe
tucked-front blouse; zippered boots, 1967. Right,
matador dress in navy and white silk linen;
hot-pink cape lining and sash, 1961.

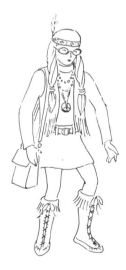

73. "Hippie" style: beaded
headband; suede bolero and
boots; shoulder bag. 1968.

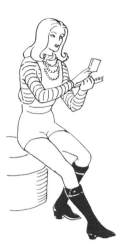

74. "Hot pants": red satin mini-overalls; striped knit shirt; tights; boots. 1971.

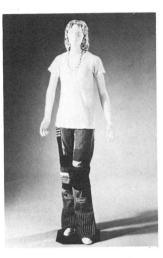

75. Faded blue jeans with patches. By Wrangler. White ribbed knit top. By Sears. Worn by student for rock concerts and other activities in New Jersey, 1970. (Division of Costume, Smithsonian Institution.)

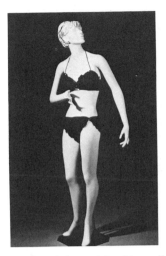

76. Blue bikini with white polka dots. By Mabs of California, early 1960s. (Division of Costume, Smithsonian Institution.)

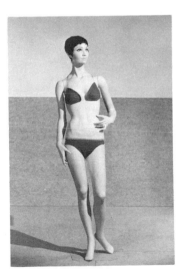

77. Wool and plastic bathing suit. Los Angeles, by Rudi Gernreich. Manufactured by Harmon Knitwear. (The Costume Institute of the Metropolitan Museum of Art. Gift of Rudi Gernreich.)

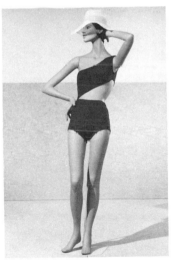

78. Nylon bathing suit. Manufactured by Sinclair Mills. New York, by Tom Brigance, 1960 – 61. (The Costume Institute of The Metropolitan Museum of Art. Gift of Sinclair Mills.)

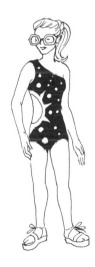

79. Cut-out swimsuit: black-and-white maillot; sandals with cork soles. 1965.

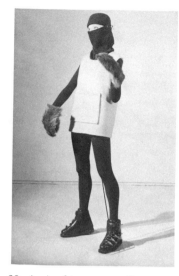

80. Après-ski costume of cotton and wool. New York, by Halston for Bergdorf Goodman, 1967. (The Costume Institute of The Metropolitan Museum of Art. Gift of Bergdorf Goodman Company.)

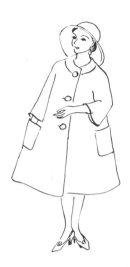

81. Tent coat in yellow tweed for spring; straw sou'wester hat by Dior. 1961.

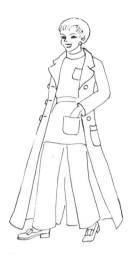

82. "Maxi-coat" over matching tunic and flared pants. 1969.

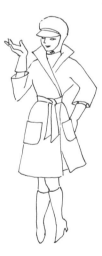

83. Vinyl raincoat with matching cap and boots. 1964.

84. Women's Fashions of the 1960s.
Left to right: Vinyl rainwear ensemble: black-and-white striped coat with matching boots, spats, and hat. American, by Jay Stone, 1965. Black alligator slacks worn with a white organdy blouse. American, by Arnold Scaasi, 1963. Electric mini-dress of black vinyl; operated by batteries that can switch it on and off at will. American, by Diana Dew for Paraphernalia, 1966. Sports costume: putty beige suede tunic; brown leather pants; white turtleneck. By Anne Klein, 1967. (The Costume Institute of The Metropolitan Museum of Art.)

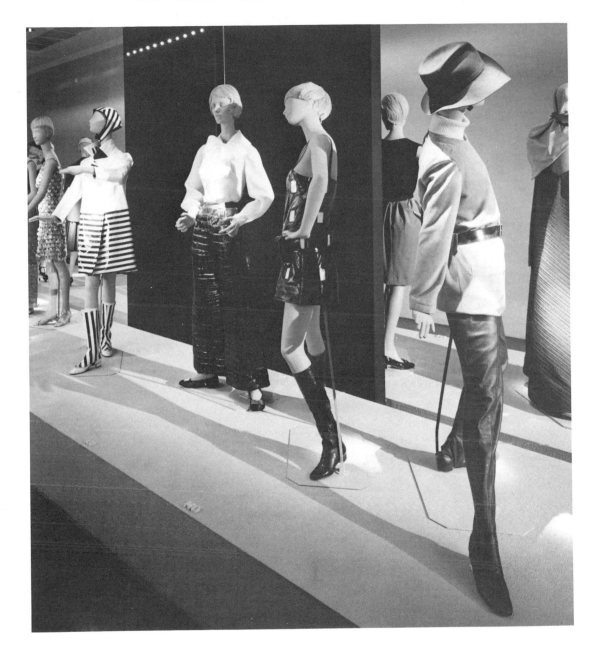

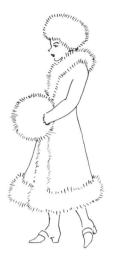

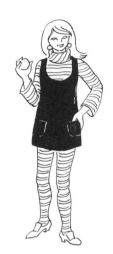

85. Russia: midi-length coat of ivory melton cloth with golden fox trim; fox toque and muff. 1967.

86. The "total look": purple mini-jumper and shoes; striped shirt and tights. 1967.

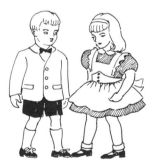

87. Party togs for six-year-olds. Left, boy's wool jacket and shorts. Right, girl's no-iron cotton dress and pinafore. 1961.

Afterword

THE COSTUME DESIGNER, in addition to having some facility in the handling of form, color, and fabric, must be an artist at distilling the essences of social climate and of character analysis and at projecting them through clothing worn by actors on stage. It is a demanding assignment, and the more understanding of history and of people that costume artists bring to their drawing boards and costume shops, the better they will be able to select and underline essential details, to use appropriate line and color, and to design effectively for the theatre. When one observes the fascinating shifts in what people wear and how they look (from inside to outside), the conviction grows that, indeed, "All the world's a stage and all the men and women merely players."

There is never a fashion with nothing to say. If one could intimately read the language of dress — a language as full of oblique reference and subtle inflection as Joyce's in *Finnegans Wake* — every pleat and pouf and button and bone would tell a tale. No fashion that hangs onto a period and stamps it is whimsical, arbitrary, or irrelevant. Whether its genesis seems inevitable or chancy, whether it comes from the couture or is set off by the popular fancy for a book, a poem, a personality, a picture at an exhibition, it has its reasons (to paraphrase Pascal) that reason knows not of. It is a capture, in dress, of a social climate, an aesthetic bent, a prevailing romantic image. The climate shifts. The image alters. It is the bold designer — or that rare, wonderful woman of spontaneous and prophetic taste — who senses the drift of the shift while it is yet a presumption in the wind, and captures it, and gives it a form *juste*.[1]

BIBLIOGRAPHY

BOOKS

Amory, Cleveland, and Bradlee, Frederick, eds. *Vanity Fair: A Cavalcade of the 1920s and 1930s*. New York: The Viking Press, 1960.

Arnold, Janet. *Patterns of Fashion*, Vol. II: 1860–1940. New York: Drama Book Specialists, 1972.

———. *A Handbook of Costume*. London: Macmillan, 1974. Distributed by S. G. Phillips.

d'Assailly, Gisèle. *Ages of Elegance: Five Thousand Years of Fashion and Frivolity*. Greenwich, Conn.: New York Graphic Society, 1968. [To 1965.]

Bakst, Léon. *Decorative Art of Léon Bakst*. Translated by Harry Melvill. New York: Dover Publications, 1973.

———. *Bakst: Collection of Costume Designs — 1909–1923*. New York: Rizzoli, 1977.

Barton, Lucy. *Historic Costume for the Stage*. Boston: Walter H. Baker, 1935. [To 1914.]

———. *Appreciating Costume*. Boston: Walter H. Baker, 1969.

Batterberry, Michael, and Batterberry, Ariane R. *Mirror, Mirror: A Social History of Fashion — from Fig Leaf to the 1970's*. New York: Holt, Rinehart and Winston, 1977.

Battersby, Martin. *The Decorative Twenties*. New York: Walker & Co., 1969.

———. *The Decorative Thirties*. New York: Walker & Co., 1971.

———. *Art Déco Fashion: French Designers 1908–1925*. New York: St. Martin's Press, 1974.

Beaton, Cecil. *The Glass of Fashion*. Garden City: Doubleday & Co., 1954.

———. *Cecil Beaton: Memoirs of the 40's*. New York: McGraw-Hill Book Co., 1972.

Bennett-England, Rodney. *Dress Optional, the Revolution in Menswear*. Chester Springs, Pa.: Dufour, 1968.

Bernard, Barbara. *Fashion in the 60's*. New York: St. Martin's Press, 1978.

Black, J. Anderson. *The Story of Jewelry*. New York: Morrow, 1974.

Blum, Daniel. *A Pictorial History of the Silent Screen*. New York: Grosset & Dunlap, 1953. [To 1929.]

Blum, Daniel, and Kobal, John. *A New Pictorial History of the Talkies*. Rev. ed. New York: G. P. Putnam's Sons, 1973.

Blum, Daniel, and Willis, John. *A Pictorial History of the American Theatre: 1860–1976*. 4th ed. New York: Crown Publishers, 1977.

Blum, Stella, ed. *Designs by Erté: Fashion Drawings and Illustrations from Harper's Bazaar*. New York: Dover Publications, 1976.

Bonner, Paul H., Jr., ed. *The World in Vogue*. New York: The Viking Press, 1963. [To 1963.]

Boucher, Francois. *20,000 Years of Fashion: The History of Costume and Personal Adornment*. New York: Harry N. Abrams, 1967. [To 1960.]

Bradfield, Nancy. *Costume in Detail, 1730 – 1930*. Boston: Plays, 1968.

————. *Historical Costumes of England: 1066 – 1968*. 3d ed. New York: Harper & Row, 1971.

Bradley, Carolyn G. *Western World Costume: An Outline History*. New York: Appleton-Century-Crofts, 1954. [To 1952.]

Braun-Ronsdorf, Margarete. *Mirror of Fashion*. New York: McGraw-Hill Book Co., 1964. [To 1930.]

Broby-Johansen, R. *Body and Clothes: An Illustrated History of Costume — from Loin Cloth to Miniskirt*. New York: Reinhold Book Corp., 1968.

Brooke, Iris. *English Costume 1900 – 1950*. London: Methuen, 1951.

————. *Footwear: A Short History of European and American Shoes*. New York: Theatre Arts Books, 1971. [Some patterns.]

————. *Dress and Undress*. Westport, Conn.: Greenwood, 1973.

Buchman, Herman. *Stage Makeup*. New York: Watson-Guptill Publications, 1972.

Carter, Ernestine. *20th Century Fashion*. London: Eyre Methuen, 1975.

Charles-Roux, Edmonde. *Chanel*. Translated by Nancy Amphoux. New York: Alfred Knopf, 1975.

Chierichetti, David. *Hollywood Costume Design*. New York: Harmony Books, 1976.

Contini, Mila. *Fashion: from Ancient Egypt to the Present Day*. New York: Crescent Books, 1965. [To 1965.]

Corey, Irene. *The Mask of Reality*. Anchorage, Ky.: The Anchorage Press, 1968. [Styles in makeup.]

Corson, Richard. *Fashions in Hair*. 3d rev. ed. Atlantic Highlands, N. J.: Humanities, 1971.

————. *Fashions in Make-up*. New York: Universe, 1973.

————. *Stage Make-up*. 5th edition. Englewood Cliffs, N. J.: Prentice-Hall, 1975. [Includes hair styles to 1973.]

Cunnington, C. Willett. *English Women's Clothing in the Present Century*. New York: Thomas Yoseloff, 1958. [To 1950.]

Cunnington, C. Willett, and Cunnington, Phillis. *The History of Underclothes*. London: Michael Joseph, 1951.

Dorner, Jane. *Fashion in the Twenties and Thirties*. London: Ian Allen, 1973.

————. *Fashion: The Changing Shape of Fashion Through the Years*. New York: Crown, 1974.

————. *Fashion in the Forties and Fifties*. New Rochelle, N. Y.: Arlington House, 1975.

Engel, Lehman. *The American Musical Theater*. New York: The Macmillan Company, 1967.

Erté. *Things I Remember*. New York: Quadrangle/New York Times Book Co., 1975. [1912 – 1973.]

————. *Erté Fashions*. New York: St. Martin's Press, 1977.

Ewing, Elizabeth. *History of Twentieth-Century Fashion*. New York: Charles Scribner's Sons, 1975.

————. *Dress and Undress: A History of Women's Underwear*. New York: Drama Book Specialists, 1978.

Garland, Madge. *Fashion*. Baltimore: Penguin Books, 1962. [To 1961.]

————. *The Indecisive Decade – The World of Fashion and Entertainment in the Thirties*. London: Macdonald, 1968.

————. *The Changing Form of Fashion*. New York: Praeger Publishers, 1970.

Glynn, Prudence. *In Fashion: Dress in the Twentieth Century*. New York: Oxford University Press, 1978. [1908–1977.]

Gold, Annalee. *75 Years of Fashion*. New York: Fairchild Publications, Inc., 1975. [1900–1975.]

Gorsline, Douglas. *What People Wore: A Visual History of Dress from Ancient Times to 20th Century America*. New York: Crown Publishers, 1951. [To 1925.]

Gottfried, Martin. *Broadway Musicals*. New York: Harry N. Abrams, 1979.

Green, Stanley, and Goldblatt, Burt. *Starring Fred Astaire*. New York: Dodd, Mead & Co., 1973.

Griffith, Richard, and Mayer, Arthur. *The Movies*. New York: Simon and Schuster, 1957.

Haedrich, M. *Coco Chanel; Her Life, Her Secrets*. Translated by Charles Lam Markmann. Boston: Little, Brown and Company, 1972.

Hansen, Henny Harald. *Costumes and Styles*. New York: E. P. Dutton, 1972. [To 1970.]

Healy, Daty. *Dress the Show: A Basic Costume Book*. Rev. ed. Rowayton, Conn.: New Plays, 1976.

Hill, Margot Hamilton, and Bucknell, Peter A. *The Evolution of Fashion: Pattern and Cut from 1066 to 1930*. New York: Reinhold Book Corp., 1968.

Horan, James D. *The Desperate Years: A Pictorial History of the Thirties*. New York: Bonanza Books, 1972.

Jackson, Sheila. *Costumes for the Stage: How to Make Costumes for Every Kind of Play*. New York: E. P. Dutton, 1978. [Greece to present day.]

The Journal of the Century. Compiled by Bryan Holme with the editors of the Viking Press and the *Ladies' Home Journal*. New York: Viking Press, 1976.

Kannik, Preban. *Military Uniforms of the World in Color*. New York: The Macmillan Company, 1968.

Keenan, Brigid. *The Women We Wanted to Look Like*. London: Macmillan London Limited, 1977.

Kidwell, Claudia B., and Christman, Margaret C. *Suiting Everyone: The Democratization of Clothing in America*. Washington, D. C.: Smithsonian Institution Press, 1974.

Kilgour, Ruth E. *A Pageant of Hats, Ancient and Modern*. New York: Robert McBride Co., 1958.

Lambert, Eleanor. *World of Fashion: People, Places, Resources*. New York: R. R. Bowker Co., 1976.

Laver, James. *Taste and Fashion*. New York: Dodd, Mead and Co., 1938.

————. *Costume in the Theatre*. New York: Hill and Wang, 1964.

————. *Women's Dress in the Jazz Age*. London: Hamish Hamilton, 1964.

————. *Modesty in Dress — from Louis XIV to Gina Lollobrigida*. New York: Houghton Mifflin, 1969.

————. *Concise History of Costume and Fashion*. New York: Charles Scribner's Sons, 1974.

Lee, Sarah Tomerlin, ed. *American Fashion: Adrian, Mainbocher, McCardell, Norell, Trigère, 1925–1975*. New York: Quadrangle/The New York Times Book Co., 1975.

Leese, Elizabeth. *Costume Design in the Movies*. New York: Frederick Ungar, 1977.

Levin, Phyllis Lee. *The Wheels of Fashion*. Garden City: Doubleday & Company, 1965.

Lynam, Ruth, ed. *Couture*. New York: Doubleday, 1972.

McConathy, Dale, and Vreeland, Diana. *Hollywood Costumes. Glamor! Glitter! Romance!* New York: Harry N. Abrams, 1976.

Mailer, Norman. *Of Women and Their Elegance*. Photographs by Milton H. Greene. New York: Simon and Schuster, 1980.

Mansfield, Alan, and Cunnington, Phillis. *Handbook of English Costume in the Twentieth Century, 1900 – 1950*. Boston: Plays, Inc., 1973.

Martin, Linda. *The Way We Wore: Fashion Illustrations of Children's Wear, 1870 – 1970*. New York: Charles Scribner's Sons, 1978.

Men's Wear Magazine. *75 Years of Fashion*. New York: Fairchild Publications, June 25, 1965.

Motley. *Designing and Making Stage Costumes*. New York: Watson-Guptill Publications, 1974.

Picken, Mary B. *Fashion Dictionary: Fabric, Sewing and Apparel as Expressed in the Language of Fashion*. Enlarged ed. New York: Funk & Wagnalls, 1972.

Prisk, Berneice. *Stage Costume Handbook*. New York: Harper & Row, 1966.

Prisk, Berneice, and Byers, Jack. *The Theatre Student: Costuming*. New York: Richard Rosen Press, 1969.

Quant, Mary. *Quant by Quant*. New York: Putnam, 1966.

Rankin, Colonel Robert H. *Uniforms of the Army*. New York: G. P. Putnam's Sons, 1967.

Robinson, Julian. *Fashion in the Forties*. New York: St. Martin's Press, 1976.

———. *The Golden Age of Style: Art Déco Fashion Illustration*. New York: Harcourt Brace Jovanovich, 1976. [1901 – 1939.]

———. *Fashion in the Thirties*. New York: Two Continents Publishing Group, 1978.

Rubin, Leonard G. *The World of Fashion: An Introduction*. San Francisco: Canfield Press (Harper & Row), 1976.

Russell, Douglas A. *Stage Costume Design*. Englewood Cliffs, N. J.: Prentice-Hall, 1973.

———. *Theatrical Style: A Visual Approach to the Theatre*. Palo Alto, Cal.: Mayfield Publishing Co., 1976.

Russell, Elizabeth. *Adaptable Stage Costume for Women*. New York: Theatre Arts Books, 1975.

Sann, Paul. *The Lawless Decade*. New York: Crown Publishers, 1957. [From World War I to the New Deal.]

———. *Fads, Follies and Delusions of the American People*. New York: Crown Publishers, 1967.

———. *The Angry Decade: The Sixties*. New York: Crown Publishers, 1979.

Schiaparelli, Elsa. *Shocking Life*. London: Dent, 1954.

Schoeffler, O. E., and Gale, William. *Esquire's Encyclopedia of Twentieth Century Men's Fashions*. New York: McGraw-Hill, 1973.

Sharaff, Irene. *Broadway & Hollywood: Costumes Designed by Irene Sharaff*. New York: Van Nostrand Reinhold, 1976.

Sichel, Marion. *Costume Reference No. 8: The Twenties and Thirties*. Boston: Plays, 1978.

Spencer, Charles. *Erté*. New York: Crown Publishers, 1971.

———. *Cecil Beaton: Stage and Film Designs*. New York: St. Martin's Press, 1976.

Spencer, Charles, and Dyer, Philip. *The World of Serge Diaghilev*. New York: P. Elek, 1974.

Springer, John. *All Talking! All Singing! All Dancing! A Pictorial History of the Movie Musical*. New York: The Citadel Press, 1966.

Squire, Geoffrey. *Dress and Society, 1560 – 1970*. New York: The Viking Press, 1974.

Thomas, Tony; Terry, Jim; and Berkeley, Busby. *The Busby Berkeley Book*. Greenwich, Conn.: New York Graphic Society, 1973.

Tilke, Max. *Costume Patterns and Designs*. (Supplement to *A Pictorial History of Costume* by Wolfgang Bruhn.) New York: Hastings House, 1974.

Tily, John C. *The Uniforms of the United States Navy*. New York: Thomas Yoseloff, 1964.

Time-Life Editors. *This Fabulous Century*. 8 volumes. New York: Time-Life Books, 1969.

———. *The Best of Life*. New York: Time-Life Books, 1973.

Torrens, D. *Fashion Illustrated: A Review of Women's Dress 1920 – 1950*. New York: Hawthorn Books, 1975.

Veronesi, G. *Style and Design 1909 – 1929*. New York: Braziller, 1968.

Waller, Jane. *A Man's Book: Fashion in the Men's World in the 20's and 30's*. London: Duckworth, 1977.

Waugh, Norah. *Corsets and Crinolines*. New York: Theatre Arts, 1954.

———. *The Cut of Women's Clothes: 1600 – 1930*. New York: Theatre Arts Books, 1968.

Westmore, Michael G. *The Art of Theatrical Makeup for Stage and Screen*. New York: McGraw-Hill, 1973.

White, Palmer. *Poiret*. New York: Potter, 1973.

Wilcox, Ruth Turner. *The Mode in Footwear*. New York: Charles Scribner's Sons, 1948.

———. *The Mode in Furs*. New York: Charles Scribner's Sons, 1951.

———. *The Mode in Costume*. New York: Charles Scribner's Sons, 1958.

———. *The Mode in Hats and Headdress*. New York: Charles Scribner's Sons, 1959.

———. *Five Centuries of American Costume*. New York: Charles Scribner's Sons, 1963.

———. *The Dictionary of Costume*. New York: Scribner's, 1969.

Williams, Colonel Dion. *Army and Navy Uniforms and Insignia*. New York: Frederick A. Stokes Company, 1918.

The World of Balenciaga. New York: The Metropolitan Museum of Art, 1973.

ARTICLES

"The Art of Fashion," *The Metropolitan Museum of Art Bulletin* 26 no. 3 (November 1967).

Baur, John I. H. "The New Whitney Museum Collection," *Art in America* 54:32 – 47 (September-October 1966).

"Change of Mind: 1900 – 1950," *Vogue* 115:96 (January 1950).

"Dior's Ideas," *Vogue* 109:145 (April 1, 1947).

"Golden Days of Style," *Life* 49:105 – 108 (December 26, 1960).

Greenberg, Clement. "America Takes the Lead: 1945 – 1965," *Art in America* 53:108 – 109 (August-September 1965).

Roshco, Bernard. "Fads and Fashion," *Redbook* 120:69 – 76 (January 1963).

Saisselin, Remy G. "From Baudelaire to Christian Dior: The Poetics of Fashion," *The Journal of Aesthetics and Art Criticism* 18:115 (September 1959).

"This Half Century," *Vogue* 115:90 (January 1950).

PERIODICALS FOR COSTUME REFERENCE

Apparel Arts
California Stylist
Delineator
Ebony
Esquire
Gentlemen's Quarterly
Glamour
Good Housekeeping
Hairdo and Beauty
Harper's Bazaar
Ingenue
Ladies' Home Journal
Life
Look

McCall's
McCall's Pattern Book
Mademoiselle
Men's Wear
The New Yorker
Pictorial Review
The Saturday Evening Post
Seventeen
Simplicity Fashion Magazine
Vanity Fair
Vogue
Vogue Pattern Book
Woman's Day
Woman's Home Companion

LIBRARY AND MUSEUM COLLECTIONS

Brooklyn Museum Costume Collection
The Fashion Institute of Technology: Library and Picture Collection
Metropolitan Museum of Art (The Costume Institute)
The Museum of the City of New York (The Costume Collection)
New York Public Library Picture Collection
The Smithsonian Institution (Division of Costume)

NOTES

I. THE FIRST WORLD WAR

1. Ernest R. May, *War, Boom and Bust*, The Life History of the United States, vol. 10:1917–1932 (New York: Time, Incorporated, 1964), p.10.

2. Ernest R. May, *The Progressive Era*, The Life History of the United States, vol. 9:1901–1917 (New York: Time, Incorporated, 1964), p.101.

3. "The New First-Aid Cover-All," *Ladies' Home Journal* 33 (February 1916):83.

4. May, *War, Boom and Bust*, pp.27–37.

5. "What He Will Wear," *Ladies' Home Journal* 34 (May 1917):105.

6. Ibid.

7. Amy La Follette Jensen, *The White House and Its Thirty-Three Families* (New York: McGraw-Hill Book Company, 1962), p.191.

8. Daniel Blum, *A Pictorial History of the Silent Screen* (New York: Grosset & Dunlap, 1953), p.122.

9. Colonel Robert H. Rankin, *Uniforms of the Army* (New York: G. P. Putnam's Sons, 1967), p.65.

10. "'There's No Place Like Home' to Wear House Gowns, Says Mrs. Ralston," *Ladies' Home Journal* 32 (October 1915):105.

11. Ibid.

12. "Now Once More for Pretty Clothes," *Ladies' Home Journal* 36 (March 1919):143.

13. Henry T. Farrar, "Ladies' Home Journal Fashions for Warm Days," *Ladies' Home Journal* 33 (July 1916):61.

14. "What He Will Wear," *Ladies' Home Journal* 34 (May 1917):105.

II. THE FLAMING TWENTIES

1. Ernest R. May, *War, Boom and Bust*, The Life History of the United States, vol. 10:1917–1932 (New York: Time, Incorporated, 1964), p.119.

2. John Canaday, *Mainstreams of Modern Art* (New York: Simon and Schuster, 1959), p.496.

3. "Change of Mind: 1900–1950," *Vogue* 115 (January 1950):96.

4. "This Half Century," *Vogue* 115 (January 1950):90.

5. Cecil Beaton, *The Glass of Fashion* (Garden City: Doubleday & Company, 1954), p.184.

6. "Fairchild's Pictured Chart of Formal Day Dress," Fairchild Company, 1922 (New York Public Library picture collection).

7. "For the Well Dressed Man," *Vanity Fair* 19 (October 1922):83.

8. "For the Well Dressed Man," *Vanity Fair* 14 (May 1920):84.

9. Ibid.

10. "Vanity Fair Makes a Selection of Correctly Cut Ready-to-Wear Clothes for the Well Dressed Man," *Vanity Fair* 22 (May 1924):72.

11. "For the Well Dressed Man," *Vanity Fair* 16 (April 1921):72.

12. "The Well Dressed Man Goes South," *Vanity Fair* 27 (January 1927):84.

13. "For the Well Dressed Man," *Vanity Fair* 19 (February 1923):74.

14. Fell Sharp, "The Clothes of Two Well Dressed English Actors," *Men's Wear* 72 (February 10, 1926):67.

15. John Chapman Hilder, "The Man and His Clothes," *Ladies' Home Journal* 37 (September 1920):172.

16. James Charlton, "What Men Wear at Weddings," *Ladies' Home Journal* 38 (April 1921):75.

17. Schuyler White, "The Boy at School," *Ladies' Home Journal* 46 (September 1929):57.

18. "For the Well Dressed Man," *Vanity Fair* 19 (October 1922):83.

19. "Some Styles That Are Being Featured in New York Shops," *Men's Wear* 76 (February 8, 1928):92.

20. "The Well Dressed Man Goes South," *Vanity Fair* 27 (January 1927):84.

21. "Every Costume Is Typical of a Pronounced Paris Fashion Note," *Ladies' Home Journal* 41 (November 1924):59.

22. "Our Paris Correspondent Cables — ," *Ladies' Home Journal* 38 (November 1921):52.

23. "Shoes Along the Bridal Path," *Vogue* 71 (February 15, 1928):66 – 67.

24. Schuyler White, "Dressing the Boy," *Ladies' Home Journal* 46 (May 1929):64.

25. "When Parisians Are Very Small," *Ladies' Home Journal* 46 (February 1929):41.

III. The Depressed Thirties

1. Marshall and Jean Stearns, "Profile of the Lindy," *Show* 3 (October 1963):114.

2. "A Basic Southern Wardrobe," *Vanity Fair* 41 (February 1934):52.

3. "For the Well-Dressed Man," *Vanity Fair* 33 (January 1930):72.

4. Ibid.

5. "A Basic Southern Wardrobe," p.52.

6. "The Wrong and Right Ways to Wear Blue," *Vanity Fair* 43 (October 1934):57.

7. L. Fellows, "June Wedding," *Esquire* 9 (June 1938):152.

8. Stewart Heidgerd, "So You're Getting Married!" *Esquire* 7 (June 1937):140.

9. Advertisement for Gunther furs, *The New Yorker* 8 (November 5, 1932):47.

10. "Pyjamas — When Are They Worn?" *Vogue* 77 (June 1, 1931):70.

11. "Line of March," *Vogue* 89 (March 1, 1937):110.

12. "Sports Girl," *Ladies' Home Journal* 56 (April 1939):28.

13. George Brooke, "Clothes for School or College," *Good Housekeeping* 105 (September 1937):115.

14. "Shophound's Spring Portfolio," *Vogue* 77 (March 15, 1931):53.

IV. The Second World War

1. "This Half Century: Shift of Tempo, Change of Dress," *Vogue* 115 (January 1950):93.

2. "Robes with Gabardine in the Lead," *Men's Wear* 101 (August 7, 1940):20.

3. Lord and Taylor advertisement for men's wear, *The New Yorker* 20 (June 10, 1944):1.

4. Arthur P. Wade, Lieutenant Colonel, United States Army, "Uniforms,

Armed Forces," *The Encyclopedia Americana*, vol. 27 (Danbury, Conn.: Americana Corporation, 1979), pp.370–72.

5. Thomas E. Griess, "Uniform," *The World Book Encyclopedia*, vol. 19 (Chicago: Field Enterprises Educational Corporation, 1968), p.18. (Modified to reflect World War II colors.)

6. "Insignia and Ranks of the Armed Forces," *Information Please Almanac* (New York: Simon and Schuster, 1967), p.238.

7. Thomas E. Griess, "Insignia," *The World Book Encyclopedia*, vol. 10 (Chicago: Field Enterprises Educational Corporation, 1968), p.225. See also Arthur P. Wade, "Insignia of Rank, Armed Forces," *The Encyclopedia Americana*, vol. 15 (New York: Americana Corporation, 1974), pp.219–20.

8. Advertisement for Chen Yu Nail Lacquer, *Ladies' Home Journal* 59 (March 1942):126.

9. Alene Bra advertisement, *McCall's* 74 (November 1946):169.

10. "Grand Gesture Gifts," *McCall's* 74 (November 1946):173.

11. "One Dress into Ten," *Vogue* 101 (April 1, 1943):71.

12. Ruth Mary Packard, "Trousers Are So Practical," *Ladies' Home Journal* 59 (February 1942):95.

13. Ogden Nash, *Face Is Familiar* (Boston: Little, Brown, and Co., 1940), p.91.

14. Information compiled from "Uniform," *The World Book Encyclopedia*, vol. 17 (Chicago: Field Enterprises Educational Corporation, 1958), p.8251, and vol. 19, 1967, p.18; and R. Turner Wilcox, *Five Centuries of American Costume* (New York: Charles Scribner's Sons, 1963), pp.97–99.

V. THE POSTWAR ERA AND THE "NEW LOOK"

1. "Dior's Ideas," *Vogue* 109 (April 1, 1947):145.

2. Christian Dior, *Christian Dior and I*, translated by Antonia Fraser (London: Weidenfeld and Nicolson, 1957), p.35.

3. "Waistliners," *Vogue* 110 (August 1, 1947):118.

4. "Celeste Holm . . . She Has a Style of Her Own," *Simplicity Pattern Book* 3 (Spring 1951):77.

VI. THE LATE FIFTIES

1. Advertisement for Du Pont Orlon acrylic fiber, *Life* 34 (April 27, 1953):8.

2. Frank Sullivan, "Go Vest, Young Man!" *Woman's Day* 18 (November 1954):28.

3. Advertisement for After Six formal wear, *Esquire* 41 (May 1954):34.

4. *New York Herald Tribune*, June 23, 1957 (New York Public Library Picture Collection: "Men's Costume — 1950's").

5. Bernard Roshco, "Fads and Fashion," *Redbook* 120 (January 1963):75.

6. Remy G. Saisselin, "From Baudelaire to Christian Dior: The Poetics of Fashion," *The Journal of Aesthetics and Art Criticism* 18 (September 1959):115.

7. Miriam Gibson French, "Project: Glamour — Experimental," *McCall's* 86 (April 1959):60–61.

8. "Beauties, Ball Gowns and Heirloom Jewels," *Life* 34 (March 30, 1953):122.

9. "Waists Rise to Gala Occasions," *Fashions of the Times*, Part 2, *The New York Times Magazine*, August 24, 1958, p.25.

10. "They Strip for Fashion!" *California Stylist* 23 (October 1959):59.

VII. THE SIXTIES

1. Calvin Tomkins, *The World of Marcel Duchamp* (New York: Time, Incorporated, 1966), p.170.

2. Marshall McLuhan and George B. Leonard, "The Future of Sex," *Look* 31 (July 25, 1967):56.

3. Elinor Lander Horwitz, "I'm Not on Your Trip," *McCall's* 94 (September 1967):140.

4. Hunter S. Thompson, "The 'Hashbury' Is the Capital of the Hippies," *New York Times Magazine*, May 14, 1967, p.120.

5. William Murray, "Hell's Angels," *Saturday Evening Post* 238 (November 20, 1965):32.

6. "Turtlenecks Come in from the Cold," *Life* 63 (November 10, 1967):113.

7. *Vogue* 154 (September 15, 1969):138.

8. Jo Ahern Zill, "Party Face Put-on," *Look* 31 (November 28, 1967):55.

9. "Hot Pants," *Life* 70 (January 29, 1971):36.

AFTERWORD

1. "This Half Century: Shift of Tempo, Change of Dress," *Vogue* 115 (January 1950):87.

Pictures

Credits have been given next to the photographs. Grateful acknowledgment is made to The Costume Institute of The Metropolitan Museum of Art, The Museum of the City of New York, and the Division of Costume of The Smithsonian Institution for permission to use photographs of costumes in their collections; and to Milton H. Greene for permission to use his photographs of costumes in Figures IV–7 and VI–1, which appeared in *Life*, December 26, 1960.

The reproductions of fashion illustrations came from the following sources: Figure I–7: *Vanity Fair*, March 1918, p.72. Copyright © 1918 (renewed 1946) by The Condé Nast Publications Inc. Figure II–73: *Vogue*, February 15, 1928, p.67. Courtesy *Vogue*. Copyright © 1928 (renewed 1956) by The Condé Nast Publications Inc. Figure III–8: *Esquire*, June 1937, p.140. Courtesy *Esquire*. Copyright © 1937 (renewed 1965) by Esquire Inc. Figure III–25: *Vogue*, June 1, 1931, pp.70–71. Courtesy *Vogue*. Copyright © 1931 (renewed 1959) by The Condé Nast Publications Inc. Figure IV–34: *Vogue*, April 1, 1943, p.71. Courtesy *Vogue*. Copyright © 1943 (renewed 1971) by The Condé Nast Publications Inc.

Quotations

Permission to quote from copyrighted material has been received from the following sources:

McCall's: Miriam Gibson French, "Project: Glamour — Experimental," April 1959, pp.60–61; Elinor Lander Horwitz, "I'm Not on Your Trip," September 1967, p.140. Courtesy *McCall's*. Copyright © 1959; 1967 by The McCall Publishing Company.

Life: "Beauties, Ball Gowns, and Heirloom Jewels," March 30, 1953, p.122; "Turtlenecks Come in from the Cold," November 10, 1967, p.113; "Hot Pants," January 29, 1971, p.36. Courtesy *Life*. Copyright © 1953; 1967; 1971 by Time Inc. All rights reserved.

Esquire: "Being a Memorandum for the Bridegroom," June 1935, p.111; L. Fellows, "June Wedding," June 1938, p.152. Courtesy *Esquire*. Copyright © 1935 (renewed 1963); 1938 (renewed 1966) by Esquire Inc.

Vogue: "Dior's Ideas," April 1, 1947, p.145; "Waistliners," August 1, 1947, p.118; "This Half Century," January 1950, pp.87, 90, 93; "Concierge hairdo," September 15, 1969, p.138. Courtesy *Vogue*. Copyright © 1947 (renewed 1975); 1947 (renewed 1975); 1950 (renewed 1978); 1969 by The Condé Nast Publications Inc.

Sources for Line Drawings

American Fabrics; American Gentleman; Apparel Arts; California Stylist; Ebony; Esquire; "Fashion," *The Americana Annual; Fashions of the Times,* Part 2, *The New York Times Magazine; Gentlemen's Quarterly; Golf Illustrated; Good Housekeeping; Harper's Bazaar; l'Homme; Ladies' Home Journal; Life; Look; Mademoiselle; McCall's; McCall's Home Catalog; McCall's Patterns; Men's Wear; Needlecraft — The Home Arts Magazine; New York Herald Tribune;* New York Public Library Picture Collection; *New York Times; New York Times Magazine; The New Yorker; Pic Pix, Inc.; The Sartorial Art Journal;* Sears, Roebuck and Company Catalog; *Simplicity Pattern Book; Vanity Fair; Vogue;* Daniel Blum, *A Pictorial History of the Silent Screen* (New York: Grosset & Dunlap, 1953);

Daniel Blum, *A Pictorial History of the Talkies* (New York: Grosset & Dunlap, 1958); Mr. and Mrs. Vernon Castle, *Modern Dancing* (New York: Harper and Brothers, 1914); Stanley Green and Burt Goldblatt, *Starring Fred Astaire* (New York: Dodd, Mead and Co., 1973); Richard Griffith and Arthur Mayer, *The Movies* (New York: Simon and Schuster, 1957); Vincent J. Esposito, ed., *The West Point Atlas of American Wars*, vol. II (New York: Frederick Praeger, 1959); Colonel Robert H. Rankin, *Uniforms of the Army* (New York: G. P. Putnam's Sons, 1967); James C. Tily, *The Uniforms of the United States Navy"* (New York: Thomas Yoseloff, Publisher, 1964); Colonel Dion Williams, *Army and Navy Uniforms and Insignia* (New York: Frederick A. Stokes Company, 1918).

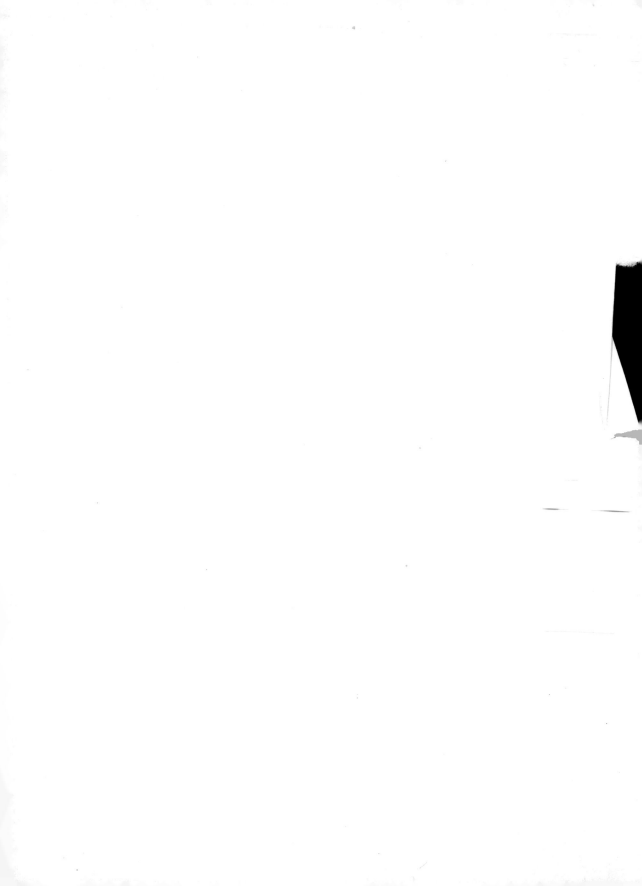